Atlas of the Ultrastructure of Diseased Human Muscle

'After all, muscle moves the world.'

SIR CHARLES SHERRINGTON

Atlas of the Ultrastructure of Diseased Human Muscle

W G P Mair MD FRCPath.

Consultant Neuropathologist, The National Hospital for Nervous Diseases, Queen Square, London. Lecturer in Neuropathology, Institute of Neurology, University of London

F M S Tomé

Neurologist, Faculty of Medicine, University of Lisbon. Lecturer in Neuropathology, Institute of Neurology, The National Hospital for Nervous Diseases, Queen Square, University of London

CHURCHILL LIVINGSTONE Edinburgh & London 1972

ISBN 0 443 00831 0

Printed in Great Britain by
Butler & Tanner Ltd, Frome and London

Foreword

Studies concerning the pathology and aetiology of muscle diseases in this country have received a considerable impetus from the Muscular Dystrophy Group of Great Britain who have donated large sums for research by prominent scientists.

Just over ten years ago an electron microscope was given by the National Fund for Research into Poliomyelitis (as it then was) to the Muscular Dystrophy Group and it was handed over to me at The Institute of Neurology, The National Hospital, Queen Square. Dr W. G. P. Mair, Consultant Neuropathologist, had the immediate opportunity of using it in diseases of muscle and was one of the earliest to undertake this type of study in this country. Since then he has taught a succession of research workers from many countries, and of these Dr F. Tomé of Lisbon is the most recent and one of the most able. Drs Mair and Tomé have devoted their time and skill during the past year or so to produce this volume which, in view of their wide experience and their most beautiful pictures, will be of the utmost importance as well as of inestimable value to all workers in this field.

Both authors, as well as myself, would desire to express our indebtedness to the Muscular Dystrophy Group of Great Britain, without whose help the work described in the volume would have been impossible.

J. N. CUMINGS, MD, FRCP, FRCPath.
Chairman, Medical Research Committee,
Muscular Dystrophy Group of Great Britain.
Emeritus Professor of Chemical Pathology,
Institute of Neurology, The National Hospital, London

Preface

A great deal of information on the ultrastructure of muscle both in experimental animals and in a wide variety of human muscular disorders is now available but is disseminated in a great many publications which are not readily accessible to the majority of workers. In this book an effort has been made to provide a concise, general view of the ultrastructure of normal and diseased human muscle: brief reference is also made to extra-ocular and cardiac muscle. In addition skeletal and cardiac muscle of the human foetus are also described.

Our main concern has been to illustrate the changes which take place in common pathological conditions, and we have tried to outline the patterns of change which occur in particular diseases. It must be stressed, however, that many of the ultrastructural changes in muscle are common to many different pathological processes.

We have provided a bibliography of the most important reports, but we are well aware that it is far from complete and the omission of any is unintentional.

We are most indebted to the Muscular Dystrophy Group of Great Britain for providing the equipment and the technical and financial assistance of their laboratory at the Institute of Neurology, The National Hospital for Nervous Diseases, Queen Square, London. It is through their generosity that this publication was made possible. We are grateful to the Calouste Gulbenkian Foundation for the Fellowship granted to one of us (F. T.) while part of the work was in progress.

The material on which the study was based consisted of some 250 biopsies. We would like to thank all the physicians and surgeons of The National Hospital, Queen Square, London, and of the Hospital de Santa Maria, Lisbon, for providing the biopsies, and the pediatricians, obstetricians and ophthalmologists of other hospitals who provided some of the material for examination. We are grateful to Drs A. Nordén and F. K.-G. Henriksson for the material from the patient with vitamin E deficiency, and to Drs J. A. Morgan-Hughes and P. M. Le Quesne for the material from rats treated with vincristine. We are indebted to Dr Ross McD. Anderson for his assistance in studying several of the biopsies and for some of the electron micrographs, and to Dr Sverrir B. Bergmann for the electron micrographs of foetal cardiac muscle. These micrographs were prepared while they worked with us.

We have been greatly assisted by Mr Brian Young who prepared all the specimens used in this publication and we are grateful to him and to Miss Alison Leigh for their goodwill, excellent technical assistance and photographic skill. We are indebted to Mr J. A. Mills for the light micrograph of Plate 9. Finally we would thank Mrs M. Beryl Bailey for her help in the preparation of the bibliography, Miss Margaret C. Wood for typing part of the manuscript, and Messrs Churchill Livingstone, particularly Mr W. G. Henderson, for their assistance and courtesy during the preparation of this atlas.

W. G. P. MAIR
F. M. S. TOMÉ

Contents

CHAPTER 1

Normal Striated Muscle

The structure of skeletal muscle has interested many workers over the past century and a considerable addition to our knowledge of its structure and function followed the introduction of electron microscopy in the pursuit of the study of normal and diseased muscle. Numerous authors studied the ultrastructure of muscle, and important amongst the reports of some of the early investigators in experimental animals are those of Draper and Hodge (1949), H. E. Huxley (1953), Bennett and Porter (1953), Ruska (1954), Hodge, H. E. Huxley and Spiro (1954), Bennett (1955), A. F. Huxley (1957a) and Hodge (1960), and in normal human muscle that of van Breemen (1960a). More recent reviews of the ultrastructure of muscle have been reported by Wilkie (1968), Price (1969) and Fardeau (1969a). The works of many important contributors to our knowledge of the ultrastructure of muscle are mentioned throughout this chapter.

SKELETAL MUSCLE FIBRES

Skeletal muscle fibres are multinucleated cells bounded successively by a plasma and a basement membrane. Collagen fibres, blood vessels and nerves lie between the muscle fibres.

Muscle fibres are fusiform in shape and of varying length depending on the length of the muscle which they form; however, individual fibres in the same muscle may also vary in length. The diameters of the muscle fibres vary between 10 and 100 μ.

The bulk of the muscle fibre consists of myofibrils (Plates 1 and 2) which are the contractile elements of muscle. They lie parallel to the long axis of the fibre and run almost its whole length. In normal human muscle the diameter of the myofibrils varies between 0·5 and 1 μ. The myofibrils display alternating dark anisotropic or doubly refractile A-bands and clear isotropic I-bands which are not doubly refractile. In the middle of the A-band is a lighter zone, the H-zone (Hensen's stripe), in the centre of which is the M-line (Mittelscheibe). Running through the centre of the I-band is the dense Z-line (Zwischenscheibe). In longitudinal sections of human muscle the Z-lines are commonly 800 Å wide. In cross section the Z-line has a lattice pattern. The ultrastructure of the Z-line has been studied by various authors including Knappeis and Carlsen (1962), Auber and Couteaux (1963), Reedy (1964), Kelly (1967) and Landon (1970). The distance between two Z-lines is called a sarcomere, which in resting human muscle measures about 2·3 μ but may vary from 2 to 3·8 μ, depending on whether the muscle is contracted or relaxed. The A-band is of fixed length about 1·5 μ, whereas the I-band varies in length according to whether the muscle is contracted or relaxed. Normally the Z-lines, and I- and A-bands of adjacent myofibrils lie in series (Plate 1). The Z-lines of adjacent myofibrils are not continuous with each other, nor do they extend to the plasma membrane except at the myotendinous junction. Myofibrils are formed of thick and thin myofilaments. The myofilaments in the I-band are thin, some 60 Å in diameter and about 1·0 μ long; they extend into the A-band, which contains also thick filaments of about 160 Å in diameter and 1·5 μ long. In the A-band the thick filaments are arranged in an hexagonal pattern, and each thick filament is also surrounded by six thin filaments. In relaxed muscle the H-zone is evident since it does not contain any of the thin filaments of the I-band. During contraction and relaxation of the muscle the thin filaments slide between the thick myofilaments (H. E. Huxley, 1953; A. F. Huxley and Niedergerke, 1954; and H. E. Huxley and Hanson, 1954). The sarcomere shortens during contraction of muscle resulting in diminution in length of the I-band and the H-zone, while in relaxation the I-band and the H-zone increase in length and consequently the whole sarcomere becomes longer. The thick filaments at the M-line are connected by short M-line bridges which are linked by thin M-line filaments which are limited to the width of the M-line (Knappeis and Carlsen, 1968; and Dos Remedios, 1970). Between each thick filament and the six thin filaments around it there occur cross bridges (H. E. Huxley, 1957), and these lie at intervals of 60–70 Å on each thick filament so that six may be seen every 400 Å along the length of the myofilaments and promote the movements of the thin filaments over the thick filaments during contraction and relaxation of the muscle (H. E. Huxley, 1960; H. E. Huxley and Brown, 1967; Miller and Tregear, 1970).

The thick filaments are formed of myosin, the thin of actin and some tropomyosin B (Hanson and Lowy, 1963), and the Z-line is similar in structure to the crystals of tropomyosin B (H. E. Huxley, 1963). H. E. Huxley (1960) stated that the total protein of myofilaments is formed of some 54 per cent of myosin, 20 per cent of actin and 10 to 20 per cent of tropomyosin: the remainder of the protein has not been clearly identified. The composition of the myofilaments was also investigated by other authors, including Hasselbach and Schneider (1951), Perry (1952), Hanson and H. E. Huxley (1953 and 1957), H. E. Huxley and Hanson (1957) and Perry and Corsi (1958). Recent reviews of the structure and composition of myofilaments have been reported by Perry (1967) and Young (1969) and a study on smooth and striated human muscle myosin was reported by Gröschel-Stewart (1971).

In addition to myofibrils the cytoplasm or sarcoplasm of the muscle fibre contains multiple nuclei, with the related Golgi apparatus, mitochondria, glycogen granules, lipid bodies, ribosomes, transverse system of tubules or T-systems and the sarcoplasmic reticulum which corresponds to the endoplasmic reticulum of other cells.

The multiple nuclei are elongated up to 11 μ long and lie immediately under the plasma membrane with their long axis running parallel to the length of the fibre (Plates 3 and 4). They vary in size and shape, depending on the functional state of the nucleus, the plane in which they have been cut and the method of fixation of the specimen. The nuclear shape in muscle cells of the rat has been studied by

Franke and Schinko (1969). Like the nuclei of other cells they are surrounded by an inner and outer membrane. The nuclear membranes are interrupted by pores 500 to 700 Å wide which are said to occupy 5 to 30 per cent of the total surface of the nuclear membranes (Toner and Carr 1968). The space between the inner and outer membranes measures generally 500 Å. The nucleus contains electron dense chromatin which is often located around the nuclear margin but may occur in dense masses or be evenly dispersed. The nucleus frequently exhibits one or more nucleoli which may be electron dense or reticulated in appearance.

Near the nucleus lies the Golgi apparatus (Plate 3 upper part), which consists of aggregates of closely applied flattened smooth tubules the ends of which may be distended and associated with vesicles. In the Golgi apparatus are located various enzymes.

Mitochondria occur between myofibrils and congregate under the plasma membrane and around the nuclei, some fibres containing more than others. In longitudinal sections (Plates 1 and 4), rounded paired mitochondria are often very apparent on either side of the Z-lines, or may extend between the myofibrils with their long axis parallel to them. The mitochondria consist of an inner and outer membrane separated by a space of about 80 Å. Infoldings of the inner membrane form the cristae within the mitochondria. The space between the membranes of the cristae is in communication with that between the inner and the outer membranes and has about the same measurements as it. The cristae may lie obliquely or in curves across part or the whole of the mitochondrion or may extend longitudinally along all its length. A matrix of fine granular material and occasional dense round particles about 500 Å in diameter may occur between the cristae of the mitochondria. The oxidative enzymes and various other enzymes are located in the mitochondria.

Glycogen granules 150 to 300 Å in diameter occur under the plasma membrane, around the nuclei and in lesser amounts between the myofibrils and the myofilaments (Plates 1 and 2). Some fibres contain more glycogen than others and the amount varies according to the physiological state of the muscle fibre (Kugelberg and Edström, 1968).

Lipid bodies 0·5 to 1 μ in diameter, some of which are bounded by a membrane, occur within the muscle fibre generally under the plasma membrane and near the mitochondria on either side of the Z-line (Plate 1) and also around the nuclei. More rarely they occur between the myofibrils. With osmium tetroxide fixation the saturated fatty acids are pale, while the unsaturated fatty acids are black (Wigglesworth, 1957). A histological study of lipid droplets of striated muscle was reported by Bullard (1912) and an ultrastructural study of lipid in normal human muscle was reported by Prineas and Ng (1967). Collections of irregular bodies of varying electron density sometimes occur in the muscle fibres, especially in the elderly, and are thought to represent the lipofuscin granules seen by light microscopy. Lysosomes, which are membrane bound bodies containing hydrolytic enzymes, occur in muscle as in the other tissues (De Duve, 1969). By electron microscopy alone it is not possible to identify them accurately in muscle but they can be identified by combined histochemical and electron microscopy techniques. Numerous authors accept lipid bodies as lysosomes.

Ribosomes, particles about 100 to 150 Å in diameter (Palade, 1956), are not usually identified in the sarcoplasm of normal adult muscle. They are generally smaller than glycogen granules, but in material fixed in glutaraldehyde and osmium tetroxide and stained by uranyl acetate and lead citrate, ribosomes cannot be easily distinguished from glycogen granules. However, if the specimen is fixed in glutaraldehyde only and stained with uranyl acetate the distinction between glycogen and ribosomes becomes easier, the ribosomes being electron dense and the glycogen granules pale (Galavazi and te Lintel Hekkert, 1968).

The endoplasmic reticulum of the muscle fibre is usually called the sarcoplasmic reticulum and consists of parallel tubules which run between the myofibrils. The adjacent tubules intercommunicate with one another. At the junction of the I- and A-bands the lateral ends of the sarcoplasmic tubules are distended and appear as rounded vesicles (Plate 1 lower part). Calcium and ATPase occur in the sarcoplasmic reticulum (Samaha and Gergely, 1965, 1969; Samaha, 1967; and Vye, Fischman and Hansen, 1969).

The sarcoplasmic reticulum is less well developed in man than in many animals and may vary in its development in different animals and in different muscles in the same animal. It is particularly abundant in the fast acting 'remotor' muscle of the lobster (Rosenbluth, 1969).

In man and other animals a transverse system of tubules usually referred to as the T-system lie near the junction of the A- and I-bands, and pass between the dilated ends of the sarcoplasmic tubules. The T-system and the two adjacent dilated ends of the sarcoplasmic reticulum form triads (Plates 1 and 4) which are concerned with excitation and contraction of the muscle fibre (A. F. Huxley, 1957b; A. F. Huxley and Straub, 1958; and A. F. Huxley and Taylor, 1958).

Lindner (1957) from his studies on the myocardium of dogs suggested that the T-systems were a prolongation of the plasma membrane into the muscle fibre. In cardiac muscle this was demonstrated in sheep by Simpson and Oertelis (1961 and 1962), in rabbit and man by Nelson and Benson (1963) and by many others including Forssmann and Gerardier (1970), who used the technique of extracellular space tracing with horseradish peroxidase. In fish muscle it was demonstrated by Franzini-Armstrong and Porter (1964 a and b). In the frog skeletal muscle H. E. Huxley (1964) and Page (1964) demonstrated that ferritin injected into the space between muscle fibres penetrates the transverse tubules but does not extend into the sarcoplasmic reticulum, showing that the T-systems and the sarcoplasmic reticulum are not in direct communication. In the skeletal muscle of the rat the continuity of the T-system with the sarcoplasmic reticulum has been reported by Walker and Schrodt (1965). Ezerman and Ishikawa (1967) demonstrated in tissue culture of chicken skeletal muscle that the T-system tubules were formed by invagination of the plasma membrane. In human skeletal muscle the continuity of the extra cellular space with the T-systems was demonstrated by Shafiq *et al.* (1966) and Jerusalem (1970).

PLASMA AND BASEMENT MEMBRANES

The muscle fibre is enclosed by a distinct *plasma membrane* (Plates 1 and 3), which is composed chiefly of lipid and in man is some 75 to 100 Å thick. In turn it is surrounded by *basement membrane* (Plates 1 and 3), which may be 300 to 500 Å thick and is much less electron dense than the plasma membrane. Some authors call the plasma membrane the sarcolemma, while others include both the plasma and basement membranes in the sarcolemma. The plasma membrane has often a wavy outline: its outer surface is frequently pitted by small indentations and small vesicles may be present along its inner surface, suggesting that it is the site of pinocytotic activity which would enable the exchange of fluid, electrolytes and protein between the muscle fibre and its environment.

SATELLITE CELLS

Mauro (1961) described in the muscle of the frog, nucleated cells situated between the plasma membrane of the muscle fibre and its basement membrane. He called them *satellite cells*. Basement membrane does not occur between the adjacent plasma membrane of the satellite cells and the muscle fibre (Plates 3 and 4 upper parts). In normal muscle, myofibrils have not been seen in the satellite cells. Mauro suggested that these cells might be dormant myoblasts capable of differentiating into muscle fibres when the muscle fibre is damaged. The satellite cells correspond to the secondary myotubes reported in embryonic muscle by Tello (1917) and Couteaux (1941). They have been described since Mauro's report by many authors both in normal and diseased human muscle, where they are much more frequent than in normal muscle and are regarded as an indication of regeneration (*see* page 57).

TYPES OF MUSCLE FIBRES

It has been known for long that two kinds of muscle are present in various animals, namely the red, slow muscles and the white, fast muscles. Dubowitz and Pearse (1960 a, c and 1961) using histochemical methods demonstrated two main types of muscle fibres in human muscle biopsies and referred to them as type I fibres and type II fibres, which correspond to the red and white fibres respectively. Stein and Padykula (1962), Guth and Samaha (1969), Samaha, Guth and Albers (1970) demonstrated that the type II fibres can be subdivided into two types, one in which the ATPase reaction is formaldehyde sensitive and the other formaldehyde resistant. Brooke and Kaiser (1970) have reported similar observations.

The ultrastructure of the different types of muscle fibres has been extensively studied in various animals by the following and other authors: Hess (1960, 1961 and 1965), Peachey and A. F. Huxley (1962), Page (1965), Bubenzer (1966), Gauthier and Padykula (1966), Padykula and Gauthier (1967 and 1970), Gauthier (1969), Shafiq, Gorycki and Milhorat (1969), Schiaffino, Hanzlíková and Pierobon (1970). The ultrastructural differences are summarised as follows. Red fibres have more mitochondria and lipid than white fibres which are rich in glycogen and have more sarcoplasmic reticulum than the red fibres. Fibres occur which have ultrastructural features intermediate between those of the red and white fibres and have been designated as intermediate type fibres. The Z-lines in the red fibres are wider than in the white fibres: this was demonstrated in the frog by Peachey and A. F. Huxley (1962), in the rat by Shafiq, Gorycki and Milhorat (1969), Landon (1970), Padykula and Gauthier (1970) and Schiaffino, Hanzlíková and Pierobon (1970).

In man the ultrastructural differences between the types of muscle fibres is much less distinct (Plate 4 upper part). Studies on their ultrastructure are reported by Shafiq *et al.* (1966) and Ogata and Murata (1969b), who found differences chiefly in the number, size and shape of the mitochondria. In diseased muscle the differentiation is still more difficult since the organelles of the fibres are often greatly altered by the pathological process affecting the muscle (Plate 4 lower part).

BLOOD CAPILLARIES, FIBROBLASTS AND COLLAGEN

Between the muscle fibres lie numerous *blood capillaries* which are formed of endothelial cells that are closely applied to each other (Plate 3 lower part). The plasma membranes of adjacent endothelial cells show zones of increased thickness and electron density which are called desmosomes. The outer aspect of the endothelial cells is covered by basement membrane of variable thickness and clefts occur in this basement membrane which lodge the pericytes. The endothelial cell may present many small depressions of its plasma membrane as well as folds of cytoplasm which project into the capillary lumen and sometimes reunite with the endothelial cell cytoplasm, having engulfed some of the capillary contents. Numerous vesicles may be seen throughout the endothelial cell cytoplasm and may collect in apposition to the plasma membrane applied to the basement membrane. These depressions, folds of cytoplasm and cytoplasmic vesicles, suggest that pinocytosis is an important activity of the endothelial cells of the blood capillaries. The pericyte cytoplasm has features similar to those of the endothelial cell and may also show evidence of pinocytosis. The ultrastructure of blood capillaries has been studied by various authors and amongst these is the report of Fernando and Movat (1964) and Vracko (1970b).

Occasional *fibroblasts* which have elongated processes also occur between the muscle fibres and in the neighbourhood of the blood capillaries. The fibroblast cytoplasm may exhibit rough endoplasmic reticulum, vesicles and fine filaments as well as the other components common to most cells. The fibroblasts are not covered by basement membrane. They elaborate *collagen* which surrounds the vessels, nerves and the muscle fibres, but only a small amount of collagen is present around these structures under normal circumstances (Plate 3).

MYOTENDINOUS JUNCTION

At the *myotendinous junction* the muscle fibre interdigitates with the collagen and fibroblasts which form the tendon (Plates 5 and 25 lower part). The collagen lies close to the muscle fibre but does not enter it. At the junction of the muscle fibre with the collagen, fine filaments als o occur in contiguity with the basement membrane. The digitations of the muscle fibre may vary a great deal in size and shape and may in random sections appear to be independent of the rest of the muscle fibre. Very often these digitations enclose pockets of collagen (Plate 5 lower part). The plasma membrane of the muscle fibre at the myotendinous junction is thickened, forming an electron dense zone of variable dimensions which corresponds to the terminal Z-line of the final sarcomere of the myofibril. At the edge of some muscle fibres there occur zebra bodies (Plate 5 upper part) which are similar to those seen in other locations such as the extra-ocular muscles (Plates 10 and 43 upper parts, *see* page 10) and muscle spindles, page 8. Rods similar to 'nemaline' rods may also occur at the myotendinous junction (Plate 25 lower part). The ultrastructure of the myotendinous junction in man and other mammals has been reported by Ishikawa (1965) who refers to earlier studies on this subject.

NERVES AND MOTOR END PLATES

Myelinated and unmyelinated *nerves* occur between the muscle fibres (Plates 6 and 7). The nerve fibres lie within Schwann cell cytoplasm, which is then surrounded by basement membrane and collagen as well as other Schwann cells containing myelinated or unmyelinated nerves, fibroblasts and collagen. All of these are in turn surrounded by several concentric layers of perineurial cells which are covered by basement membrane. Groups of collagen fibres occur between and around the outer aspect of the perineurial cells. The nuclei of the perineurial cells are not strikingly different from other cell nuclei but the cytoplasm of the perineurial cells is very rich in vesicles, much more so than the cytoplasm of the Schwann cells (Thomas, 1963).

Before the nerve contacts the muscle fibre to form the *motor end plate* (Plate 8) the axon loses its myelin sheath but retains a covering of Schwann cell cytoplasm. The terminal axon lies in a depression, the primary synaptic cleft or gutter on the surface of the muscle fibre. The nerve is covered on its outer aspect by a crescent of Schwann cell cytoplasm and the part lying in the primary synaptic gutter is separated from the muscle fibre by basement membrane. The surface of the muscle fibre at the synaptic gutter has several indentations arranged in a palisade manner, referred to as the subneural apparatus which can be readily demonstrated by histochemical methods for cholinesterase activity. The subneural apparatus is formed by extensions of the primary synaptic cleft which indent the surface of the muscle to form the secondary synaptic clefts: these also contain basement membrane. They are bounded by the plasma membrane of the muscle fibre. Continuity of the primary and secondary synaptic clefts may not be apparent in some sections and the secondary synaptic clefts may appear to lie independently within the muscle fibre. The terminal axon contains mitochondria, filaments, tubules and synaptic vesicles which are said to contain acetylcholine. In the muscle fibre around the secondary synaptic clefts there are numerous mitochondria and small vesicles.

The cholinesterase is localised in the primary and secondary synaptic clefts (Lehrer, 1962) and also at the plasma membrane and in the vesicles of the terminal axon and in the plasma membrane of the muscle fibre covering the synaptic clefts (Barrnett, 1962). Teräväinen (1969c) demonstrated that the reaction for acetylcholinesterase is more intense in the neighbourhood of the plasma membrane of the muscle bounding the synaptic clefts.

The ultrastructure of the motor end plate was first described in animals by Beams and Evans (1953) and subsequently by Reger (1954, 1955 and 1959), Palade (1954), Robertson (1954 and 1960), Andersson-Cedergren (1959), Birks, H. E. Huxley and Katz (1960), Lehrer (1960) and later by many other authors. Zacks (1964) and Coërs (1967) reported extensively on the structure of the motor end plate. In man the ultrastructure of the motor end plate was first studied by De Harven and Coërs (1959) and Coërs and De Harven (1962). The ultrastructure of the developing motor end plate was reported by Hirano (1967) in the chick, by Kelly and Zacks (1969) and Zacks and Saito (1970) in the rat and mouse, and by Lentz (1969 and 1970) in regenerating limbs of the newt triturus.

The ultrastructure of the motor end plates in the various types of muscle fibres of animals was reported by Ogata and Murata (1969a), Padykula and Gauthier (1970) and Fardeau and W. K. Engel (1970) and in human muscle by Murata and Ogata (1969).

MUSCLE SPINDLES

Muscle spindles, being small, are not commonly found in the small biopsies of human muscle prepared for electron microscopy. The spindles (Plate 9) consist of a capsule formed by concentric layers of cells which surround 3 to 12 small muscle fibres, numerous myelinated and unmyelinated nerves, some small blood vessels and collagen fibres.

The cells of the capsule have an elongated electron dense nucleus and a relatively small amount of cytoplasm. Numerous slender processes which may communicate with each other extend from the cells and are arranged concentrically around the spindle. They may also extend into the spindle and surround some of its contents. The cytoplasm of these cell processes are fairly electron dense and contain a large number of clear vesicles. Basement membrane covers the capsule cells and their processes which are structurally similar to perineurial cells. Bundles of collagen fibres and occasional groups of myelinated and unmyelinated nerve fibres lie between the concentric cell layers (Plate 9 lower part).

Two types of muscle fibres occur in the spindle. The longer, thicker—nuclear bag—fibres which run the length of the spindle and are attached at either end to the collagen outside the poles of the spindle. In the equatorial zone the nuclear bag fibres are distended with collections of nuclei; nuclei occur in addition along the length of the fibre. The shorter, thinner—nuclear chain—fibres lie entirely within the spindle. Their nuclei are distributed in the long axis of the fibre. Both types of muscle fibres have the same structural features as the extra-fusal fibres. Satellite cells are said to be more frequent in intra-fusal muscle fibres than in the extra-fusal fibres. Within the muscle fibres of the spindle there occur zebra bodies which lie mainly at the surface of the muscle fibre and are perpendicular to its long axis. The zebra bodies consist of electron dense bars like Z-lines with thin filaments extending between them. They may vary in shape and size. The dense bars of the zebra bodies are in places continuous with the plasma membrane of the muscle fibre. Zebra bodies were described in muscle spindles of the extensor longus digitorum IV of the frog by Katz (1961), who referred to them as 'ladder-like' structures and thought that they may possibly form intracellular 'microtendons' between the myofilaments and sensory endings. Such zebra bodies were illustrated in the human muscle spindle by Gruner (1961) and in the muscle spindle of man and the rat by Rumpelt and Schmalbruch (1969). They were described in the muscle spindle of the rat by Landon (1966a) and in the frog by Karlsson and Andersson-Cedergren (1968). They occur in extra-fusal muscle fibres in the latissimus dorsi of the thrush (Ruska and Edwards, 1957) and also in the myocardium of sheep (Caesar, Edwards and Ruska, 1958), mice (Theones and Ruska, 1960) and macacus rhesus (Virágh, 1968), in the ciliary muscle of the chick (Zenker and Krammer, 1967) and in human extra-ocular muscle (Mukuno, 1966). They are illustrated in human extra-ocular muscle in Plates 10 and 43 (upper parts) and at the myotendinous junction of the first dorsal interosseous muscle of the foot in man (Plate 5).

Bundles of collagen fibres, collections of fine fibrils, myelinated and unmyelinated nerves and small blood vessels are seen within the spindle (Plate 9 upper part). Two types of nerve ending occur in the intra-fusal fibres: the sensory and motor endings. The sensory endings are not covered by Schwann cell cytoplasm: they lie inside the basement membrane of the muscle fibre: no basement membrane separates the adjacent plasma membranes of the nerve ending and the muscle fibre. The sensory nerve endings contain neurofilaments, tubules, vesicles and mitochondria. The motor nerve endings resemble the motor end plates of extra-fusal muscle fibres and are covered by Schwann cell cytoplasm: basement membrane separates the plasma membrane of the axon from that of the muscle fibre.

The structure of muscle spindles and their innervation have been studied by light microscopy by various authors including Barker (1948), Boyd (1962) and Cooper and Daniel (1963). Histochemical studies of muscle fibres of the muscle spindle have been reported by various authors and amongst the recent reports is that of Spiro and Beilin (1969).

The ultrastructure of the muscle spindle has been reported in man by Gruner (1961) and in man and the rat by Rumpelt and Schmalbruch (1969), in frogs by Robertson (1960), Katz (1961) and Karlsson and Andersson-Cedergren (1966 and 1968), Karlsson, Andersson-Cedergren and Ottoson (1966), in the rat by Merrillees (1960) and Landon (1966 a and b) and in the cat by Adal (1969) and Barker, Stacey and Adal (1970).

EXTRA-OCULAR MUSCLE

Extra-ocular muscle is composed of muscle fibres of small diameter, the average being between 17·5 and 20 μ (Adams, Denny-Brown and Pearson, 1962), and contains numerous myelinated and unmyelinated nerves (Plate 11 upper part). In man they are very rich in spindles (Cooper and Daniel, 1949), but spindles have not been found in the extra-ocular muscles of many other species.

A striking feature of extra-ocular muscle is the presence within it, and often usually near the plasma membrane, of ellipsoid or fan-shaped collections of alternating light and dark parallel bands (Plates 10 and 43 upper part). The dark bands are similar in appearance to the Z-lines and sometimes are continuous with the plasma membrane of the muscle cell. The light bands are formed of fine filaments perpendicular to the dark lines. Both the light and dark bands may be continuous with the myofilaments and the dark bands may extend to the plasma membrane (Mukuno, 1966). Similar structures have been described in the muscle spindles and at the myotendinous junction: we refer to them as zebra bodies.

Filamentous bodies (Plate 10 lower part) may also be found fairly frequently in extra-ocular muscle and generally near the nucleus.

Rods similar to those described in nemaline myopathy have been described in normal and diseased human extra-ocular muscle by Mukuno (1969). We found them in the extra-ocular muscles of three patients (Plate 26).

Two types of muscle fibres occur in extra-ocular muscle which are often referred to as having 'Fibrillenstruktur' and 'Feldenstruktur' respectively: they correspond to the twitch and slow fibres. In different muscles of different species Krüger (1929 and 1949) described these two types of muscle fibres. They differ in their ultrastructure. The 'Fibrillenstruktur' fibres or twitch fibres are about 25 to 50 μ in diameter, have a large amount of sarcoplasm, many mitochondria between the myofibrils and the sarcoplasmic reticulum and the T-systems are very evident. Their motor end plates resemble those of skeletal muscle (Plate 11 lower part). The 'Feldenstruktur' fibres or slow fibres are about 9 to 15 μ in diameter with less sarcoplasm and mitochondria: their myofibrils are closely packed and less well demarcated: their sarcoplasmic reticulum and T-systems are less evident than in the twitch fibres. The slow fibres have many nerve endings in relation to them but only a few rudimentary synaptic clefts. The ultrastructure of the motor end plates of human extra-ocular muscle was reported by Mukuno (1968b), who classified them into six different types, some of which he regarded as being peculiar to extra-ocular muscle.

The ultrastructure of human extra-ocular muscle and its innervation was reported by Dietert (1965), Brandt and Leeson (1966) and Mukuno (1966, 1968 a and b), and of the guinea pig by Hess (1962), the cat by Hess and Pilar (1963), Chèng and Breinin (1965), Peachey (1966) and Pilar and Hess (1966), the rat by Namba *et al.* (1968), Teräväinen (1968, 1969 a, b and c) and in the monkey by Cheng and Breinin (1966).

FOETAL SKELETAL MUSCLE

Muscle cells arise from undifferentiated mononucleated cells, the myoblasts which fuse to form multinucleated cells and differentiate into adult muscle fibres. In the same muscle of the foetus from early stages of development, there occur simultaneously cells at different stages of differentiation (Plates 12 and 13).

Myoblasts are rounded undifferentiated cells with a large rounded nucleus, the chromatin of which is fairly dense and more concentrated at its periphery. Nucleoli may be prominent in the nucleus. Myoblasts have a relatively large amount of cytoplasm which contains a prominent Golgi apparatus, centrioles, rough and smooth endoplasmic reticulum, glycogen granules, some ribosomes and mitochondria. They have a fine plasma membrane and may or may not exhibit a thicker, less electron dense layer of basement membrane. Myoblasts multiply by mitotic division (Plate 14). They fuse to form multinucleated cells which at early stages of development are sometimes referred to as myocells. The multinucleated cells so formed elaborate well-differentiated myofibrils which are situated at the periphery of the cell with rows of nuclei surrounded by glycogen granules in the centre. These cells are the myotubes. They contain also rough and smooth endoplasmic reticulum, ribosomes, polysomes, mitochondria and lipid droplets. These multinucleated cells have not been observed to multiply by mitotic division. Basement membrane surrounds the myotube and in the same common basement membrane of the myotube may occur cells at early stages of differentiation (Plates 12 and 13), including myoblasts in mitosis (Ochoa and Mair, 1968).

The histogenesis of skeletal muscle was studied extensively by light microscopy by several authors, including Tello (1917) and Couteaux (1941).

The ultrastructure of human foetal skeletal muscle was reported by Ishikawa (1966 and 1970), Ochoa and Mair (1968), Larson, Hudgson and Walton (1969), Hudgson, Jenkison and Larson (1970) and Conen and Bell (1970) and has been fairly well investigated in experimental animals by van Breemen (1952), Bergman (1962), Shafiq (1963), Allen and Pepe (1965), Heuson-Stiennon (1965), Dessouky and Hibbs (1965), Konigsberg (1965), Przybylski and Blumberg (1966), Fischman (1967), Church (1969), Kelly and Zacks (1969) and Hudgson, Jenkison and Larson (1970).

The ultrastructure of the development of chick embryo muscle has been reported by Ezerman and Ishikawa (1967), Ishikawa, Bischoff and Holtzer (1968), Larson, Jenkison and Hudgson (1970) and Shimada (1970).

CARDIAC MUSCLE. ADULT AND FOETAL

Cardiac muscle resembles skeletal muscle in that the myofibrils of both are striated. Cardiac muscle fibres are, however, shorter and smaller in diameter than skeletal muscle fibres. Interdigitation of the myocardial fibres occurs, but numerous clefts also exist between adjacent cells. Contiguous myocardial fibres present thickened zones of increased electron density without any intervening basement membrane between their plasma membranes. These are the intercalated discs and are illustrated in the lower part of Plate 15, where it is seen that they may be very tortuous and may correspond to the terminal Z-lines of myofibrils of contiguous fibres. The ultrastructure of the intercalated disc was reviewed and studied in detail in a recent report by McNutt (1970). Myocardial fibres contain large amounts of glycogen granules and numerous large mitochondria. Abundant osmophilic granules are particularly prevalent throughout the sarcoplasm of the atrial muscle fibres and these were reported by Jamieson and Palade (1964) as specific granules in the atrium of various animals and man. The sarcoplasmic reticulum is not well developed. The T-system in the ventricle is very apparent and larger than in skeletal muscle. The T-tubules run straight from the plasma membrane at the level of the Z-line and penetrate deeply into the myocardial fibre, where they lie in relation to only one lateral sac of the sarcoplasmic reticulum, forming a diad and not a triad as in skeletal muscle.

There are numerous reports on the ultrastructure of cardiac muscle of various animals and amongst these are the recent reports of Fawcett and McNutt (1969) and McNutt and Fawcett (1969). In man the ultrastructure of myocardium was first reported by Kisch, Grey and Kelsch (1948), later by Smith, Burford and Chiquoine (1960), Battig and Low (1961), Nelson and Benson (1963), Poche and Ohm (1963), Richter and Kellner (1963) and by Burdette and Ashford (1965) and other authors.

The development of cardiac muscle has been studied in animals by various authors including Hibbs (1956), Wainrach and Sotelo (1961), Manasek (1968 and 1970) and Weinstein and Hay (1970). In man it has been studied by Leak and Burke (1964) and Bergmann and Mair and the following description is based on the latter study.

At 16 weeks development (Plate 15 upper part) the myocardial cells occur in groups bounded by a common basement membrane with frequent spaces between the adjacent cell groups. Basement membrane does not penetrate between the plasma membranes of adjacent cells. Collagen fibres and fibroblasts separate the myocardial cells from the endocardial cells lining the cardiac chambers. Numerous small vesicles may be present under the plasma membrane of some myocardial cells. Frequent zones of electron dense thickening, which are the intercalated discs, are found on the plasma membrane of adjacent cells and as in adult myocardium they may lie at the site of the terminal Z-line of myofibrils of contiguous cells. Well-differentiated myofibrils are situated at the periphery of the fibre and are similar in structure to the myofibrils of adult muscle. Large accumulations of glycogen granules are present throughout the cells as well as numerous mitochondria. Many osmophilic granules about 180–250 μ in diameter are found in the myocardial cells of the auricle. The nucleus occupies the centre of the cell and may have prominent nucleoli. Prominent flattened tubules of the Golgi apparatus and vacuoles are numerous around the nucleus. Smooth and rough endoplasmic reticulum are prominent in some cells. Centrioles (Plate 16 upper part) with their typical structural pattern (Fawcett, 1966), are found fairly frequently in the neighbourhood of the nucleus and the Golgi apparatus. In addition there occur myocardial cells undergoing mitosis; they are rich in granular material and mitochondria and possess at their periphery well-differentiated myofibrils (Plate 16 lower part). Myocardial cells undergoing mitosis and containing well-developed myofibrils were reported in the developing chick by Manasek (1968) and by Weinstein and Hay (1970).

PLATE 1. LONGITUDINAL SECTION OF NORMAL MUSCLE

UPPER. Part of a muscle fibre is illustrated: it is limited by a plasma membrane covered by basement membrane immediately adjacent to which lie strands of collagen. The muscle fibre is composed of myofilaments which lie in parallel rows forming myofibrils which exhibit recurring light and dark bands, the I- and A-bands. In the middle of the I-band is the very dense broad Z-line: the distance between two Z-lines is called a sarcomere. The thin filaments which form the I-bands extend from the Z-line into the A-band interdigitating with the thick filaments which are confined to the A-bands. In the middle of the A-band is a lighter zone, the H-zone, in which only thick filaments occur. In the centre of the H-zone is a dense thick line, the M-line. The length of the sarcomere varies according to the state of contraction or relaxation of the muscle. The length of the A-band is fairly constant, about 1·5 μ, but the length of the I-band is variable. In relaxed muscle as here the I-band is long, about 1·7 μ, but in contracted muscle it shortens due to the fine filaments sliding between the thick filaments of the A-band. The myofibrils are separated by glycogen granules, mitochondria, some triads and occasional lipid bodies.

MAGNIFICATION 15,000 ×.

LOWER. Higher magnification of a muscle fibre cut near its surface shows the basement membrane of the fibre and overlying it strands of collagen. The plasma membrane is not clearly defined in all its course. The Z-lines of the myofibrils are not attached to the plasma membrane nor are they continuous between neighbouring myofibrils. Occasional glycogen granules are apparent between the fine filaments of the I-bands but are more numerous under the plasma membrane and between the myofibrils. Related to the Z-lines, mitochondria occur between the myofibrils. Near the junction of the I- and A-bands lie the triads which consist of a clear central tubule of the T-system bounded on either side by the electron dense lateral sac of the sarcoplasmic reticulum.

MAGNIFICATION 35,500 ×.

A	A-band	Mf	Myofibril
BM	Basement membrane	Mi	Mitochondria
C	Collagen	PM	Plasma membrane
G	Glycogen	Sa	Sarcomere
H	H-zone	SR	Sarcoplasmic reticulum
I	I-band	T	T-system
LB	Lipid body	Tr	Triad
M	M-line	Z	Z-line

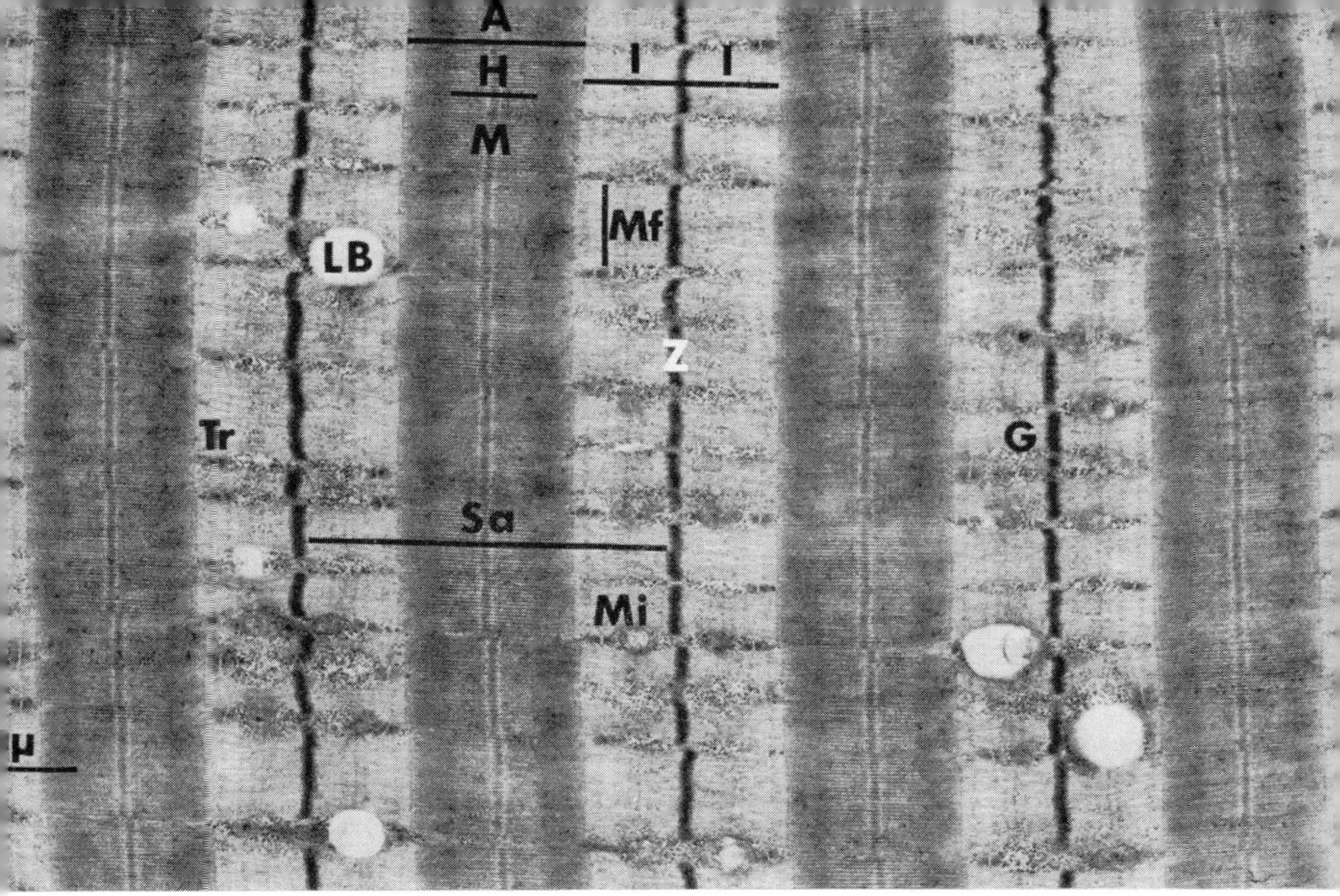
A
H
M
I I
Mf
LB
Z
Tr
G
Sa
Mi
μ

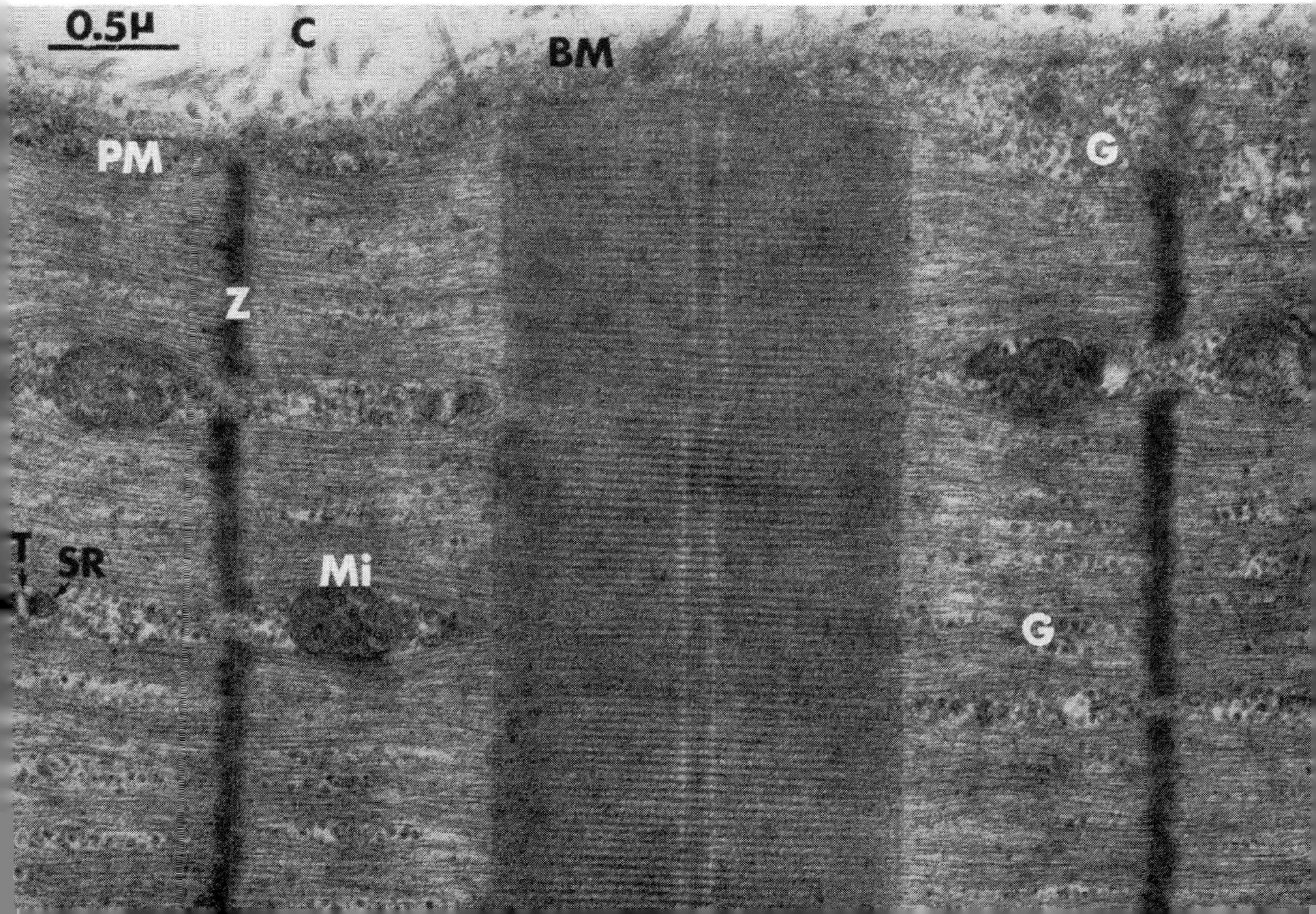
0.5μ
C
BM
PM
G
Z
T
SR
Mi
G

PLATE 2. TRANSVERSE SECTION OF NORMAL MUSCLE

UPPER. Several myofibrils are cut through the Z-lines and the I- and A-bands. Glycogen granules and occasional mitochondria occur between the myofibrils.

MAGNIFICATION 25,000 ×.

LOWER LEFT. This illustrates at higher magnification the lattice appearance of the Z-line and the fine filaments of the I-bands surrounding it. Glycogen granules lie between the Z-line and the various I-bands around it.

MAGNIFICATION 50,000 ×.

LOWER RIGHT. The *upper part* shows that the A-band consists of one thick and six thin filaments in hexagonal distribution as indicated within the rings.

In the centre of the A-band is the H-zone which consists of thick filaments only.

The *lower part* illustrates the M-line which lies in the centre of the H-zone and consists of thick filaments with interconnecting bridges.

MAGNIFICATION 100,000 ×.

A	A-band	Mf	Myofibril
G	Glycogen	Mi	Mitochondria
H	H-zone	Z	Z-line
I	I-band		

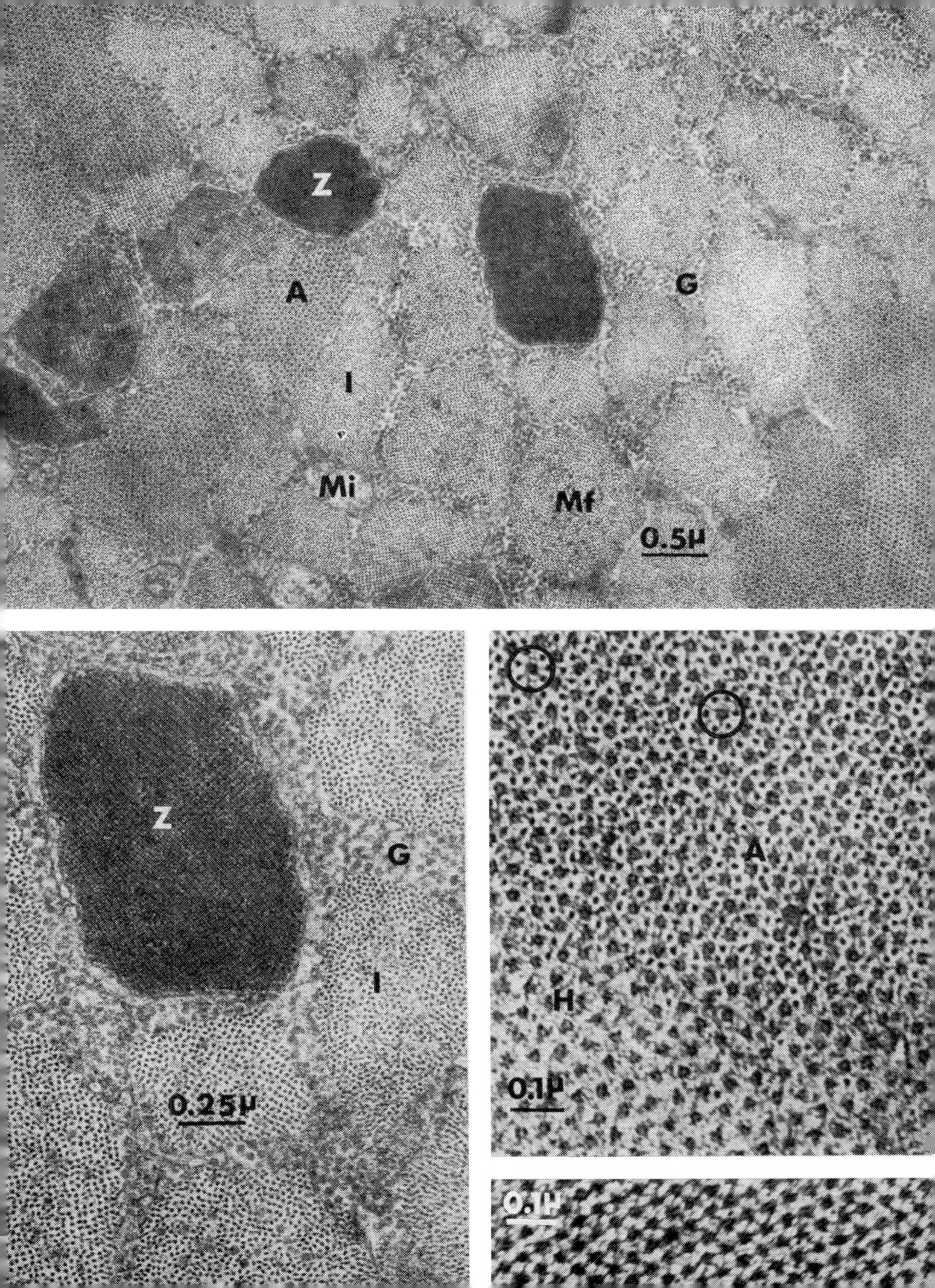
Z
A
G
I
Mi
Mf
0.5µ
Z
G
I
0.25µ
A
H
0.1µ
0.1µ

PLATE 3. TRANSVERSE SECTION OF NORMAL MUSCLE SATELLITE CELL. INTRAMUSCULAR BLOOD CAPILLARY

UPPER. Two adjacent muscle fibres are cut in cross section. Collagen lies between them. Their nuclei lie just under the plasma membrane. The lower fibre shows the chromatin in electron dense masses throughout the nucleus and around its margin. At either pole of the nucleus lie the flattened tubules of the Golgi apparatus. Within the basement membrane of the fibre is part of a satellite cell containing mitochondria, rough endoplasmic reticulum and numerous small electron dense granules. No basement membrane occurs between the plasma membranes of the muscle fibre and the satellite cell. The I- and A-bands and the H-zones of the myofibrils are indicated. Mitochondria and glycogen granules lie between the myofibrils.

MAGNIFICATION 19,000 ×.

LOWER. Between adjacent muscle fibres there lie a blood capillary, strands of collagen and processes of fibroblasts. The blood capillary is lined by endothelial cells which in turn are surrounded by basement membrane. In the lumen of this capillary only plasma occurs. No spaces occur between adjacent endothelial cells: where two cells lie in close apposition their plasma membranes show electron dense thickenings which are termed desmosomes. The nucleus of the endothelial cell has electron dense chromatin scattered throughout its substance and around its edge. The outer nuclear membrane is distinct. Many vesicles are present in the endothelial cell cytoplasm. In the basement membrane around the capillary are clefts which contain pericyte processes.

MAGNIFICATION 12,500 ×.

A	A-band
BM	Basement membrane
BC	Blood capillary
D	Desmosome
E	Endothelial cell
F	Fibroblast
Go	Golgi apparatus
H	H-zone
I	I-band
L	Lumen
Mf	Myofibril
MF	Muscle fibre
N	Nucleus
Pe	Pericyte
PM	Plasma membrane
S	Satellite cell

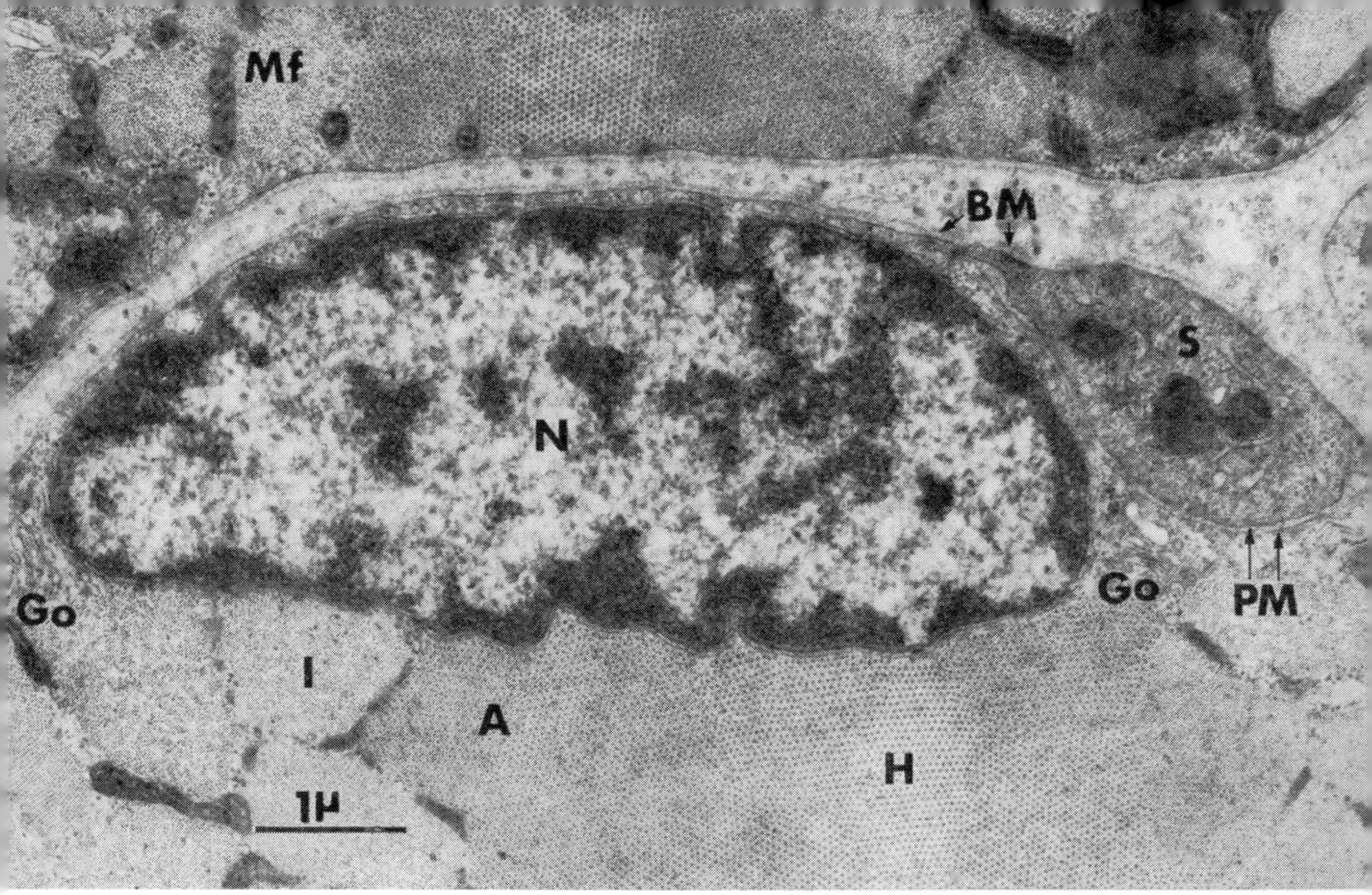
Mf
BM
S
N
Go
Go
PM
I
A
H
1μ

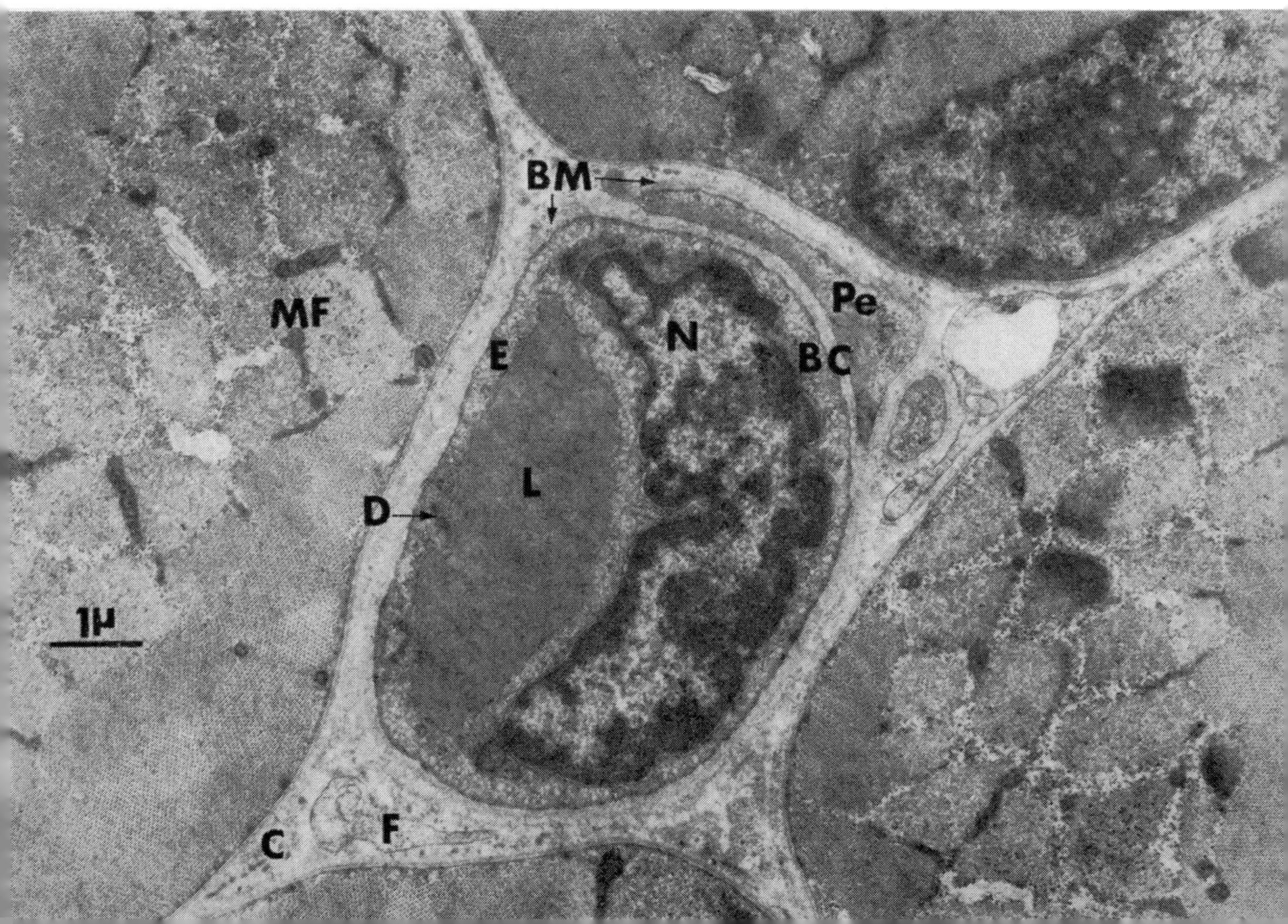
BM
MF
Pe
N
E
BC
L
D
1μ
C
F

PLATE 4. TYPES OF MUSCLE FIBRES

UPPER. It is difficult in electron micrographs of normal human muscle to distinguish the type of a fibre. Red fibres have thicker Z-lines, more mitochondria, less glycogen granules and more compactly arranged myofibrils than white fibres. In both types of fibres, the triads can be distinguished readily. Lipid bodies occur more frequently in red fibres. The upper fibre is white and the lower fibre red. As the muscle is stretched the I-band is long: consequently the sarcomere is long— 3·1 μ (Z-line to Z-line). In the middle of the A-band, the H-zone is evident with the M-line in its centre. The lower fibre which is red is rich in mitochondria and contains a satellite cell with a prominent nucleus which is more electron dense than that of the muscle fibre. The plasma membranes of both cells are distinct (arrowed).
Red fibres = Type I fibres. White fibres = Type II fibres.

MAGNIFICATION 9,000 ×.

Normal human muscle.

LOWER. In diseased muscle it is still more difficult to decide the type of a muscle fibre: it may, however, be possible. Here the upper fibre is white and the lower red. In the lower fibre the Z-line is slightly thicker and the myofibrils are more compact than in the upper fibre, where more glycogen granules are present between the myofibrils. The mitochondria are numerous in both fibres and cannot be used as a criterion to distinguish the type of these particular fibres. As the muscle is contracted the sarcomere measures only 2 μ long. In the upper and lower illustrations the A-bands are the same length, but in the lower the I-band is very short.

MAGNIFICATION 9,500 ×.

From a patient with limb girdle muscular dystrophy.

A	A-band	Mi	Mitochondria
G	Glycogen	N	Nucleus
H	H-zone	Tr	Triads
I	I-band	S	Satellite cell
LB	Lipid body	Z	Z-line

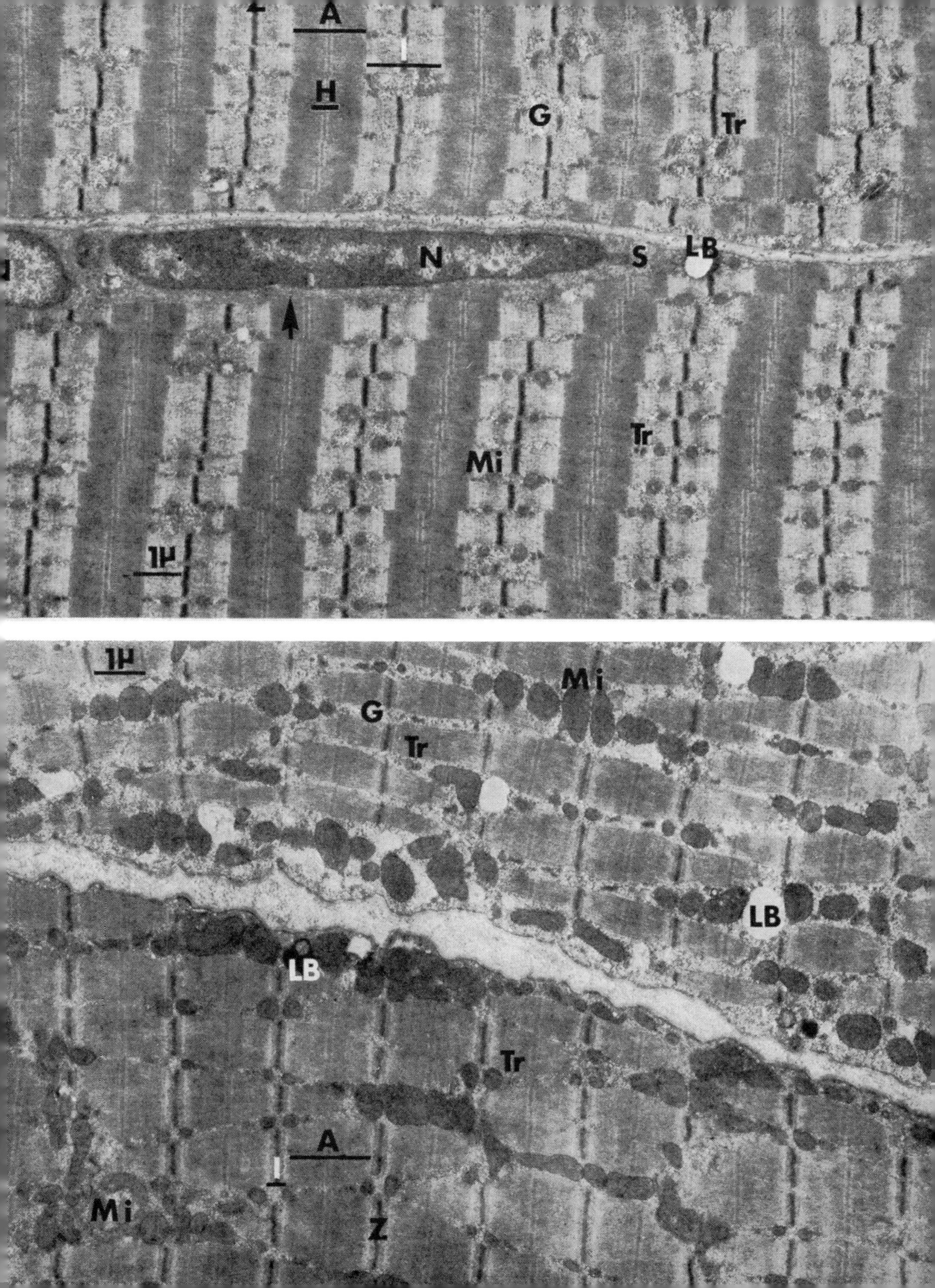
A
I
H
G
Tr
N
S
LB
Tr
Mi
1μ
1μ
Mi
G
Tr
LB
LB
Tr
A
I
Mi
Z

PLATE 5. MYOTENDINOUS JUNCTION

UPPER. On the top lie collagen fibres and some processes of fibroblasts. Below them are terminal portions of muscle fibres covered by a thick layer of basement membrane beneath which lies a broadened electron dense zone in place of the thin electron dense plasma membrane. These terminal parts of the muscle fibre surround rings of basement membrane which represent the indentations of the muscle by the tendon. The lower central part of the muscle shows that the terminal Z-line of the myofibrils corresponds to the broadened electron dense zone underlying the basement membrane. On the left a zebra body lies near the surface of a muscle fibre.

MAGNIFICATION 8,000 ×.

The *inset* shows the zebra body at higher magnification: fine filaments stretch between the very electron dense lines forming it. This structure is similar to those in extra-ocular muscle in Plate 10.

MAGNIFICATION 40,000 ×.

LOWER. A fibroblast, collagen and processes of fibroblasts lie to the left. Amongst the collagen, in the centre, are terminal digitations of the muscle fibres. They are surrounded by basement membrane and have a broad electron dense zone replacing the usual, thin, plasma membrane which, however, can be identified in some regions at the margin of this broadened zone. Some terminal parts of the muscle present central collections of collagen enclosed by rings of basement membrane: these correspond to the interdigitations of the muscle and the collagen of the myotendinous junction. On the right the muscle fibre is cut obliquely and illustrates the variable thickness of the plasma membrane at the myotendinous junction.

MAGNIFICATION 28,000 ×.

All from the first dorsal interosseous muscle of the foot.

BM Basement membrane
C Collagen
DZ Dense zone
F Fibroblast
MF Muscle fibre
PM Plasma membrane
ZB Zebra body

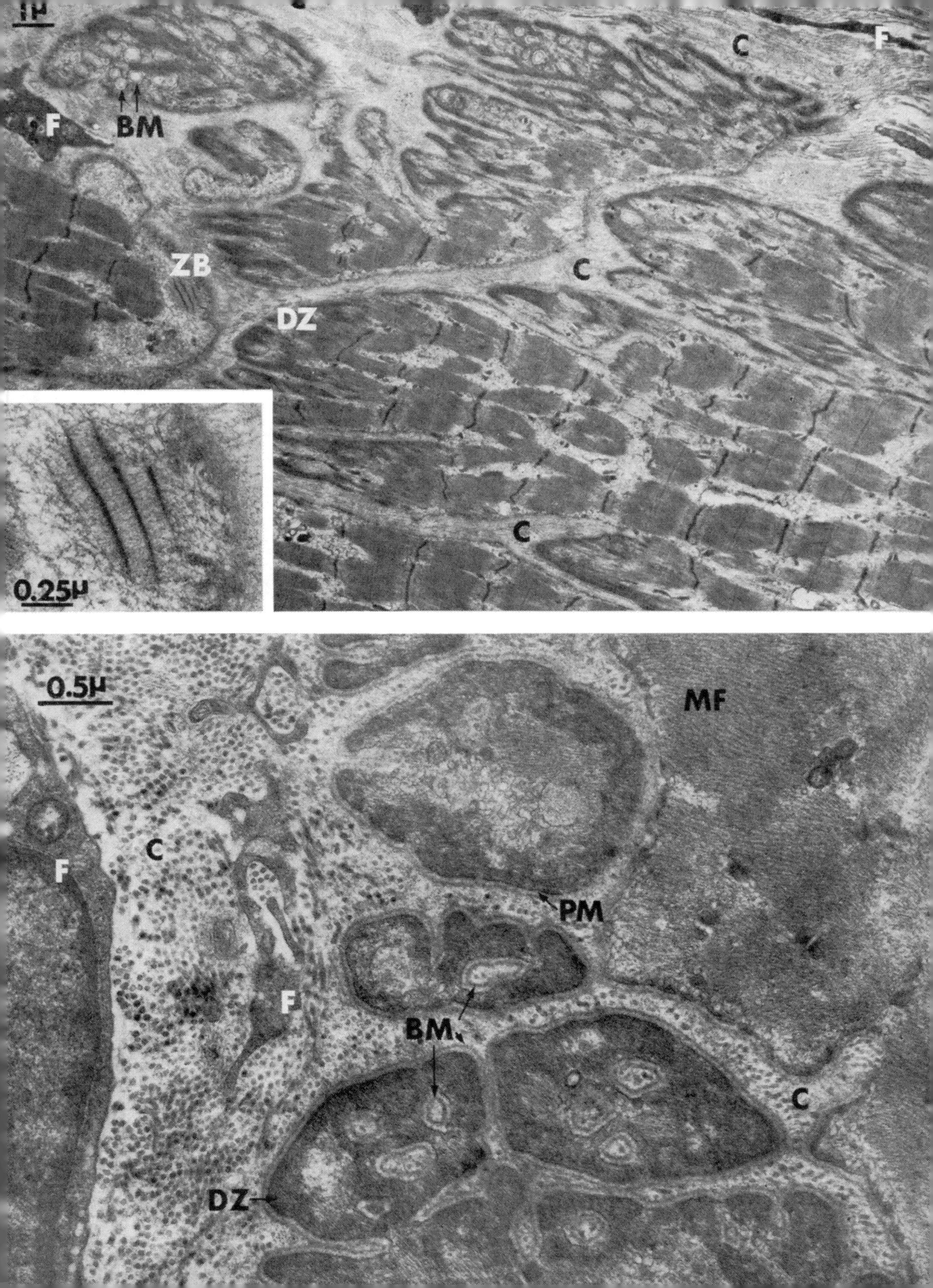
1μ
BM
F
C
F
ZB
C
DZ
C
0.25μ
0.5μ
MF
C
F
PM
F
BM
C
DZ

PLATE 6. NORMAL NERVE FIBRES IN SKELETAL MUSCLE

The central myelinated axon lies within its Schwann cell cytoplasm which is surrounded by basement membrane, bundles of collagen and processes of fibroblasts. To the left of the myelinated fibre is part of a Schwann cell enclosing an unmyelinated axon: a pocket of collagen fibres is almost completely surrounded by the Schwann cell cytoplasm as frequently happens with Schwann cells containing unmyelinated nerve fibres. Surrounding all the above structures are layers of perineurial cells, the innermost of which is cut through its nucleus and presents a prominent Golgi apparatus. Basement membrane surrounds the perineurial cells, the concentric processes of which are separated from one another by bundles of collagen. A myelinated nerve fibre surrounded by its perineurial cells lies to the top of the illustration and bottom left is another nerve containing a myelinated fibre, Schwann cell and fibroblast processes and collagen, all being surrounded by perineurial cells. Part of a muscle fibre lies to the bottom right of the illustration.

MAGNIFICATION 12,000 ×.

Ax Axon
BM Basement membrane
C Collagen
F Fibroblast
MF Muscle fibre
MN Myelinated nerve
N Nucleus
PN Perineurial cell
SCC Schwann cell cytoplasm

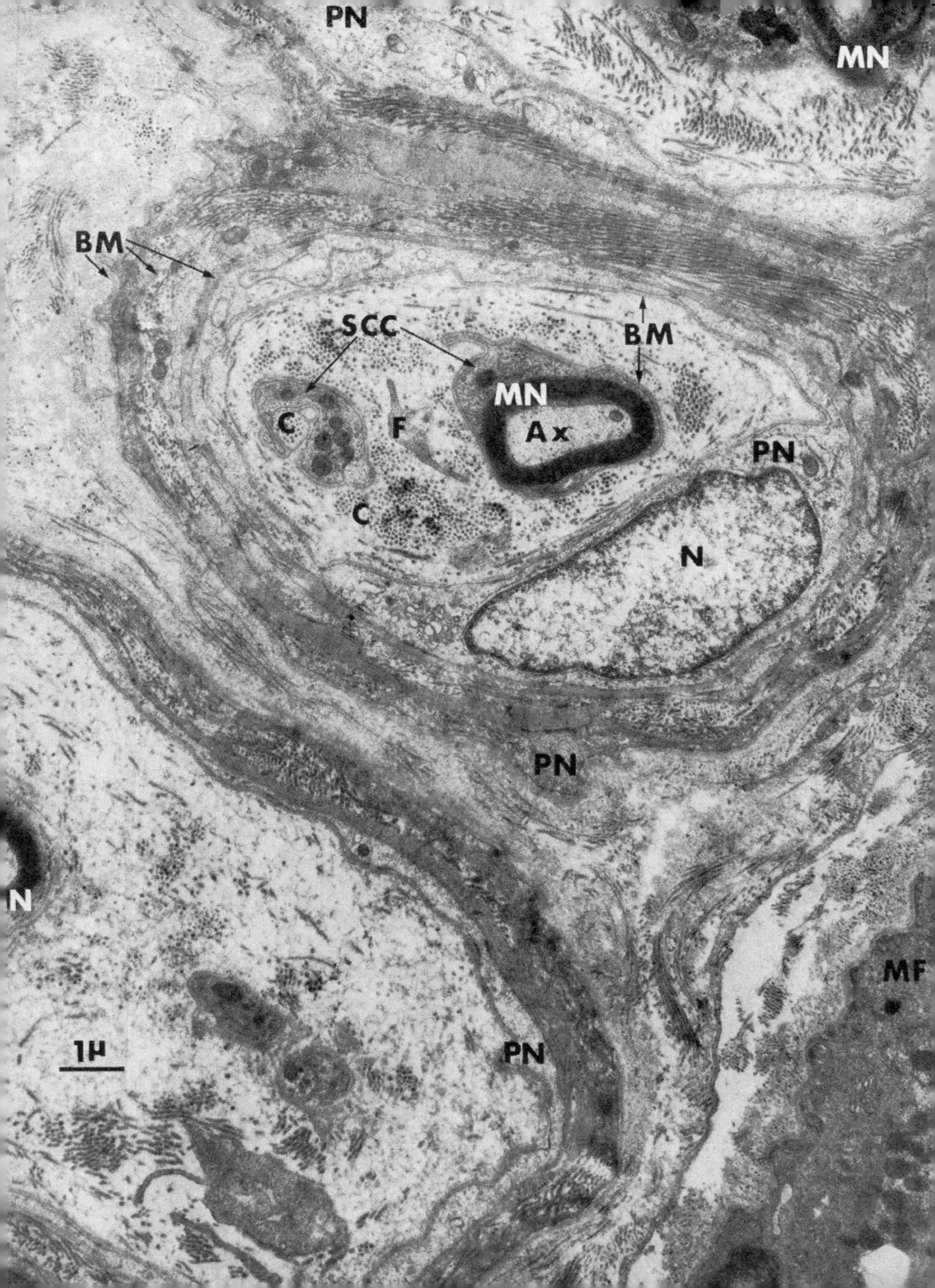

PN
MN
BM
SCC
BM
MN
C
F
Ax
PN
C
N
PN
N
MF
1μ
PN

PLATE 7. NORMAL NERVE FIBRES IN SKELETAL MUSCLE

UPPER. This myelinated nerve within the muscle is cut through the node of Ranvier and is covered by Schwann cell cytoplasm and a layer of basement membrane. The myelin lamellae as they become separated at the node are arrowed. The axon contains obvious neurofilaments and some swollen mitochondria. Above lies a nucleated Schwann cell and a Schwann cell process whose cytoplasm is different from the vesicle rich cytoplasm of the perineurial cells around the nerve. Basement membrane surrounds each perineurial cell: collections of collagen lie between and around them. Fibroblast processes and collagen lie between the perineurial cells and the muscle fibre at the top of the illustration.

MAGNIFICATION 22,000 ×.

LOWER LEFT. One myelinated nerve eventually remains within the perineurial cells of the nerve fibre before it loses its layers of myelin and terminates on the muscle fibre. The single myelinated nerve fibres are surrounded by Schwann cells, collagen and processes of the same or neighbouring Schwann cells. Collagen and processes of fibroblasts surround the nerve fibre. The axon contains numerous neurofilaments.

MAGNIFICATION 18,000 ×.

LOWER RIGHT. Besides a myelinated nerve (top right) the nerve fascicle may contain unmyelinated axons as seen in the nucleated Schwann cell in the centre. Bundles of collagen fibres may be surrounded by the processes of these Schwann cells containing unmyelinated axons. A large amount of collagen surrounds the Schwann cell: a fibroblast and related collagen lie at the bottom of the illustration.

MAGNIFICATION 26,000 ×.

Ax Axon
BM Basement membrane
C Collagen
F Fibroblast
MF Muscle fibre
MN Myelinated nerve
N Nucleus
PN Perineurial cell
SC Schwann cell
SCC Schwann cell cytoplasm
SCP Schwann cell process

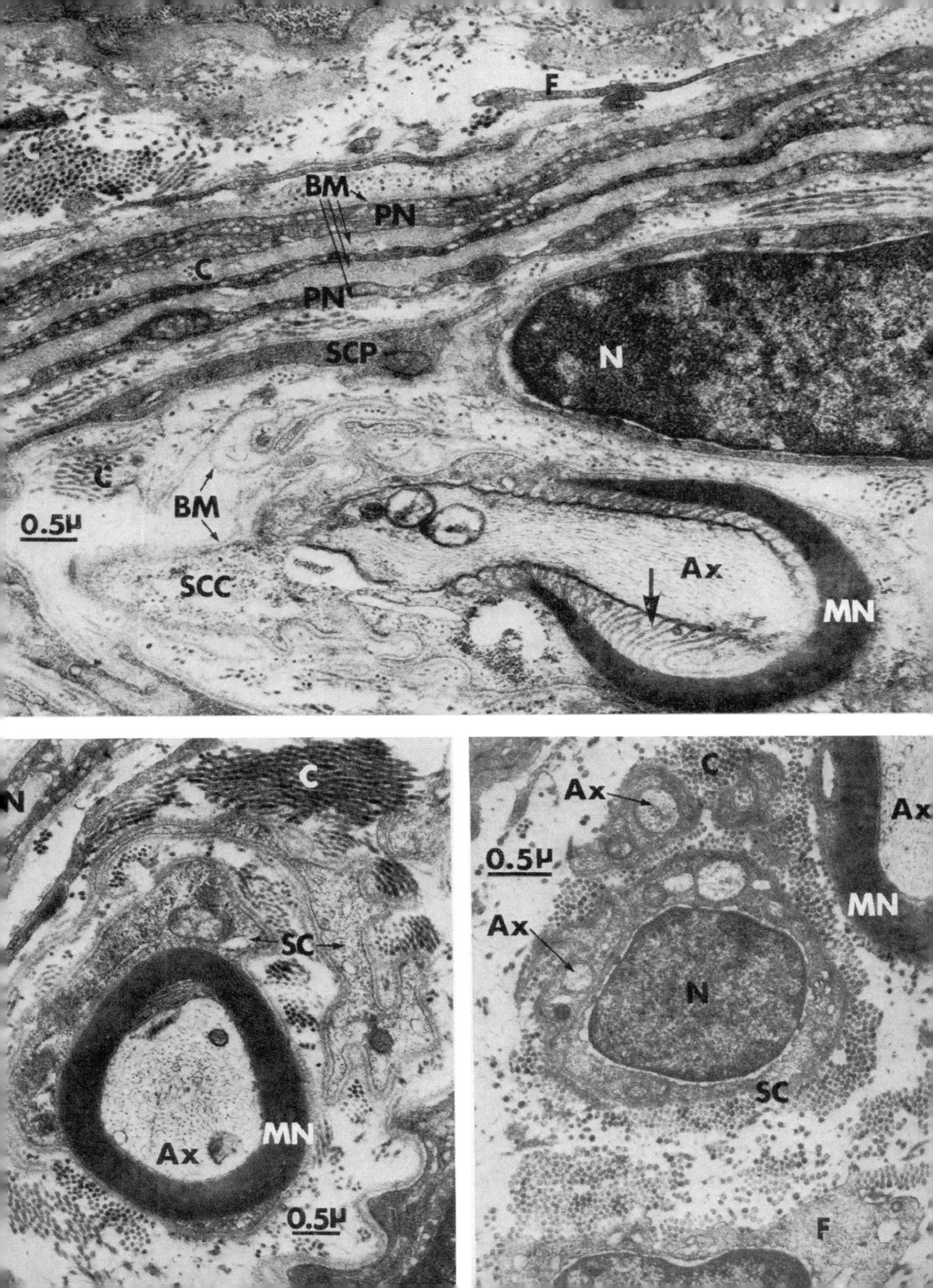
F
C
BM
PN
C
PN
SCP
N
C
BM
0.5µ
BM
SCC
Ax
MN
N
C
SC
SC
MN
Ax
0.5µ
C
Ax
Ax
0.5µ
MN
Ax
N
SC
F

PLATE 8. NORMAL MOTOR END PLATE

Three sections of a terminal axon lie in the primary synaptic cleft on the surface of this muscle fibre. Cytoplasm of the Schwann cell with its layers of plasma and basement membrane cover the outer aspect of the axon. Within the axon are mitochondria, synaptic vesicles and tubules. A layer of basement membrane lies between the axon and the muscle fibre. Numerous secondary synaptic clefts extend from the primary synaptic cleft to indent the surface of the muscle fibre. Basement membrane lies within these secondary synaptic clefts. In the sarcoplasm around the secondary synaptic clefts occur numerous vesicles and granules as well as mitochondria. Portions of two sarcolemmal nuclei and myofilaments of a myofibril lie below the secondary synaptic clefts.

MAGNIFICATION 18,000 ×.

Ax	Axon	PM	Plasma membrane
BM	Basement membrane	PSC	Primary synaptic cleft
Mi	Mitochondria	SCC	Schwann cell cytoplasm
My	Myofilaments	SSC	Secondary synaptic clefts
N	Nucleus	V	Vesicles

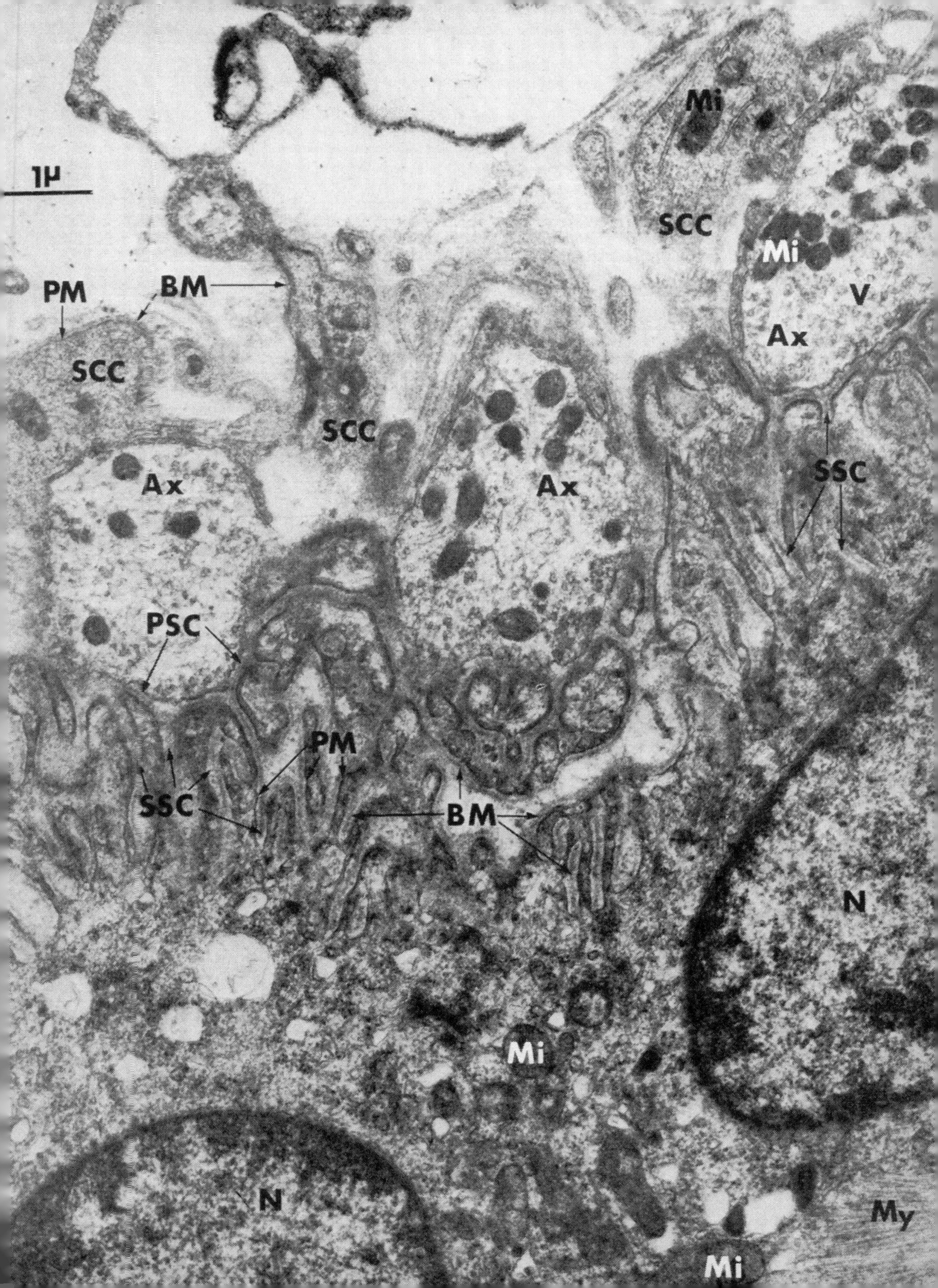
1μ
Mi
SCC
Mi
V
Ax
PM
BM
BM
SCC
SCC
Ax
Ax
SSC
PSC
PM
SSC
BM
N
Mi
N
My
Mi

PLATE 9. MUSCLE SPINDLE

UPPER LEFT. Here is a cross section of a muscle spindle containing muscle fibres with related slender cell processes which are derived from the capsule of the spindle. In addition there are nerve fibres within the spindle and between the multiple layers of cells which form its capsule. Blood vessels occur in the capsule and around it as well as collagen.

MAGNIFICATION 550 ×. Toluidine Blue.

UPPER RIGHT. A cross section of the spindle contains small muscle fibres (intrafusal fibres) in which are numerous mitochondria between the myofibrils. The two smaller muscle fibres correspond to the nuclear chain fibres and the larger to the nuclear bag fibre. Processes of cells from the capsule (arrowed) lie around the muscle fibres as well as a small amount of collagen. Numerous myelinated and some unmyelinated nerve fibres are present inside the spindle. The relatively large space between the constituents of the spindle is filled with fluid.

MAGNIFICATION 1,900 ×.

LOWER LEFT. Myelinated nerve fibres, a Schwann cell cut through its nucleus and numerous surrounding collagen fibres are seen between the concentric cell layers forming the capsule of the spindle. The capsule cells have an elongated electron dense nucleus.

MAGNIFICATION 2,500 ×.

LOWER RIGHT. Unmyelinated axons in Schwann cell processes are present between the multiple cell layers of the capsule of the muscle spindle. The thin electron dense cytoplasmic processes of these cells contain numerous, clear, relatively large vesicles. The cells are covered on either side by basement membrane and separated from each other by small bundles of collagen. These cells are similar in appearance to perineurial cells. Top right is an extrafusal fibre: a process of a fibroblast is situated between it and the capsule of the spindle.

MAGNIFICATION 9,000 ×.

Ax Axon
BM Basement membrane
BV Blood vessel
C Collagen
Ca Capsule
F Fibroblast
MF Muscle fibre
MN Myelinated nerve
N Nucleus
NB Nuclear bag fibre
NC Nuclear chain fibre
SC Schwann cell
UN Unmyelinated nerve

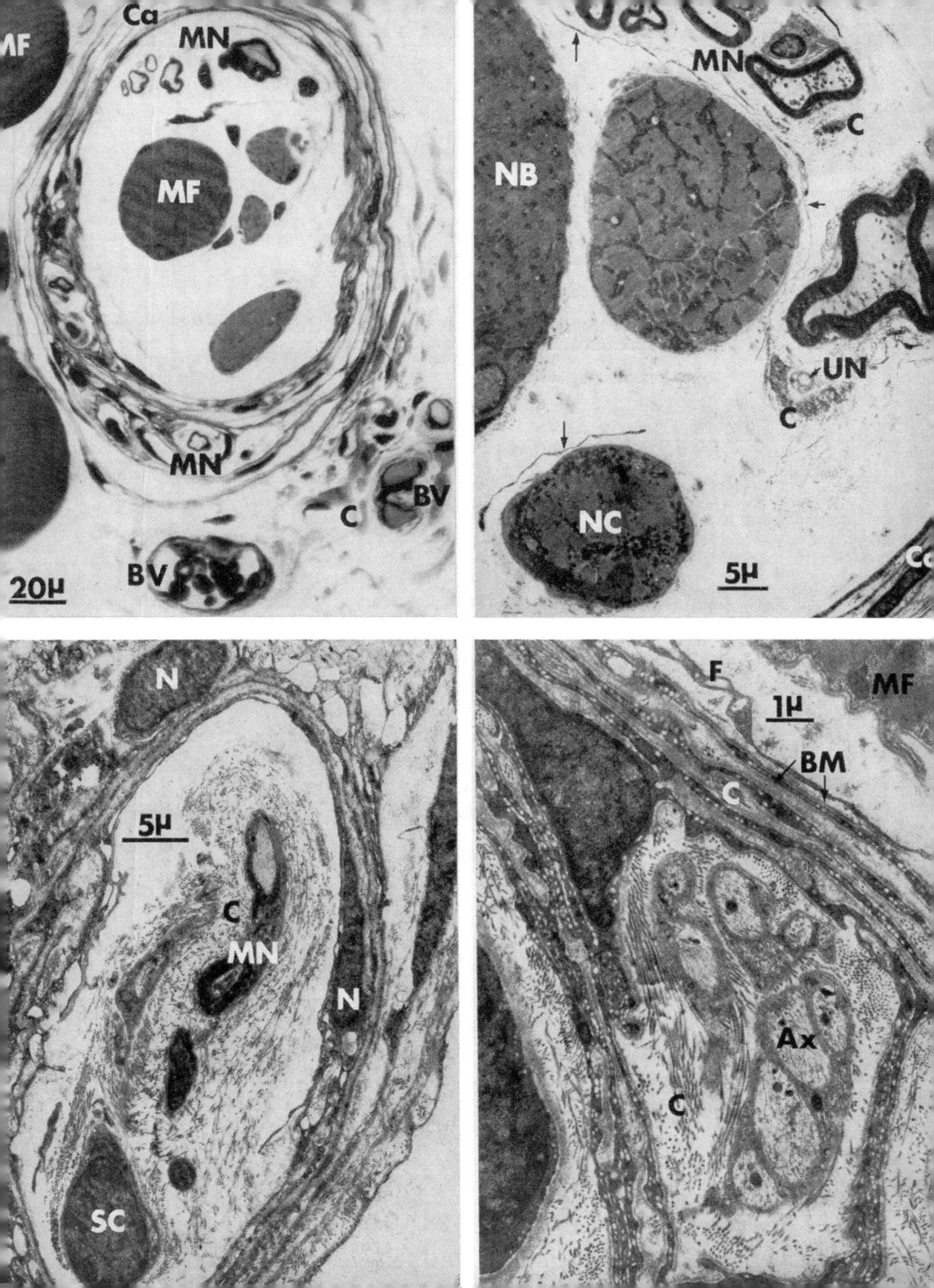
Ca
MN
MF
MF
MN
BV
C
BV
20μ
MN
C
NB
UN
C
NC
5μ
Ca
N
5μ
C
MN
N
SC
F
MF
1μ
BM
C
Ax
C

PLATE 10. EXTRA-OCULAR MUSCLE

UPPER. This muscle fibre shows curious zebra striped bodies consisting of light and electron dense filaments. They occur between the surface of the muscle fibre and the nucleus, mitochondria and myofilaments. The dense parts of these zebra bodies are continuous sometimes with the plasma membrane.

MAGNIFICATION 16,500 ×.

LOWER. Near the nucleus of another fibre are mitochondria, a rounded filamentous body, lipid and membranous bodies and masses of glycogen granules.

MAGNIFICATION 20,000 ×.

C	Collagen	Mi	Mitochondria
FB	Filamentous body	My	Myofilaments
G	Glycogen	N	Nucleus
LB	Lipid body	ZB	Zebra body
Mf	Myofibrils		

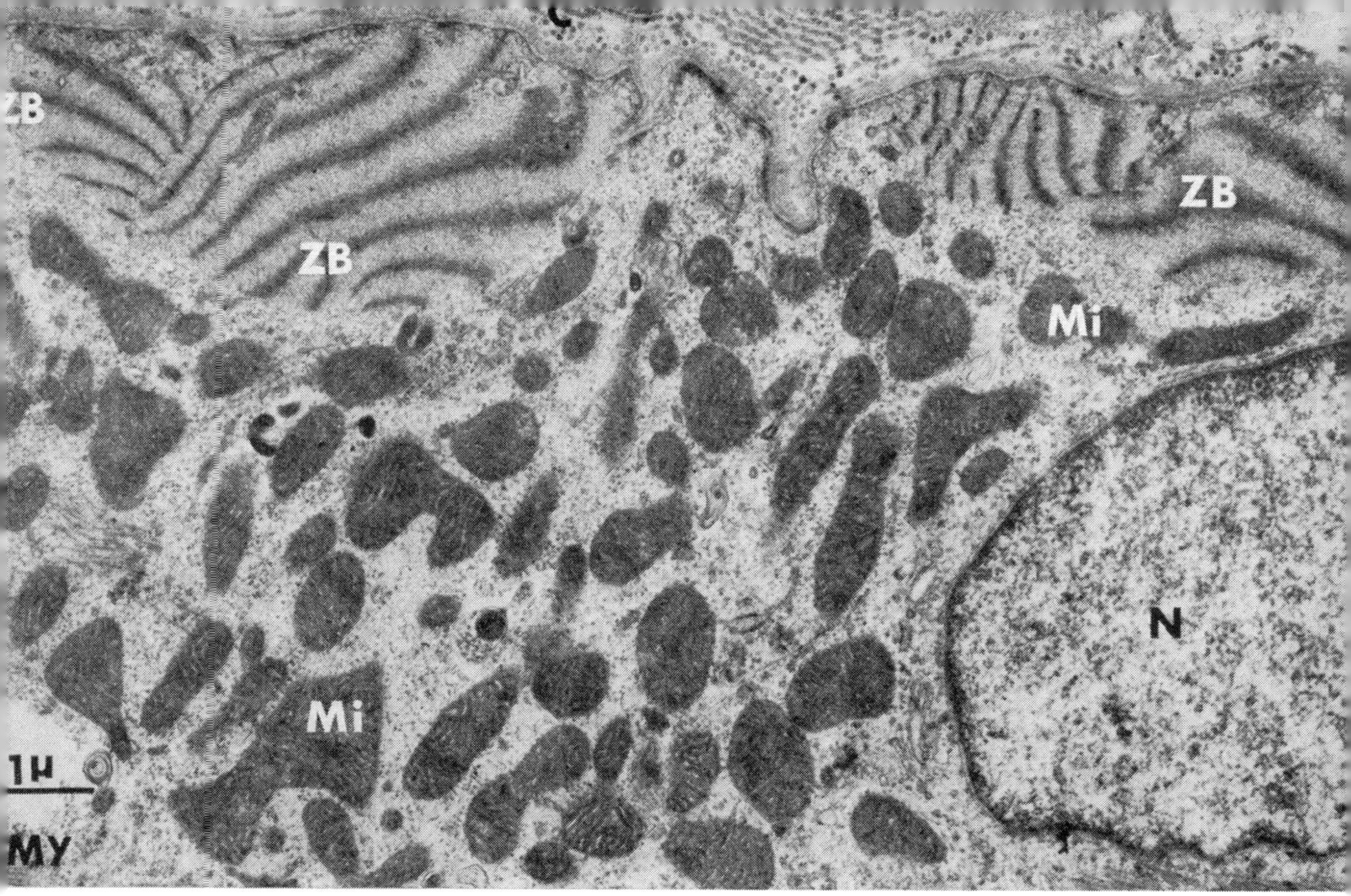
ZB
ZB
ZB
Mi
Mi
N
1μ
MY

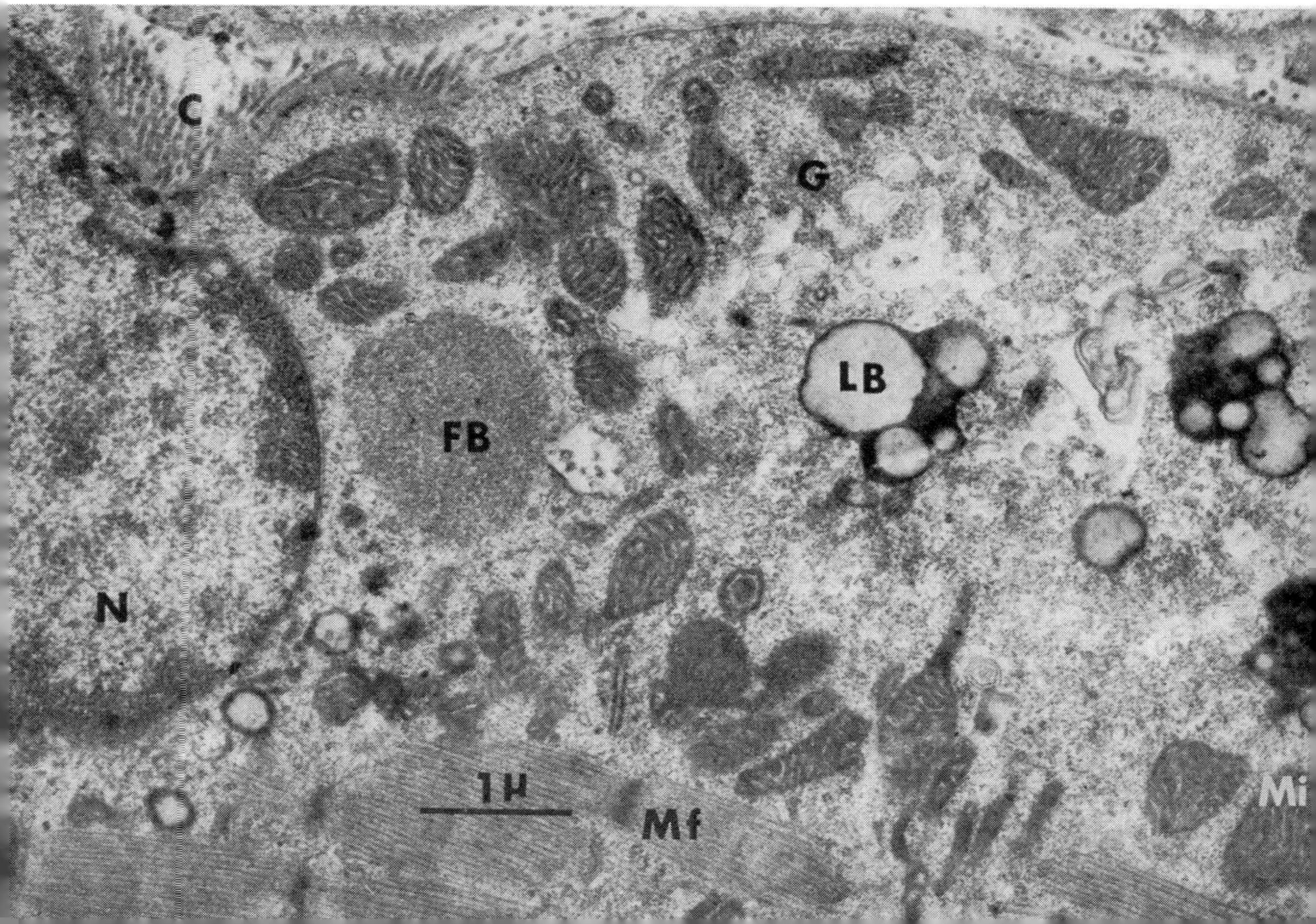
C
G
FB
LB
N
1μ
Mf
Mi

PLATE 11. NERVES AND MOTOR END PLATE IN EXTRA-OCULAR MUSCLE

UPPER. Myelinated nerve fibres are frequent in extra-ocular muscle. They are surrounded by concentric layers of perineurial cells which are covered by basement membrane and have some collagen fibres around them. Collagen and fibroblasts which have no covering of basement membrane lie between the perineurial cells and the myelinated nerve fibres. Both nerve fibres contain filaments and mitochondria in their axons. The fibre upper right has a prominent nucleus in its Schwann cell. The nerve is cut through the node of Ranvier. To the left lies a muscle fibre.

MAGNIFICATION 9,000 ×.

LOWER. Here is a motor end plate on the surface of the muscle fibre. Several portions of the terminal axon without any myelin sheath are enclosed in the nucleated Schwann cell. Distended mitochondria with broken cristae and numerous synaptic vesicles are present in the axon which lies in the primary synaptic cleft on the surface of the muscle fibre. In the primary synaptic cleft basement membrane lies between the plasma membranes of the axon and the muscle fibre and extends into the indentations, the secondary synaptic clefts, on the surface of the muscle fibre. The plasma membrane of the muscle fibre along the secondary synaptic clefts is thickened. Numerous mitochondria lie in the sarcoplasm between the secondary synaptic clefts and the myofibrils. Collagen lies outside the muscle fibre.

MAGNIFICATION 13,500 ×.

Ax Axon
BM Basement membrane
C Collagen
F Fibroblast
Mf Myofibril
Mi Mitochondria
MF Muscle fibre
MN Myelinated nerve
N Nucleus
NSC Nucleus of Schwann cell
PM Plasma membrane
PN Perineurial cell
PSC Primary synaptic cleft
SCC Schwann cell cytoplasm
SSC Secondary synaptic cleft
V Vesicles

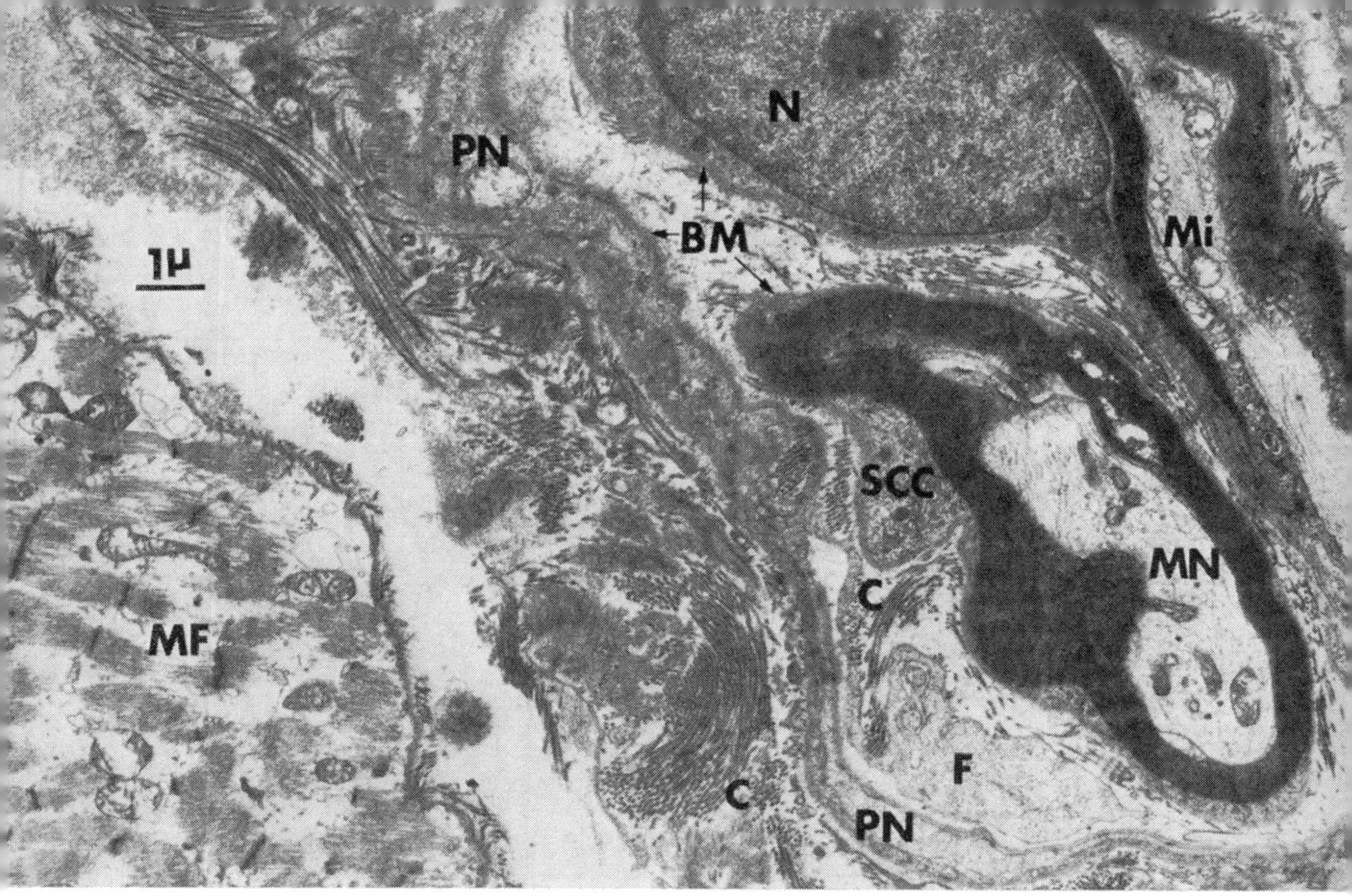
N
PN
BM
Mi
1μ
SCC
MN
C
MF
F
C
PN

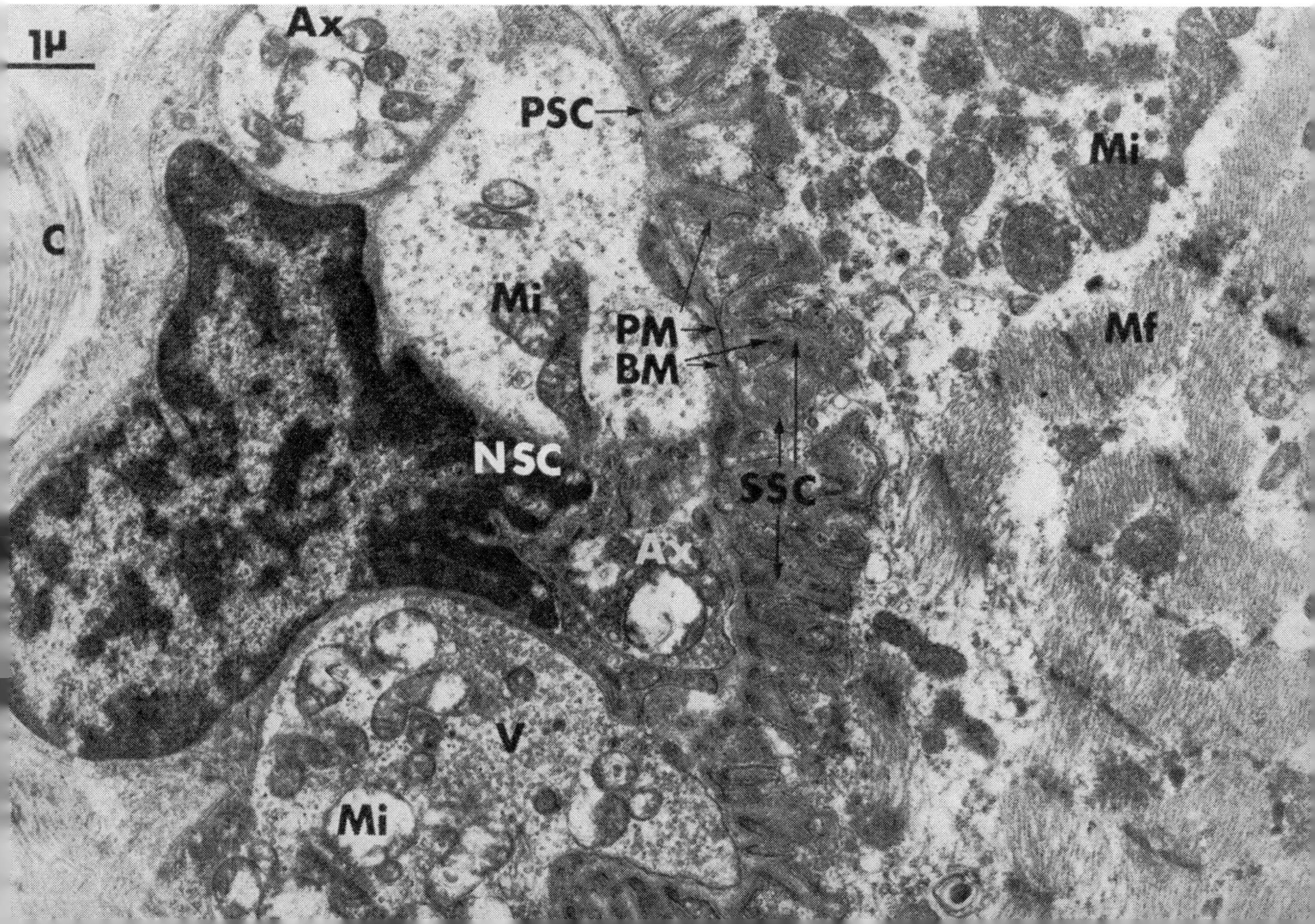
Ax
1μ
PSC
Mi
C
Mi
PM
BM
Mf
NSC
SSC
Ax
V
Mi

PLATE 12. HUMAN FOETAL MUSCLE

A cross section of muscle from a foetus of 12 weeks shows cells at different stages of development. A few strands of collagen and scanty numbers of fibroblast processes lie between the muscle cells. A thin layer of basement membrane surrounds the muscle cells and more than one cell may lie within the same basement membrane. The plasma membranes of the cells may show short interruptions. Most of the cells are myotubes and their nuclei are central and large in size: the chromatin is dispersed in granules throughout the nucleus with a narrow rim of electron dense chromatin at the margin. Nucleoli may occur in them. Collections of glycogen granules lie around the nuclei and between the well-differentiated myofibrils which occupy a large part of the myotubes. The myofibrils exhibit distinct I- and A-bands as well as well-formed Z-lines. Mitochondria are present between the myofibrils.

Cells of smaller size occur in the same basement membrane as the myotubes and the myofilaments present in them are less well organised into myofibrils. Mitochondria and some granules occur in these cells which are at an earlier stage of development and are sometimes referred to as myocells.

More primitive cells or myoblasts also occur: they may lie independently of the myotubes or occur within the same basement membrane as cells at a more advanced stage of development. The myoblasts have a dense nucleus and their cytoplasm contains prominent rough endoplasmic reticulum and numerous fine granules.

MAGNIFICATION 7,000 ×.

A	A-band
BM	Basement membrane
C	Collagen
G	Glycogen
I	I-band
Mb	Myoblast
Mf	Myofibril
MC	Myocell
N	Nucleus
PM	Plasma membrane
RER	Rough endoplasmic reticulum
Z	Z-line

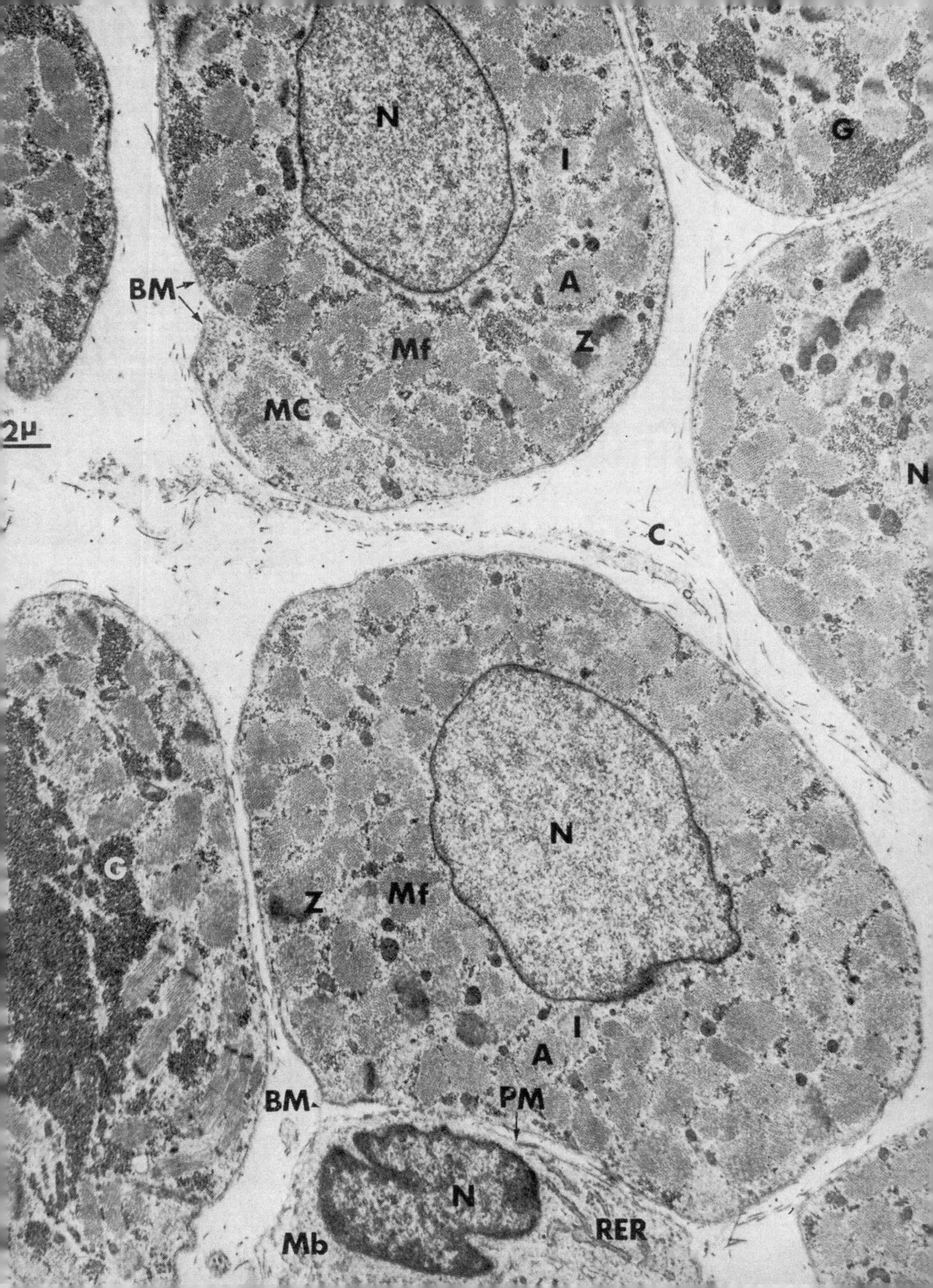
N
G
I
A
BM
Z
Mf
MC
2μ
N
C
G
N
Z
Mf
I
A
BM
PM
N
Mb
RER

PLATE 13. HUMAN FOETAL MUSCLE

A longitudinal section of muscle from a foetus of 12½ weeks shows muscle cells in different stages of development. Several myotubes are illustrated. The uppermost exhibits a nucleus with a prominent nucleolus and nearby part of a Golgi apparatus and surrounding glycogen granules. The myofibrils lie at the periphery of the myotube. The plasma membrane is surrounded by a thin layer of basement membrane. Below this myotube are three cells within a common basement membrane. The nucleated cell is a myoblast which has prominent rough endoplasmic reticulum, numerous polysomes and ribosomes and some mitochondria. Parts of its plasma membrane are very distinct: it is not covered by basement membrane. A prolongation of the cytoplasm of the myoblast (arrowed) lies between the two myotubes which have well-differentiated myofibrils showing exactly the same features as adult muscle. The sarcoplasm is rich in polysomes, ribosomes and glycogen granules and in addition mitochondria, vacuoles and lipid bodies. The cells at the bottom of the illustration are a myoblast on the left, and on the right a myotube containing myofibrils, mitochondria and numerous glycogen granules.

MAGNIFICATION 10,000 ×.

BM	Basement membrane	N	Nucleus
G	Glycogen	Po	Polysomes
LB	Lipid body	PM	Plasma membrane
Mb	Myoblast	RER	Rough endoplasmic reticulum
Mf	Myofibril	Va	Vacuoles
Mi	Mitochondria		

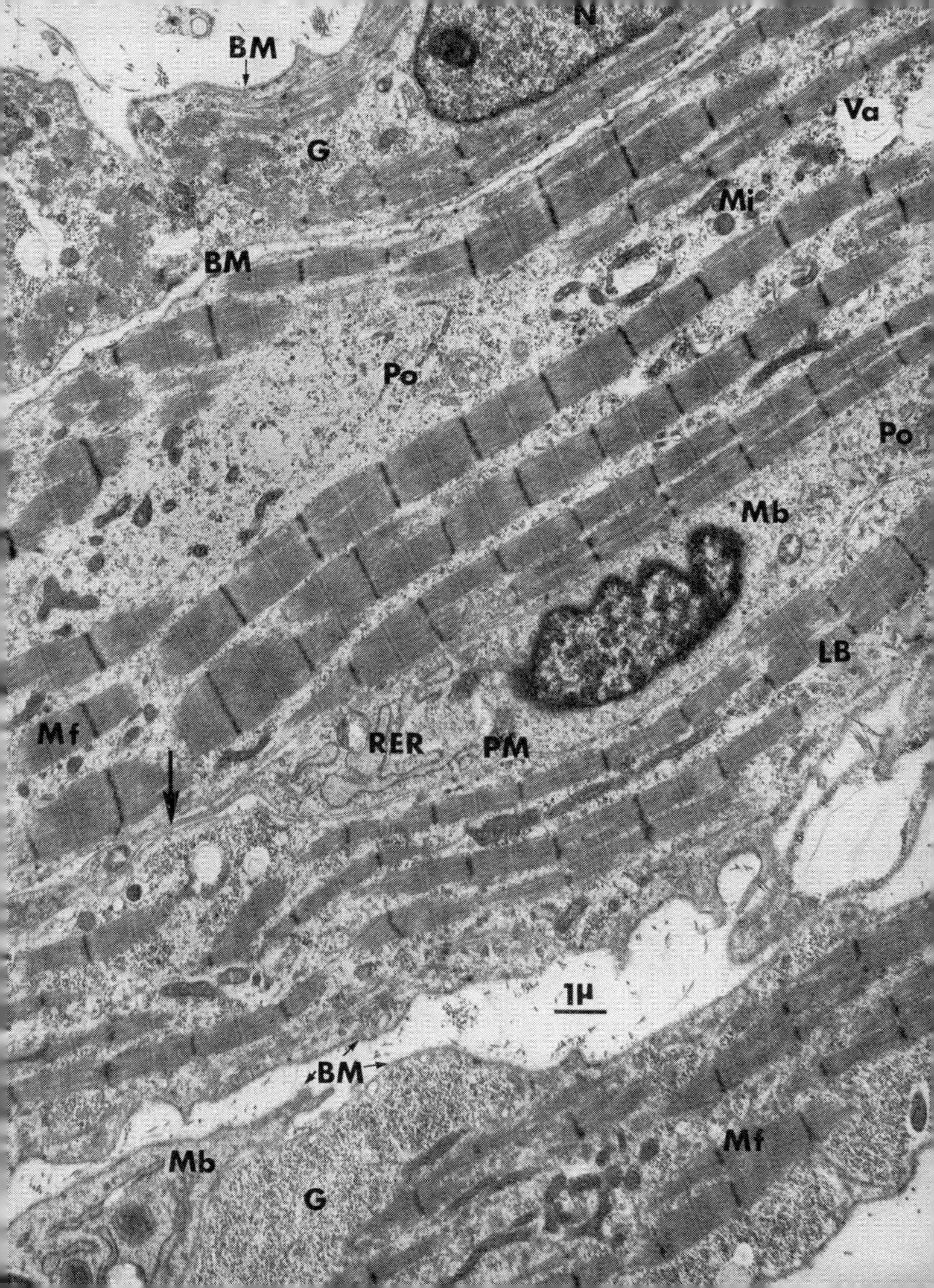

N
BM
Va
G
Mi
BM
Po
Po
Mb
LB
Mf
RER
PM
1μ
BM
Mb
Mf
G

PLATE 14. HUMAN FOETAL MUSCLE MYOBLAST IN MITOSIS

In developing human muscle mitosis occurs in the myoblasts as illustrated in the muscle from a foetus of 12½ weeks development. The chromosomes are distributed throughout the cell cytoplasm which contains numerous small granules, ribosomes, polysomes and some rough endoplasmic reticulum. A distinct layer of basement membrane surrounds this myoblast, but basement membrane is not always present around the myoblast. Strands of collagen and processes of unidentified cells without basement membrane lie in the neighbourhood of the cell in division. A muscle cell in an advanced stage of development lies at the bottom of the illustration.

MAGNIFICATION 23,000 ×.

BM Basement membrane
Ch Chromosomes
MF Muscle fibre
RER Rough endoplasmic reticulum

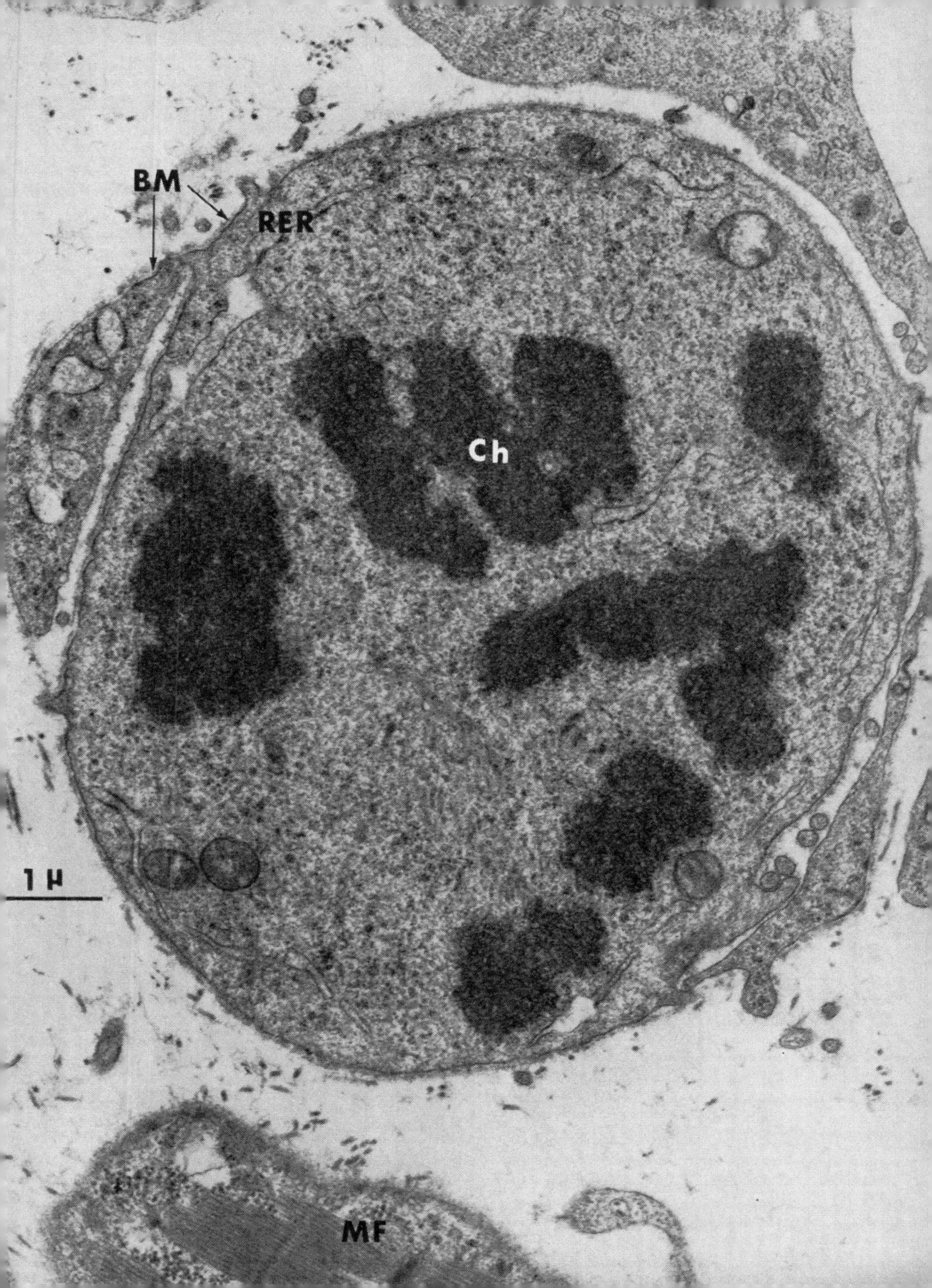
BM
RER
Ch
1 μ
MF

PLATE 15. HUMAN CARDIAC MUSCLE

UPPER. Foetal.
Developing human cardiac muscle shows groups of muscle fibres with distinct plasma membranes enclosed in a common layer of basement membrane with a few strands of collagen around it. No basement membrane separates the individual myocardial cells within the group. Well-formed myofibrils, some cut obliquely and some longitudinally, display distinct Z-lines and A- and I-bands and they lie mainly at the periphery of the muscle fibres, the more central parts of which contain a large amount of glycogen granules and fairly numerous mitochondria. Some fibres contain rounded osmophilic bodies. Parts of the Golgi apparatus and parallel arrays of rough endoplasmic reticulum are present in some cells. At the margins of adjacent muscle fibres which are not separated by basement membrane dense zones occur: these are the intercalated discs. The muscle fibre to the left of the illustration has numerous vesicles under its plasma membrane.

MAGNIFICATION 12,500 ×.

From the auricle of a human foetus of 16 weeks development.

LOWER. Adult.
In the adult heart the intercalated discs between adjacent myocardial cells are very extensive and the contiguous surfaces of the cells are very tortuous, without any basement membrane intervening between the cells. The broadened zones of electron dense material in the adjacent cells correspond to the Z-lines of the sarcomere. The mitochondria are swollen and the space between the myofibrils is fairly wide due perhaps to post mortem change.

MAGNIFICATION 26,000 ×.

Human auricle obtained post mortem.

BM Basement membrane
G Glycogen
Go Golgi apparatus
ID Intercalated disc
Mf Myofibril
Mi Mitochondria
O Osmophilic bodies
PM Plasma membrane
RER Rough endoplasmic reticulum
Z Z-line

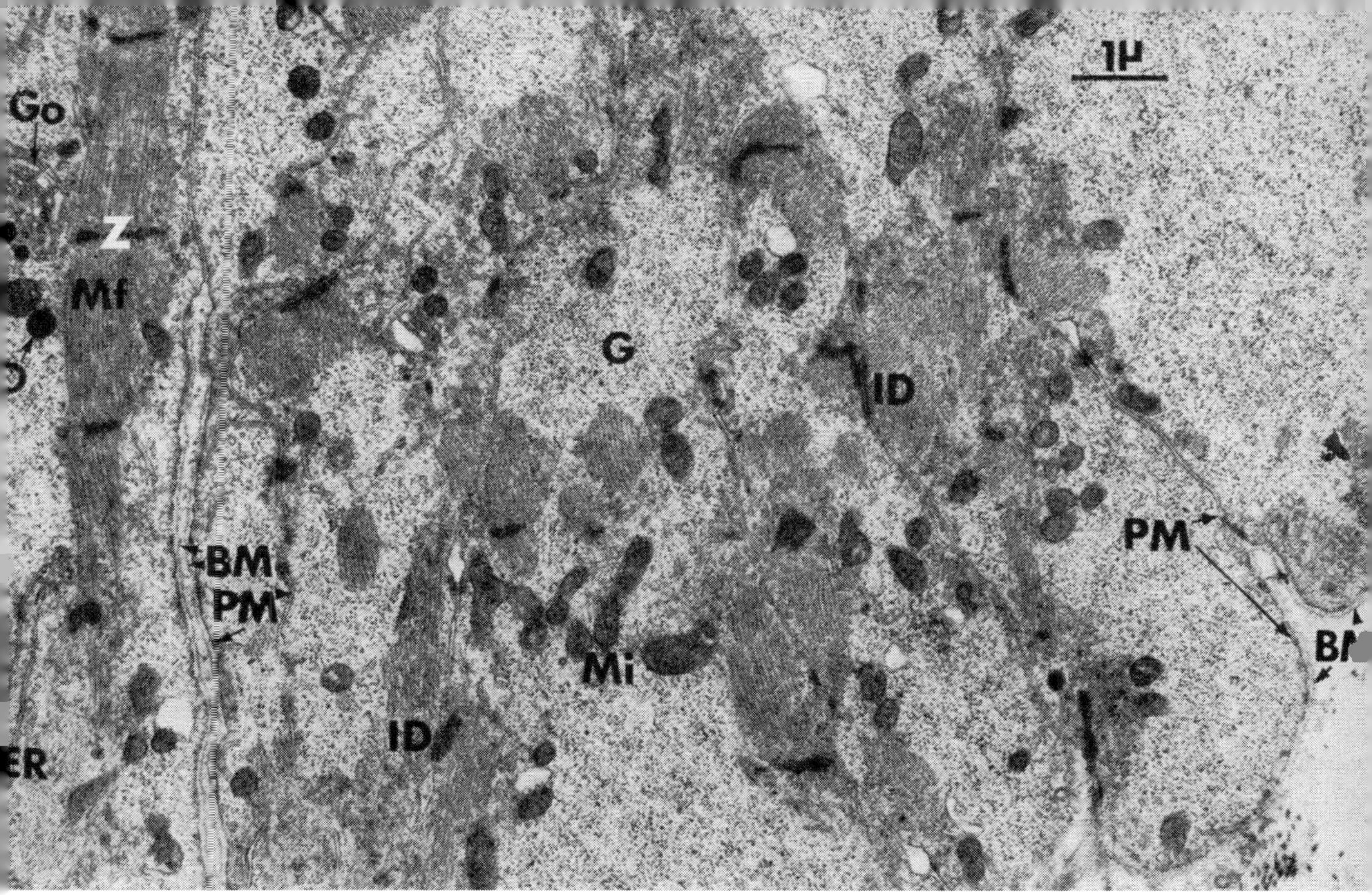
1μ
Go
Z
Mf
G
ID
BM
PM
Mi
ID
ER
PM
BM

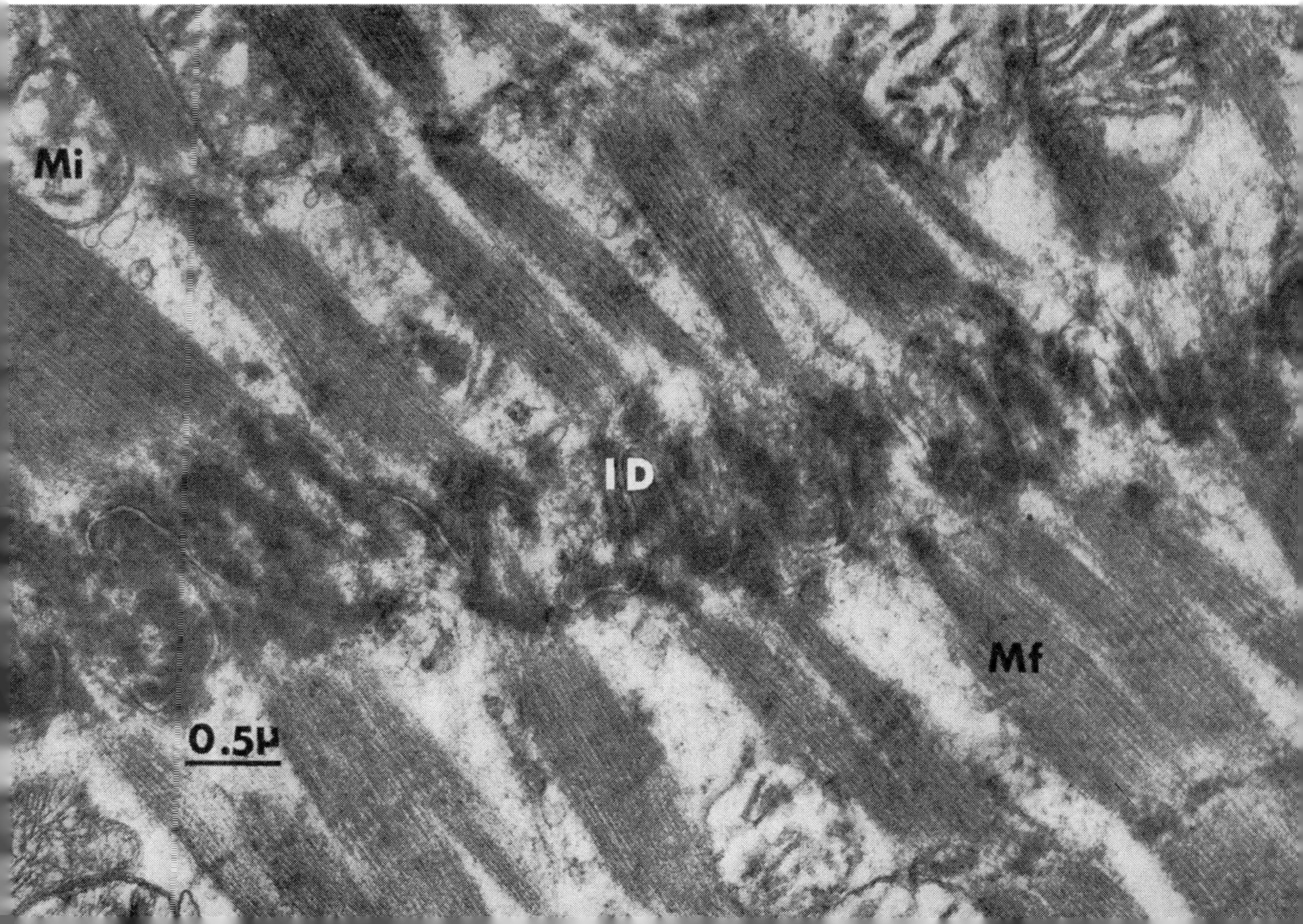
Mi
ID
Mf
0.5μ

PLATE 16. HUMAN FOETAL CARDIAC MUSCLE
CENTRIOLES AND A MITOTIC FIGURE IN MYOCARDIAL CELLS

UPPER. This myocardial cell exhibits portions of well-differentiated myofibrils, some rough endoplasmic reticulum, a large amount of glycogen granules, some mitochondria and numerous round osmophilic bodies around the nucleus of the cell. Near the nucleus and between flattened tubules of the Golgi apparatus lie two centrioles, one cut longitudinally and the other more transversely.

MAGNIFICATION 13,000 ×.

The *inset* shows the centrioles within the rectangle above at higher magnification. To the right can be seen the tubules of the centriole cut slightly obliquely and to the left the longitudinally cut centriole.

MAGNIFICATION 55,000 ×.

LOWER. A myocardial cell in mitotic division displays, in addition to the chromosomes, differentiating myofibrils around the margin of the cell. A large amount of glycogen granules, some mitochondria and collections of flattened tubules are also present in the cell cytoplasm. The cell undergoing mitosis lies in close apposition to other myocardial cells. To the left is a cleft lined by basement membrane between several myocardial cells.

MAGNIFICATION 7,500 ×.

Both are from the auricle of a human foetus of 16 weeks development.

Ce	Centriole	Mi	Mitochondria
Ch	Chromosomes	N	Nucleus
G	Glycogen	O	Osmophilic body
Go	Golgi apparatus	RER	Rough endoplasmic reticulum
Mf	Myofibrils		

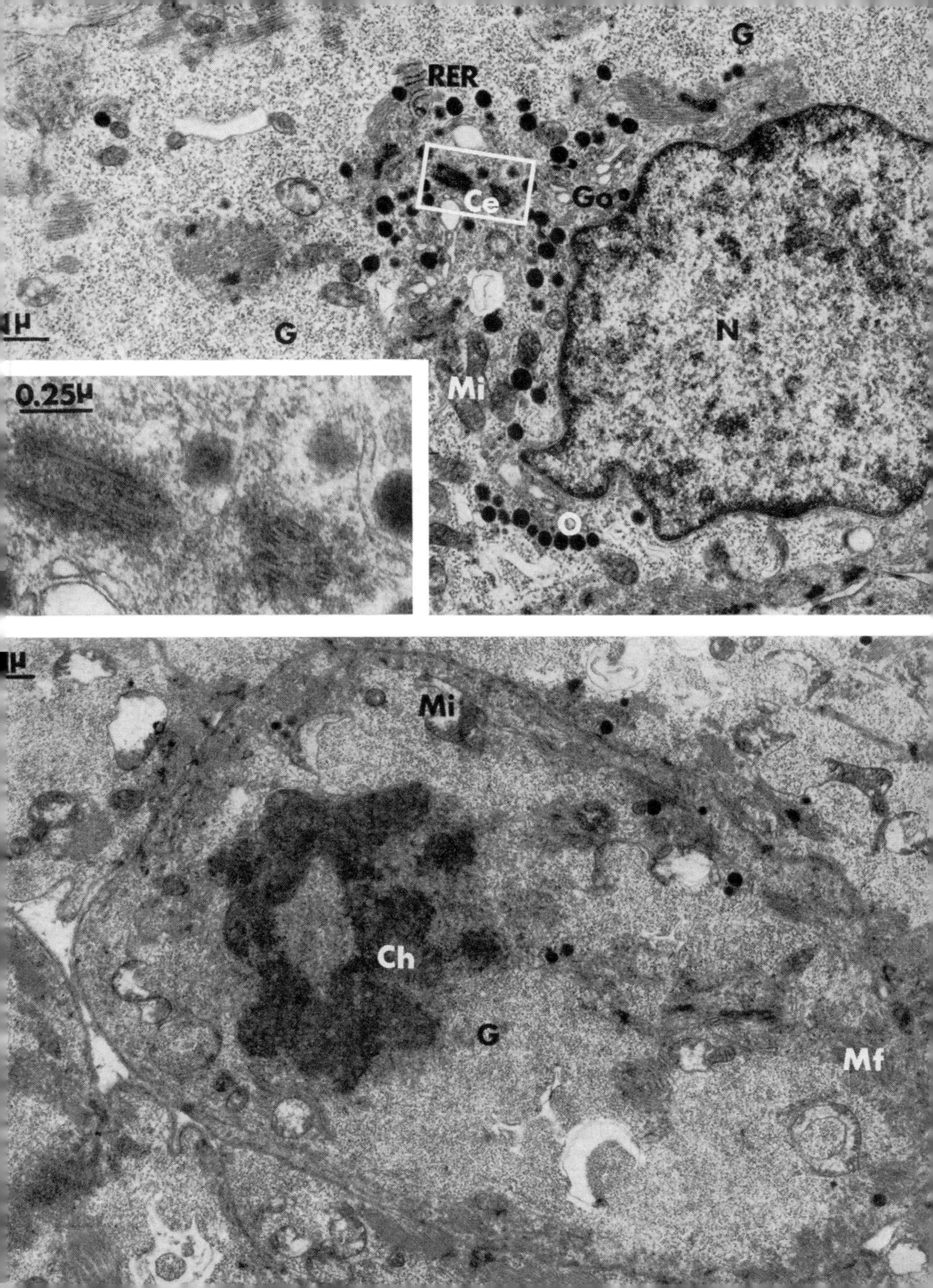
G
RER
Ce
Go
1μ
G
N
0.25μ
Mi
O
1μ
Mi
Ch
G
Mf

CHAPTER 2

Changes in Muscle Fibres

The changes which occur in diseased muscle have been extensively investigated by light microscopy. Important contributions in this field are the works of Adams, Denny-Brown and Pearson (1953 and 1962), Greenfield, Shy, Alvord and Berg (1957) and those edited by Walton (1964 and 1969). These authors give, in addition to their own observations, a review of the reports of the very numerous authors who have studied normal and diseased muscle. The book edited by Walton deals also with the ultrastructure of normal and diseased muscle.

Muscle biopsies of numerous muscle disorders have been investigated by electron microscopy and the information which has accumulated from these studies has added significantly to our knowledge of the changes which may occur when the muscle is affected by some disease process. Some of the ultrastructural changes would be little expected from examination of the muscle by light microscopy. The alterations which occur in the muscle cannot usually be related to specific clinical conditions, but in some instances the changes tend to follow a pattern which would imply a particular disorder.

All the structures forming the muscle fibres and the tissues around them, namely the nerves, blood vessels, fibroblasts and collagen, may participate in the pathological process. The changes which take place in the muscle fibre involve the myofibrils, nuclei, mitochondria, and the other elements of the sarcoplasm and the membranes surrounding the fibres.

MYOFIBRILS

Regarding changes which may affect the *organisation of the myofibrils* reference must be made to the *ring fibres*, which are so called because they exhibit a peripheral ring of myofibrils running obliquely or at right angles to a central longitudinal core of myofibrils. In cross section of a ring fibre, the myofibrils at the periphery of the fibre run longitudinally while the central ones are seen in cross section as illustrated in Plate 17 and in the upper part of Plate 18. In longitudinal section, the myofibrils at the periphery of the ring fibre appear in cross section and the central ones in longitudinal section as seen in the lower part of Plate 18. No membrane separates the peripheral from the central myofibrils.

Ring fibres occur in many disorders of muscle but are said to be more common in dystrophia myotonica. Ring fibres were first reported by Bataillon (1891) in the tail musculature of amphibians and have since been reported by numerous authors in other animals and man in normal and pathological conditions. The ultrastructure of ring fibres in human skeletal muscle has been studied by several authors including Milhaud, Fardeau and Lapresle (1964), Lapresle, Fardeau and

Milhaud (1966), Schotland, Spiro and Carmel (1966), Lapresle and Fardeau (1968), Schroeder and Adams (1968) and Hayward and Mair (1970).

Degenerative changes of the myofibrils involve the myofilaments and the Z-lines. The myofibrils often become reduced in diameter with a relative increase of the intervening sarcoplasm. Loss of myofilaments may involve one or more sarcomeres (Plate 19) and is sometimes more apparent in the I-band, especially in muscular dystrophy (Plate 70). Part of the Z-line may persist after the filaments of the I-band have disappeared (Plate 19). These degenerative changes of the myofibrils may be reflected in the configuration of the muscle fibre, the surface of which often becomes very indented or presents sarcoplasmic projections (Plate 20). Degeneration of the myofibrils may also result in the formation of a sarcoplasmic mass at the edge of the fibre (Plate 21 upper part). The sarcoplasmic masses may contain many glycogen granules, mitochondria, occasional nuclei and remains of degenerate myofibrils. Eventually the myofibrils may disappear from a considerable extent of the fibre with consequent diminution in their size (Plate 21 lower part).

Disarray and loss of myofibrils are accompanied by changes in the shape and size of the muscle fibre (Plate 22).

The Z-lines frequently exhibit structural changes and become irregular in shape and size and as often happens appear to extend into the I- and A-bands, a change which is generally referred to as *streaming of the Z-lines* (Plate 23). It is impossible in the myofibrils showing this abnormality to assess by visual inspection alone whether this change is in fact extension of the Z-line material into the I- and A-bands or whether it arises as a result of condensation of the myofilaments. Streaming of the Z-lines has been reported in various pathological conditions of muscle by numerous authors.

Another change in the muscle fibre which is related to streaming of the Z-line is that seen in *target fibres*, where the sarcomeres of several adjacent myofibrils are replaced by electron dense material (Plate 24). This material may result from condensation of the myofilaments as well as extension of the Z-line into the I- and A-bands. Target fibres are usually described as exhibiting three concentric zones: central, intermediate and outer zones. In the central zone the lesion is most severe; the severity diminishes towards the periphery. Sometimes the three zones are not well defined. In the central zone, the accumulation of electron dense material is devoid of glycogen and mitochondria. Collections of triads (Plate 36), vacuoles and tubules may occur, however, in this zone.

Target fibres were illustrated in amyotrophic lateral sclerosis by Buzzard and Greenfield in 1921, although these authors made no reference to this particular feature. Target fibres were reported by W. K. Engel (1961), who thought that they were a sign of denervation. However, they may be found in disorders of muscle other than denervation.

The ultrastructure of target fibres was reported by Resnick and W. K. Engel (1967), Shafiq, Milhorat and Gorycki (1967b), Schotland (1969), Tomonaga and Sluga (1969 and 1970) and others.

Other interesting changes which are thought to derive from the Z-lines are the dense *rods* which were first described in nemaline myopathy. Such bodies have also been found in other muscular disorders such as muscular dystrophy (Plate 25 upper part), in denervation (Plate 69) and in polymyositis (Plate 77): in the latter condition they were reported by Cape, Johnson and Pitner (1970). Rods also occur in normal muscle (Schmalbruch, 1968), in muscle fibres at the myotendinous junctions (Plate 25 lower part), in extra-ocular muscle (Mukuno, 1969) in which they are illustrated in Plate 26, in rhabdomyoma (Cornog and Gonatas, 1967) and in cardiac muscle of tom cats (Fawcett, 1968). In the muscle fibres of the muscle spindle, rods were observed by light histology in a case of nemaline myopathy (Shafiq, Dubowitz *et al.*, 1967).

The rods may be small or large, up to 5 μ long and 1 μ in diameter: they occur usually in aggregates forming palisades and generally at the periphery of the muscle fibre. The rods are devoid of enzyme activity (W. K. Engel, 1962; Shy *et al.*, 1963; Gonatas, Shy and Godfrey, 1966; Shafiq, Dubowitz *et al.*, 1967, etc.).

By electron microscopy the rods have an irregular margin and display a filamentous structure, the filaments being continuous sometimes with those of the I-bands (Plate 26 lower part). According to Price *et al.* (1965) the filaments lie either perpendicular to the long axis of the myofibrils and have a periodicity of 180 to 200 Å or may run parallel to the myofilaments and the periodicity is 80 to 100 Å: however, they may lie at right angles to one another, forming a lattice similar to that of the Z-lines. The filamentous nature of the rods may not always be apparent. The periodicity of the filaments of the rods as stated by different authors varies and this may be due either to the method of fixation and embedding or to the plane of sectioning. Price *et al.* (1965), Gonatas *et al.* (1966) and Gonatas (1966) demonstrated that the rods arise from the Z-lines, a view that had already been suggested by Afifi, Smith and Zellweger (1965) and has been adopted by subsequent authors. In fact the ultrastructural characteristics of the rods and particularly their lattice pattern is identical to that of the Z-lines with which the rods are sometimes continuous (Plates 25 and 26 upper parts).

The Z-lines may exhibit other changes such as thickening and distortion (as seen in central core disease and other conditions) and in some circumstances the Z-lines may be fragmented or disappear. Occasionally the Z-lines may be doubled, as illustrated in Plate 71, in muscular dystrophy. This change was reported by Grabow and Chou (1968) and A. G. Engel and Macdonald (1970). We have observed reduplication of the Z-line also in muscle fibres at the myotendinous junction and in extra-ocular muscle.

The pathological reactions of the Z-lines have been described by various authors, particularly by A. G. Engel (1967).

Another structure which sometimes is observed in diseased muscle is the '*cytoplasmic body*' reported by Macdonald and A. G. Engel (1969) as a structural anomaly of the Z-line. Cytoplasmic bodies were first described in light microscopy in human skeletal muscle and in tissue cultures of chicken embryo muscle by W. K. Engel (1962).

By electron microscopy the cytoplasmic body is seen to be formed of filaments, those in the centre being closely packed and electron dense while those at the periphery are more loosely arranged and less electron dense. The peripheral filaments appear to be continuous with the myofilaments of the myofibrils: a lighter halo separates the electron dense central part from the myofilaments. These bodies occur in denervation atrophy of muscle, inflammatory conditions of muscle (Shafiq, Milhorat and Gorycki, 1967a, and Macdonald and A. G. Engel, 1969), dystrophia myotonica (Schroeder and Adams, 1968) and muscular dystrophy (Macdonald and A. G. Engel, 1969). They are illustrated in denervation and in muscular dystrophy in Plate 27. A similar structure was demonstrated by Serratrice, Roux, *et al.* (1970) in a patient with myopathy associated with arthropathic psoriasis.

Nakashima *et al.* (1970) illustrated in a muscle biopsy of a patient with a neuromuscular disorder 'cytoplasmic bodies' as well as other oval bodies with a filamentous structure. These are similar to the *filamentous bodies* demonstrated in Plate 28 in skeletal muscle and in Plate 10 in extra-ocular muscle. They consist of filaments of similar diameter and electron density and may run in different directions. They occur usually near the nucleus and under the plasma membrane. They have been illustrated in publications by Revel (1962) in the crico-thyroid muscle of the bat, Odor, Patel and Pearce (1967) in hypokalaemic periodic paralysis, Hurwitz *et al.* (1967) in muscular dystrophy, Macdonald, Rewcastle and Humphrey (1968) in hyperkalaemic periodic paralysis, Shafiq *et al.* (1966) and Schmalbruch (1968) in normal muscle, Reger and Craig (1968) in hypertrophied deltoid muscle, Hayward and Mair (1970) in muscular dystrophy and Morgan-Hughes, Mair and Lascelles (1970) in a patient with myopathy with tubular aggregates. We have observed them in denervation, muscular dystrophy and dystrophia myotonica.

NUCLEI AND GOLGI APPARATUS

The ultrastructural changes of the *nuclei* of the muscle fibres in diseased human muscle have not been well studied. They have been studied in experimental animals by Lee and Altschul (1963) and others.

By light microscopy, it is well known that the muscle nuclei may vary in size and their capacity of staining and that they may appear to be increased in number and occur in rows at the periphery or in a more central part of the muscle fibre (Plate 29) or may accumulate in groups filling the whole width of the muscle fibre. The enlarged nuclei are often vesicular with the chromatin situated chiefly at the nuclear margin and they contain one or more prominent nucleoli. It is difficult to assess whether the number of nuclei is increased or is only apparently so in consequence of the accompanying degeneration and atrophy of the fibre. There is no evidence, in electron microscope studies, of mitotic division of adult skeletal muscle fibres, but they were reported in the satellite cells of the muscle in rats by Shafiq, Gorycki and Mauro (1968). Frequently the surface of the nuclei are indented. The nuclear membranes may show localised distensions (Plates 77 and 82 lower part). The nuclei of the muscle fibre, like all the other constituents of the fibre, may undergo degeneration and disintegration (Plate 82 lower part), even to the extent of necrosis, so that only the basement membrane of the muscle fibre may remain.

The significance of the changes which occur in the nucleus in diseased muscle is far from being clearly understood and may be more important than has been attributed to them. More information concerning the biochemical and the ultrastructural changes of the nuclei in normal and pathological conditions is required to appreciate what the changes imply.

Closely associated with the nuclei is the *Golgi apparatus* which in diseased muscle often presents more flattened tubules with terminal expansions than in normal muscle. Since enzymes are localised in the membranes of the Golgi apparatus its proliferation may be very significant in disease.

MITOCHONDRIA

Mitochondria play an important part in the metabolism of the muscle fibre and it is not surprising that mitochondria frequently exhibit changes in the various muscle disorders. These changes are difficult to assess since even in normal muscle the site, number, size, shape and internal structure of the mitochondria may vary.

The commoner mitochondrial changes are the variation in their number, size and shape. Often their ultrastructure may be altered. The number of mitochondria may be increased or severely reduced in number. An increase in number occurs in the early stages of any muscle disorder and particularly in muscular dystrophy, while in degenerating fibres their number is reduced and eventually the mitochondria disappear from the very atrophied muscle fibres.

Ultrastructural changes of the mitochondria affect the cristae, which may become less electron dense and undergo fragmentation and eventually disappear. Sometimes the mitochondria become swollen and their matrix may be more or less electron dense than normal. Some of the changes in the mitochondria, especially fragmentation of the cristae, increased electron density and distension, are frequently attributed to artefact in the preparation of the tissue, but sometimes these changes are undoubtedly of pathological significance and may be seen in some mitochondria adjacent to others which are normal in structure. The normal electron dense mitochondrial granules may also increase in number. Glycogen granules may also be seen in the mitochondria. Vesicles, vacuoles, tubular structures, membranous and myelin bodies may appear in mitochondria, but how these various abnormal structures arise in them is imperfectly understood. More rarely inclusions may occur in mitochondria. They have been reported by several authors in a great number of muscle disorders (*see* page 179). Three types of inclusions are described: a. Round bodies of moderate electron density; b. Rectangular, irregular shaped or round bodies of much greater electron density; c. Laminated quadrilateral bodies which may be rectangular, square or rhomboid and are thought to be crystalline in nature (Plate 32). Other mitochondrial abnormalities are seen in Plates 30 and 31.

GLYCOGEN

In most disorders of muscle the *glycogen* is often increased, particularly in glycogenosis, but the increase may be very marked in some conditions of obscure nature (Slotwiner, Song and Maker, 1969). The glycogen granules accumulate throughout the muscle fibres but especially between the myofibrils and under the plasma membrane (Plate 33). Glycogen granules may appear in the mitochondria (Plate 30), in autophagic vacuoles (Plate 39) and other membrane bound bodies, but how they arise in these structures is difficult to understand. In muscle fibres undergoing degeneration only the nucleus and the glycogen granules may be seen: in fibres in advanced stages of degeneration the glycogen granules, however, disappear along with the other organelles (Plate 84).

LIPID BODIES

Lipid bodies occur in normal muscle but appear in increased amount in diseased muscle (Plate 34) and are found in large numbers in some myopathies (Prineas *et al.*, 1968 and Bradley *et al.*, 1969).

Lipofuscin is not usually seen in skeletal muscle fibres in light microscopy: in electron micrographs, lipofuscin cannot be differentiated with accuracy from other lipid bodies (Plate 79 lower right).

SARCOPLASMIC RETICULUM AND T-SYSTEM (HONEYCOMB STRUCTURES)

The *sarcoplasmic reticulum* in normal human muscles is not very striking, but the lateral sacs of the tubules forming it are electron dense and are often easily identified as they lie next to the T-tubules with which they form triads. In diseased muscle the triads are often displaced from their normal relationship with the other elements of the muscle fibre at the junction of the I- and A-bands and may be increased in number (Plate 35). Many triads may lie in rows in close apposition to one another: sometimes the T-system is dilated (Plate 36).

The sarcoplasmic reticulum may also be distended and contain electron dense, granular material (Plate 37). Dilatation of the sarcoplasmic reticulum has been emphasised in periodic paralysis, but may also be seen in other conditions. In diseased muscle besides being more numerous than normal, the *T-systems* are sometimes unusually long, extending over several myofibrils as seen in Plate 35 and Plate 79 lower left.

In some pathological conditions the T-systems are thought to proliferate, producing a *honeycomb structure* of varying size (Plate 38) formed of numerous tubules of 250 to 400 Å in diameter separated from each other by electron dense material. Evidence in support of their origin from the T-systems has been provided in electron micrographs of tissue cultures of breast muscle of the chicken, where ferritin introduced into the culture medium entered the T-systems and the honeycomb structures but did not enter the sarcoplasmic reticulum (Ishikawa, 1968). In human muscle the continuity of the honeycomb structures with the T-tubules has been demonstrated by Jerusalem (1970) and is illustrated in the lower right of Plate 38.

Honeycomb structures have been found in human muscle in many disorders, namely, muscular dystrophy (Hülsmann *et al.*, 1967 and Fardeau, 1970), dystrophia myotonica (Schroeder and Adams, 1968; Schotland, 1968 and 1970; Mussini, Di Mauro and Angelini, 1970 and Fardeau, 1970), acid maltase deficiency (A. G. Engel and Dale, 1968 and A. G. Engel, 1970a and b), hyperkalaemic periodic paralysis (Macdonald, Rewcastle and Humphrey, 1968), thyrotoxic hypokalaemic periodic paralysis (Schutta and Armitage, 1969), chloroquine myopathy (Fardeau, 1970), polymyositis (A. G. Engel and Macdonald, 1970), paroxysmal idiopathic myoglobinuria (Schutta, Kelly and Zacks, 1969), Cushing's myopathy (Jerusalem, 1970), alcoholic polyneuropathy (Tomé and Mair, 1970) and in rhabdomyoma (Cornog and Gonatas, 1967). The honeycomb structures were first reported by Pellegrino and Franzini (1963) in denervated muscle of rats and have been reported subsequently in experimental animals by other authors. They are very numerous in the muscle of rats treated with vincristine sulphate (Morgan-Hughes, LeQuesne and Mair).

VACUOLES. AUTOPHAGIC VACUOLES

Vacuoles of varying size may occur in muscle fibres in many muscular disorders. They may be very prominent in periodic paralysis. The vacuoles are bounded by a single membrane and lie usually under the plasma membrane or between myofibrils. Some contain slightly electron dense material or tubules and vesicles while others are clear. It is difficult to say how these vacuoles arise, but they may be derived from any membranous component of the muscle fibre such as the mitochondria, sarcoplasmic reticulum, T-systems and the Golgi apparatus. Spaces also occur in muscle which are not bound by a membrane.

Vacuoles thought to be derived from lysosomes and containing hydrolytic enzymes are termed *autophagic vacuoles* (Plate 39). They are bound by a single or double membrane and enclose material of varying size, shape and electron density. Some of the material in these vacuoles consists of glycogen granules and some membranous and myelin bodies of varying complexity. A. G. Engel and Macdonald (1970), A. G. Engel (1970 a and b) and Macdonald and A. G. Engel (1970) regard the membranes of the autophagic vacuoles as being derived from the T-systems or the Golgi apparatus and have demonstrated in them acid phosphatase which is a hydrolytic enzyme. Autophagic vacuoles were described in the muscle of rats in vitamin E deficiency (Howes, Price and Blumberg, 1964), and chloroquine myopathy (Macdonald and A. G. Engel, 1970). In the muscle of man they were reported in a variety of conditions including chloroquine myopathy (Humphrey and Rewcastle, 1963; Garcin, Rondot and Fardeau, 1964 and Rewcastle and Humphrey, 1965), muscular dystrophy (Milhorat, Shafiq and Goldstone, 1966 and Santa, 1969), polymyositis (Shafiq and Milhorat, 1967) and in acid maltase deficiency (A. G. Engel and Dale, 1968; A. G. Engel and Macdonald, 1970 and A. G. Engel, 1970 a and b). The autophagic vacuoles are extruded from the muscle fibre and their content may then accumulate in the basement membrane (Plates 39 and 40). In this location they were described in acid maltase deficiency (A. G. Engel and Dale, 1968 and A. G. Engel and Macdonald, 1970) and in polymyositis (A. G. Engel and Macdonald, 1970). They occur also in the phagocytes in diseased muscle and have been illustrated in the endothelial cells and pericytes of blood capillaries in human chloroquine myopathy by Garcin, Rondot and Fardeau (1964) and by Rewcastle and Humphrey (1965). We have found them in human muscle in chloroquine myopathy (Plate 81 lower part), polymyositis and dystrophia myotonica and also in experimental vincristine myopathy in rats. The autophagic vacuoles arise in the muscle fibre as a result of degradation of the various sarcoplasmic components and are a non-specific finding of many disorders of muscle.

MYELIN AND MEMBRANOUS BODIES

Myelin bodies (Plates 40, 41 and 81) occur in any diseased muscle and may be rare or frequent. They are most often seen under the plasma membrane and between myofibrils of degenerating fibres and often lie within large membrane-bound vacuoles, some of which are autophagic vacuoles. Sometimes they are extruded from the muscle fibre into the basement membrane around it (Plate 40 lower part). The structure of the myelin bodies is variable. Some are formed of thick electron dense rings or ellipsoids: clear zones are often found within them. Some lie inside mitochondria (Plate 31) but many do not give any indication of their origin.

Membranous bodies (Plates 42, 43, 78 and 80) are often found in degenerating muscle fibres including extra-ocular muscle. They occur under the plasma membrane, between myofibrils and within mitochondria (Plate 31 lower part and Plate 42 lower right), from which some of them appear to be derived as the illustration in Plate 78 suggests. Their structure is variable, some being formed of concentric laminae of similar thickness and electron density while others are irregular in shape and the laminae forming them vary in thickness and electron density.

CONCENTRIC LAMINATED BODIES

In diseased muscle various unusual laminar structures of doubtful origin and pathological significance may be encountered. Striking amongst these are *concentric laminated bodies* (Plate 44) which appear in the sarcoplasm of the muscle fibre and are formed of successive layers of lamellae 60 to 80 Å thick and with a periodicity of about 75 Å. The diameter of these bodies varies from 0·3 to 0·7 μ. They may be formed of 3 to 14 lamellae. In longitudinal sections these bodies have a cylindrical appearance, while in oblique sections they are formed of interrupted electron dense lines as can be seen in the lower part of Plate 44. Glycogen granules may occur in the centre of many of these concentric bodies, groups of which are found in degenerating muscle fibres near the plasma membrane or in some instances filling a great part of the degenerating fibre. They were first described in hypermetabolism of nonthyroid origin (Luft *et al.*, 1962) and subsequently in neurogenic atrophy (Thiébaut *et al.*, 1963; Tomé and Mair, 1970 and Roy, Dubowitz and Wolman, 1971), in nemaline myopathy (Shafiq, Dubowitz *et al.*, 1967), in glycogenosis (A. G. Engel and Dale, 1968), in hypokalaemic periodic paralysis of nonthyroid origin (Schutta and Armitage, 1969), in hypothyroid myopathy (Bergouignan, Vital and Bataille, 1967), in central core disease (Dubowitz and Roy, 1970), in the muscle of a patient with spongy degeneration of the brain (Gambetti, Mellman and Gonatas, 1969) and in another patient with infantile neuroaxonal dystrophy or Seitelberger's disease (Toga *et al.*, 1970). Some dubiety exists concerning the origin of these concentric laminated bodies; Luft *et al.* express the view that they arise from the mitochondria and Toga *et al.* from the myofilaments.

Structures which resemble these concentric laminated bodies have been reported in tissues other than muscle, namely in the spermatids of snails (André, 1959), in the lung (Policard *et al.*, 1961), in haemangioblastoma of the cerebellum (Cancilla and Zimmerman, 1965) and in the cerebral cortex in the neighbourhood of a glioma (Ramsey, 1967).

TUBULAR STRUCTURES

Another interesting feature of diseased muscle is the occurrence of various *tubular structures* of doubtful origin and significance. Amongst these are the parallel and concentric arrays of tubules illustrated in Plate 45. Two up to 20 such tubules may occur together, most frequently near the plasma membrane and the nucleus but sometimes more centrally in the fibre. They consist of tubules 20 to 100 mμ in diameter lying at variable distances from one another. Each tubule has electron dense walls of about 75 Å thick. Groups of glycogen granules may lie in the centre of these concentric arrays of tubules and also between the individual tubules. They occur in alcoholic polyneuropathy (Tomé and Mair, 1970) and in familial myopathy of uncertain type (Banerjee and Mair). Structures of somewhat similar morphology have been described in: neurogenic atrophy by Shafiq, Milhorat and Gorycki (1967b), dystrophia myotonica by Schroeder and Adams (1968), hyperkalaemic periodic paralysis by Macdonald, Rewcastle and Humphrey (1968), hypokalaemic periodic paralysis by Macdonald, Rewcastle and Humphrey (1969) and chronic polymyositis by Stoebner *et al.* (1970). Tubules in concentric and parallel arrangement occur also in human muscle in Vitamin E deficiency (Plate 83). They were reported in experimental denervation in rats by Lee (1963), Schrodt and Walker (1966) and by Miledi and Slater (1969). It seems likely that these concentric and parallel arrays of tubules are derived from the sarcoplasmic reticulum.

Tubules of a different type are illustrated in Plates 46 and 47. These occur in aggregates, in parallel and hexagonal array, one tubule being surrounded by six others. In the case illustrated in Plate 46 the tubules are mainly under the plasma membrane and around the nuclei: more rarely they were in the centre of the fibre. In the case illustrated in Plate 47, the tubules occur frequently between the myofibrils running parallel, obliquely or transversely to them. These tubules are usually 400 to 500 Å in diameter but may be smaller or may even reach 800 Å in diameter. They contain a central mass 250 to 300 Å in diameter with a clear zone 70 to 120 Å wide between the central mass and the outer wall of the tubule which is about 80 Å thick. The ultrastructure of these tubules was first reported by Gruner (1966) in a case of hypokalaemic periodic paralysis. Similar structures were reported by W. K. Engel (1970) who had earlier (1964) reported the histochemical changes in the muscle fibre. More detailed studies of these tubules were reported by W. K. Engel, Bishop and Cunningham (1970), who found them in 24 of more than 1500 patients who had muscle biopsies and most frequently in the cases of hypo- and hyperkalaemic periodic paralysis. They found them also in a case of phorphyria cutanea tarda and in individuals who had taken drugs for prolonged periods. Histochemical studies by these authors showed that the tubules occurred in type II fibres which presented areas of increased activity of DPNH and TPNH tetrazolium reductase and other enzymes but lacked ATPase. Histochemical and electron microscope studies on similar structures were reported by Pearse and Johnson (1970) and Morgan-Hughes, Mair and Lascelles (1970) in cases of myopathy of difficult classification. Their ultrastructure was reported by Mussini, Di Mauro and Margreth (1968), Bergman *et al.* (1970) and Dunkle *et al.* (1970) in cases of hypokalaemic periodic paralysis. The origin and significance of these tubules remain obscure, although some regard them as arising from the sarcoplasmic reticulum and others from the nuclear membrane.

Other types of tubules may occur in the muscle fibres as illustrated in Plate 48, in the upper part of which are tubules from a case of alcoholic myopathy where they occurred around the nuclei and near the surface of the muscle fibre (Morgan-Hughes, Anderson and Mair). These structures were about 500 to 800 Å in diameter.

Still another type of tubule is illustrated in the lower part of Plate 48, where the tubules are seen to lie amongst filaments in the muscle fibre of a patient with rheumatoid arthritis treated with steroids. The tubules were 500 to 700 Å in diameter and contained a central dense mass separated from the wall of the tubule by a clear zone. Their origin and pathological significance are again unknown.

Other tubules have been reported in the muscle, in patients with periodic paralysis by Odor, Patel and Pearce (1967) and Bradley (1969), in a girl with familial facio-scapulo-humeral muscular dystrophy by Hurwitz *et al.* (1967), in a patient with spinal progressive muscular atrophy (Sato and Tsubaki, 1968), in paramyotonia of Eulenberg by Castaigne *et al.* (1970) and in a young healthy male student by Riske-Nielsen and Harmsen. Tubules have been reported also in the muscle fibres of rats whose muscle was exposed to injury by severe cold by Price, Howes and Blumberg (1964a).

CRYSTAL AND VIRUS-LIKE PARTICLES

Crystals may be found in muscle fibres. Electron micrographs of crystalline deposits were demonstrated by Shafiq, Milhorat and Gorycki (1968) in two patients with diabetic amyotrophy and neuropathy and by Bradley *et al.* (1969) in a patient suffering from myopathy associated with abnormal lipid metabolism. Chalmers *et al.* (1969) demonstrated xanthine crystals in the muscle of a patient with myopathy.

Schmalbruch (1967) illustrated aggregates of crystals 140 Å in diameter in the muscle of two patients but did not regard them as having any pathological significance.

Virus-like particles have been described both in the nucleus and the cytoplasm of human muscle fibres. In the sarcoplasm of degenerate muscle fibres of a case of polymyositis Palmeiro, Behrend and Wechsler (1966) illustrated tubular structures which they postulated might be altered virus particles, but they lacked definite evidence of this. Myxomatous-like tubular filaments were described by Chou (1967b and 1968) in the muscle of a patient with chronic polymyositis. Crystalline groups of rounded virus-like particles 190 Å in diameter were described by Burch *et al.* (1968) in the skeletal muscle of a patient dying of heat stroke. In addition dense rounded virus-like particles 250 to 300 Å in diameter were reported by Caulfield, Rebeiz and Adams (1968) in the extra-ocular muscle of a patient dying of a ruptured thoracic aneurysm and by Norris *et al.* (1969) in skeletal muscle of two patients with myositis accompanying herpes zoster: in the latter case the particles were in hexagonal array. Slightly larger particles, 350 to 400 Å in diameter, also in hexagonal array are illustrated in Plate 74, in a degenerated muscle fibre from a patient with long standing muscular dystrophy: we have, however, no evidence to suggest that they may be virus in nature. More recently Chou and Gutmann (1970) reported in two patients dying of dermatomyositis the presence of numerous crystalline structures 170 to 200 Å in diameter which were similar to picorna virus and most likely belonged to the coxsakie group, and Mastaglia and Walton (1970) described particles 160 to 240 Å in diameter resembling the picorna virus in a patient with subacute polymyositis.

PLASMA AND BASEMENT MEMBRANES

The plasma membrane which is electron dense and surrounds each muscle fibre has often a wavy outline and may exhibit electron dense beading when the fibre is affected by some pathological process (Plates 20 and 76). Frequently the plasma membrane exhibits interruptions in its continuity or may be separated from the basement membrane (Plate 49). Small indentations of the plasma membrane are often observed (Plate 58) and may produce a villiform appearance at the edge of the sarcoplasm. Rows of tiny vesicles may also occur just under the plasma membrane and these indentations and vesicles suggest that pinocytotic activity takes place at the plasma membrane. In degenerating muscle fibres the plasma membrane may have disappeared, leaving only the basement membrane around the degenerating fibre (Plates 49, 63 lower part and 73). The changes in the plasma membrane reflect changes within the muscle fibre and are not specific to a particular disease process.

Changes in the *basement membrane* may accompany those taking place in the plasma membrane. Generally the basement membrane follows closely the wavy contour of the undulating plasma membrane of the pathological muscle fibre (Plate 20). The basement membrane may be thickened and contain electron dense bodies of varying size and shape which are extruded from autophagic vacuoles in the muscle fibre (Plate 40). More often in atrophied muscle fibres, loose folds of basement membrane which may be of considerable dimensions project from several points on the surface of the muscle fibre as is illustrated in Plates 22, 50 and 72. In inflammatory lesions when phagocytes attack the degenerating muscle fibre its basement membrane may disappear at the areas of contact with the phagocyte (Plate 63 upper part) while the plasma membrane of the two apposed cells remains intact. In advanced stages of degeneration a scanty amount of degenerate sarcoplasm and a nucleus may remain in the fibre, or phagocytes only may be seen within the basement membrane tube of the fibre. Eventually only collapsed basement membrane tubes with a loose undulating outline persist (Plate 84).

Projections of basement membrane from atrophied fibres were first reported by Birks, Katz and Miledi (1959) in denervated muscle of the frog but have since been observed by numerous authors.

SATELLITE CELLS AND REGENERATION OF MUSCLE

Satellite cells are found frequently in diseased muscle (Plate 51), and more than one may be present in the same muscle fibre (Plate 55). They do not usually contain well-differentiated myofilaments and are shorter than the parent muscle fibre. Random sections of muscle fibres may not pass through the nucleus of the satellite cell, so that only the cytoplasm may be apparent, which contains rough endoplasmic reticulum, prominent ribosomes and some mitochondria (Plates 53 lower part and 55). Centrioles have not been described in human muscle satellite cells, but have been reported by Muir, Kanji and Allbrook (1965) in the satellite cells of the muscle of the fruit-bat and in the guinea pig by Hess and Rosner (1970). Lipid material may also occur in some satellite cells but its significance is not understood. Satellite cells are common in polymyositis and allied conditions, especially in young patients where regeneration of muscle fibres would be expected. They occur also in muscular dystrophy (Laguens, 1963), particularly in the early stages of the disease (Plate 19), in denervated muscle (Plate 44) and in various other muscle disorders. Why the satellite cells become more frequent in diseased muscle is not known, nor is it clear why in normal muscle the satellite cells remain in a stationary stage of development.

Regarding the *regeneration of muscle*, it is well known, especially in inflammatory diseases, that some muscle fibres with well-formed myofibrils exhibit in addition numerous fine filaments and large numbers of ribosomes and polysomes scattered throughout an abundance of sarcoplasm as illustrated in Plate 52. These particular changes in the sarcoplasm suggest regeneration rather than degeneration of the muscle fibres.

In other instances some muscle fibres with well-developed myofibrils present large numbers of polysomes and flattened tubules in their sarcoplasm (Plate 53 upper part) and these occur also in the cytoplasm of active satellite cells (Plate 53 lower part). Such similar features in the mature muscle fibres and in the satellite cell tend to suggest that the muscle fibre may be in a stage of regeneration. Another possible explanation of these changes in the muscle fibre may be that it was damaged by some pathological agent and may be undergoing repair.

Even if the appearances just described in the muscle fibres are not accepted as evidence of regeneration, regeneration of the muscle is generally assumed to originate from the satellite cells. Under certain conditions, satellite cells are seen more frequently and show evidence of increased activity. They enlarge, the cytoplasm increases in amount and the Golgi apparatus, rough endoplasmic reticulum, ribosomes and polysomes become very apparent (Plate 53 lower part) and the number of mitochondria is increased. At this stage of development the satellite cell resembles the myoblast of foetal muscle. Fine filaments may be scattered throughout the cytoplasm and eventually thick and thin filaments appear and become aligned to form myofibrils (Plate 54). In the early stage of regeneration these cells with the newly formed myofibrils lie in the same basement membrane as the parent muscle fibre. The newly formed muscle fibre may in time dissociate from the parent fibre, although for some time they may share the same basement membrane tube and are sometimes associated with a more primitive satellite cell (Plate 55). Later the developing muscle fibre acquires its own basement membrane. The parent muscle fibre sometimes presents evidence of degenerative changes while the satellite cell is evolving into a mature muscle fibre.

The ultrastructure of regeneration of human muscle has been studied by various authors including Shafiq, Gorycki and Milhorat (1967) and Mastaglia, Papadimitriou and Kakulas (1969a and 1970). In experimental animals the regeneration of skeletal muscle has been widely investigated by a large number of authors. These include Allbrook (1962), Price, Howes and Blumberg (1964b), Shafiq and Gorycki (1965), Church, Noronha and Allbrook (1966), Larson, Hudgson and Walton (1969), Reznik and W. K. Engel (1970), Teräväinen (1970) and Jerusalem and Schick (1970). The recent publication edited by Mauro, Shafiq and Milhorat (1970) deals with the regeneration of striated muscle both in man and animals.

PLATE 17. RING FIBRE

A ring fibre fills most of the illustration. The nucleus lies near the surface of the fibre (bottom left). A thin layer of longitudinally disposed myofibrils at the edge of the fibre surround a mass of myofibrils running transversely. The Z-lines, I- and A-bands are apparent in all the myofibrils. The H-zone with the M-line in its centre occupies the middle of the A-band. Mitochondria and glycogen granules lie under the plasma membrane. Blood capillaries and collagen separate the ring from adjacent muscle fibres. No obvious degenerative change is noted in the ring fibre.

MAGNIFICATION 7,500 ×.

From a patient with muscular dystrophy.

A A-band
BC Blood capillary
I I-band
M M-line
N Nucleus
RF Ring fibre
Z Z-line

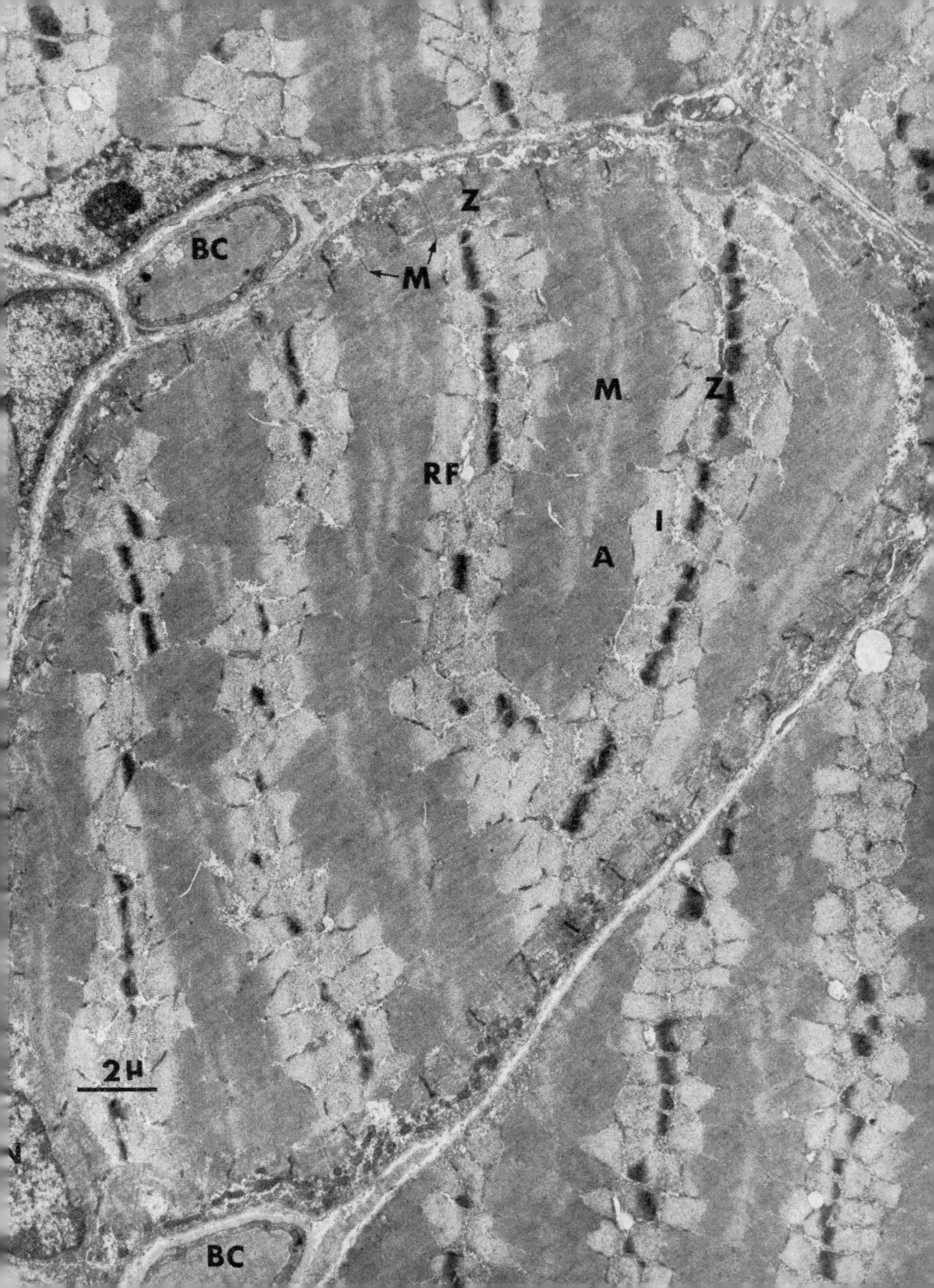
BC
Z
M
M
Z
RF
I
A
2μ
BC

PLATE 18. RING FIBRES

In both illustrations the Z-lines, I- and A-bands and the triads can be identified readily. The M-line in the centre of the H-zone lies in the middle of the A-band. Glycogen granules occur between the myofibrils. No plasma membrane separates the longitudinal from the transverse myofibrils.

UPPER. A ring fibre cut in transverse section shows longitudinally disposed myofibrils at the edge of the fibre around the transverse central myofibrils.

MAGNIFICATION 21,000 ×.

From a patient with muscular dystrophy.

LOWER. A ring fibre cut longitudinally shows the peripheral myofibrils lie transversely around the central longitudinal myofibrils.

MAGNIFICATION 25,000 ×.

From a patient with periarteritis nodosa.

A	A-band	M	M-line
G	Glycogen	Tr	Triads
H	H-zone	Z	Z-line
I	I-band		

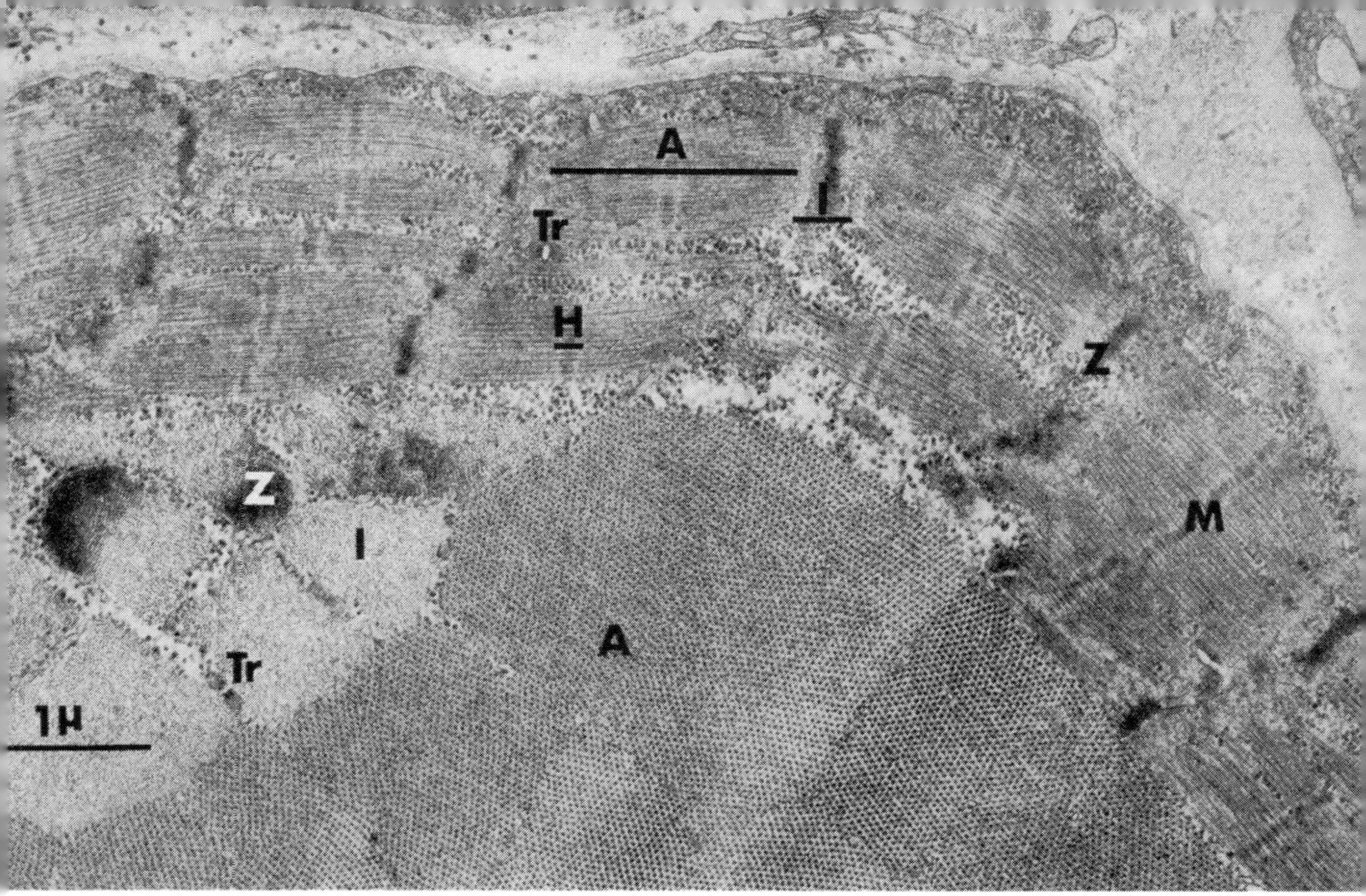
A
I
Tr
H
Z
Z
I
M
A
Tr
1μ

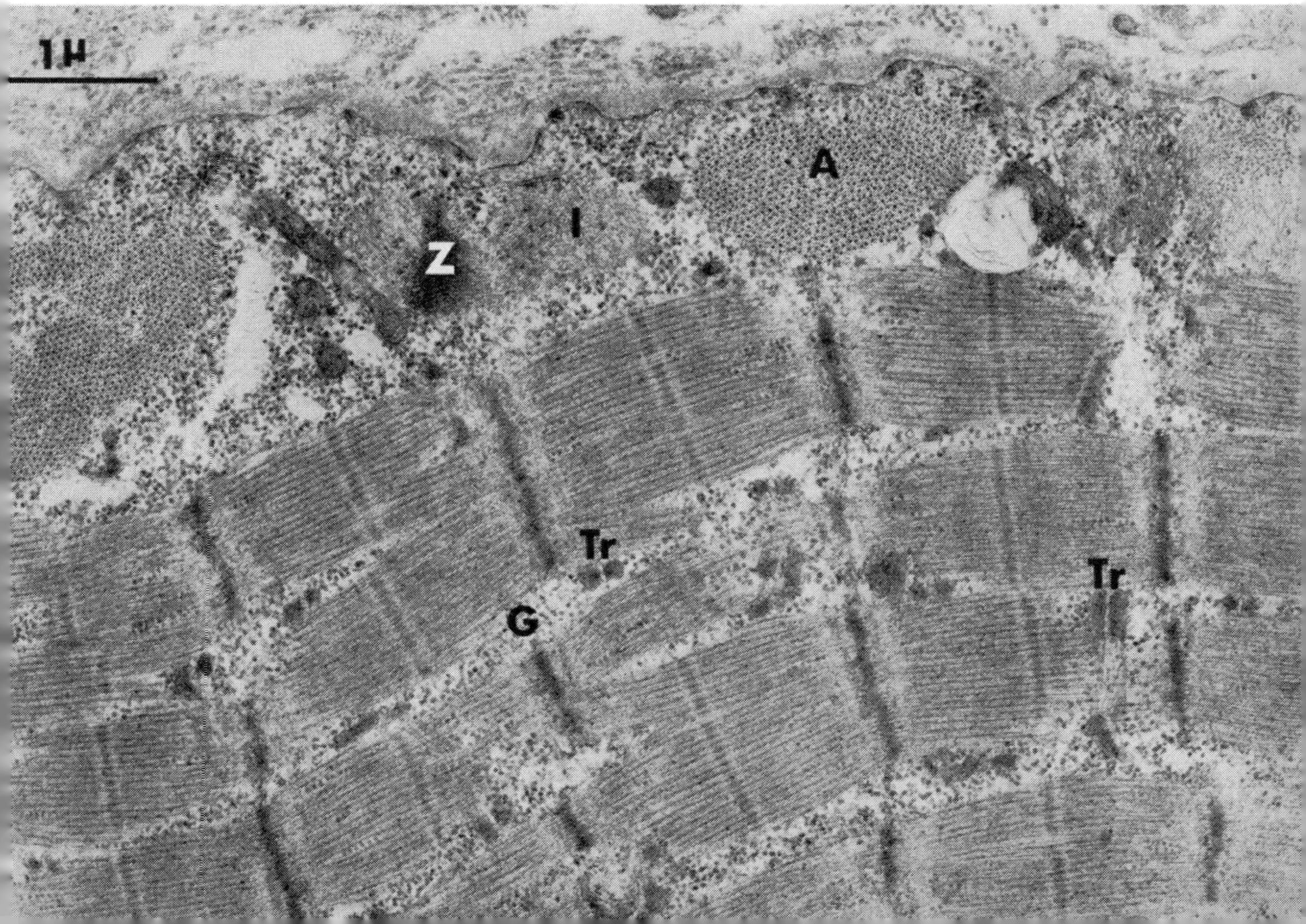
1μ
A
I
Z
Tr
G
Tr

PLATE 19. MYOFIBRILLARY DEGENERATION

UPPER. Loss of myofilaments is an early change in some of the muscle fibres affected by muscular dystrophy. The loss of myofilaments is often very apparent in the I-band while the Z-line may persist (arrowed). The myofibrils are often widely spaced and between them and in the regions from which the myofilaments disappear glycogen and other granules and large numbers of small mitochondria occur.

MAGNIFICATION 11,000 ×.

LOWER. A satellite cell from which a mature muscle fibre may develop occurs in a muscle fibre showing loss of myofilaments and widely spaced myofibrils. No basement membrane occurs between the adjacent plasma membranes of the satellite cell and the muscle fibre.

MAGNIFICATION 14,500 ×.

Both from a patient with muscular dystrophy.

G Glycogen
Gr Granules
Mi Mitochondria
N Nucleus
S Satellite cell

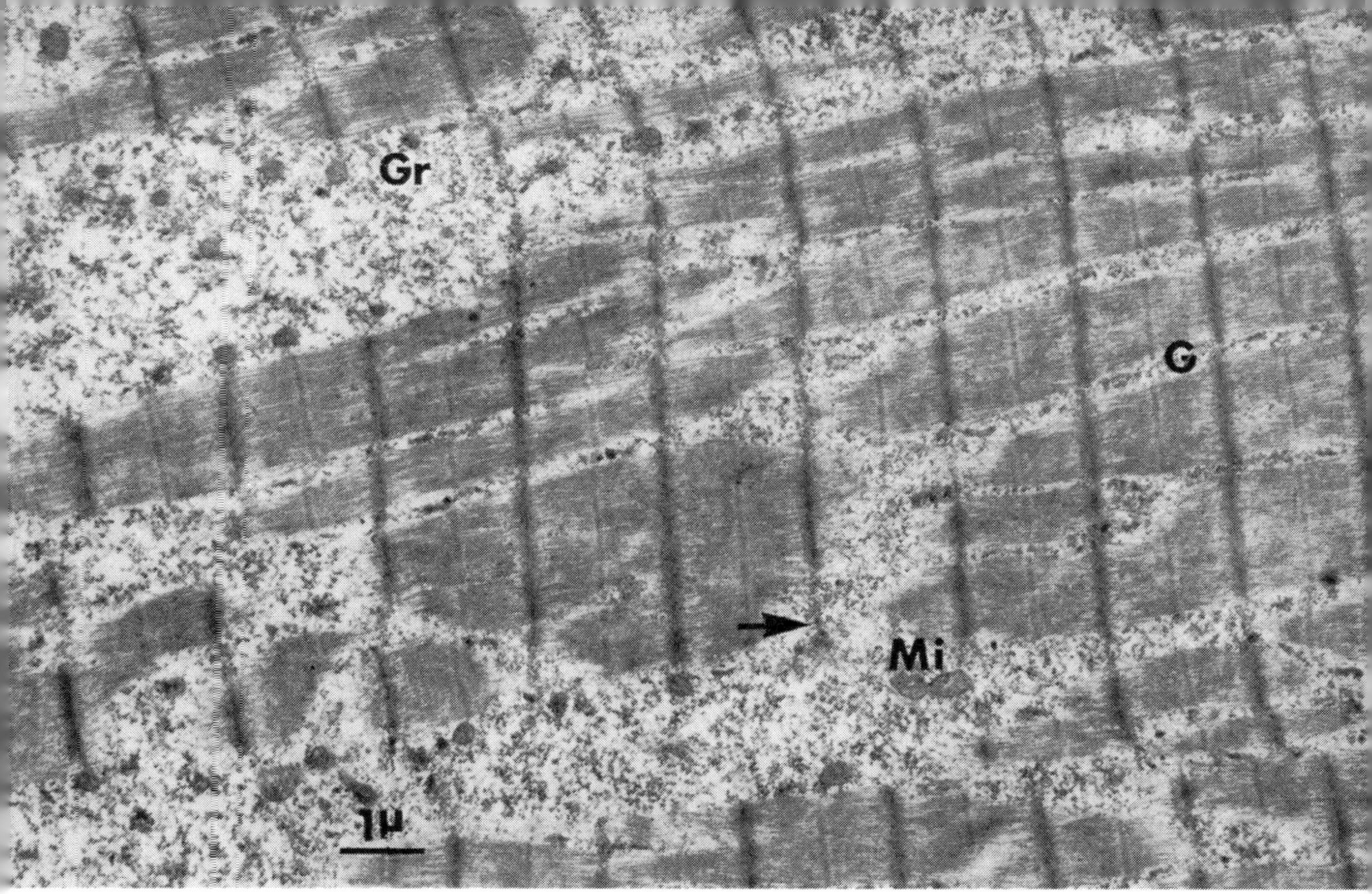

Gr
G
Mi
1μ

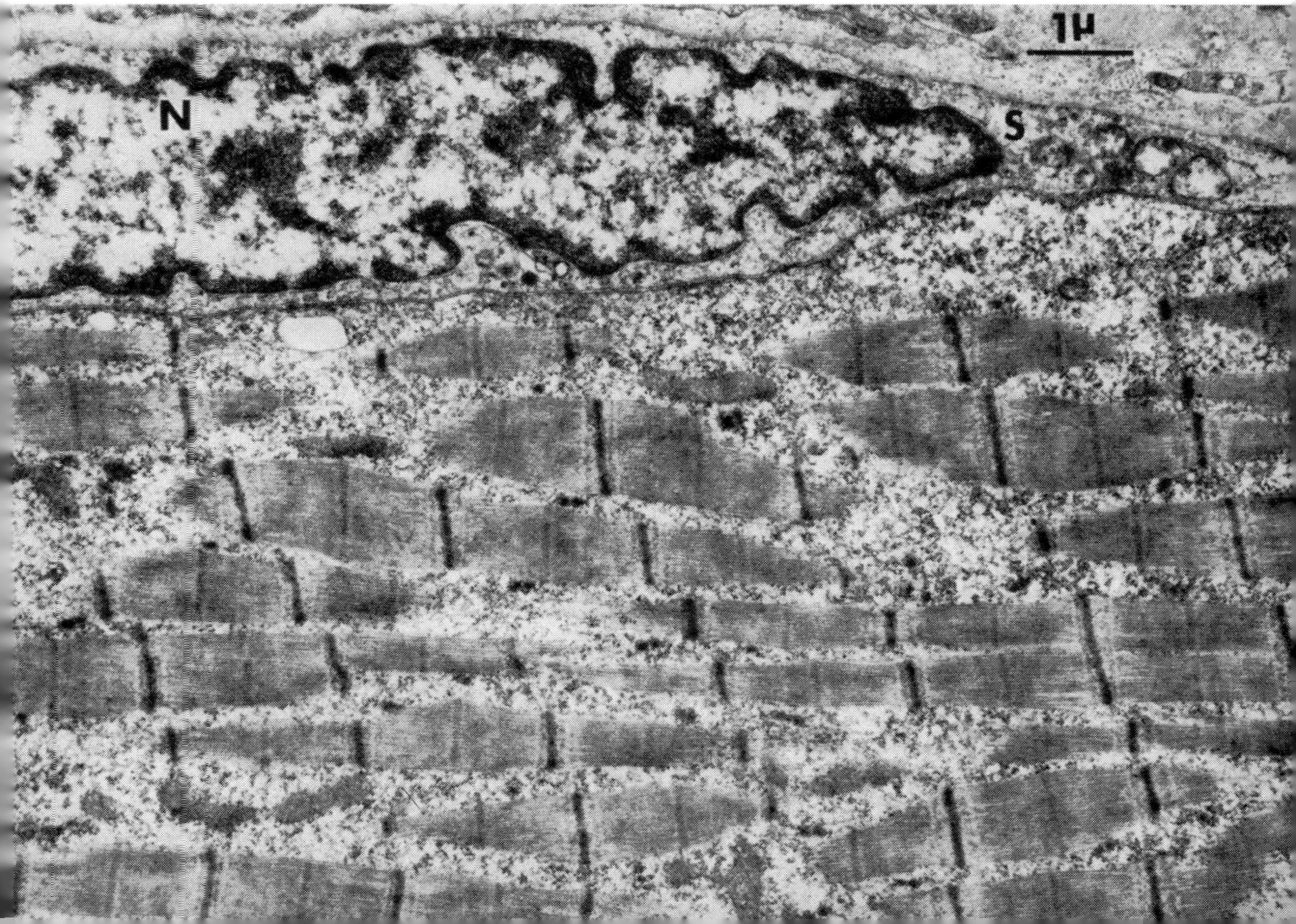

1μ
N
S

PLATE 20. MYOFIBRILLARY DEGENERATION
UNDULATIONS OF THE SURFACE OF MUSCLE FIBRES

UPPER. The undulating surface of this degenerating muscle fibre shows electron dense beading of the plasma membrane. The sarcoplasm contains a large amount of granular material, mitochondria and numerous vacuoles. Some myofibrils are intact: others are undergoing degenerative changes. Top right is a blood capillary containing a leucocyte.

MAGNIFICATION 8,000 ×.

From a patient with polymyositis.

LOWER. In some muscle fibres isolated, thin projections of sarcoplasm extend into the collagen surrounding the muscle fibres. These projections contain numerous vesicles and granules. Processes of fibroblasts and collagen lie alongside them.

MAGNIFICATION 10,000 ×.

From a patient with polyneuropathy.

BC Blood capillary
C Collagen
F Fibroblast
Le Leucocyte
Mf Myofibril
PM Plasma membrane

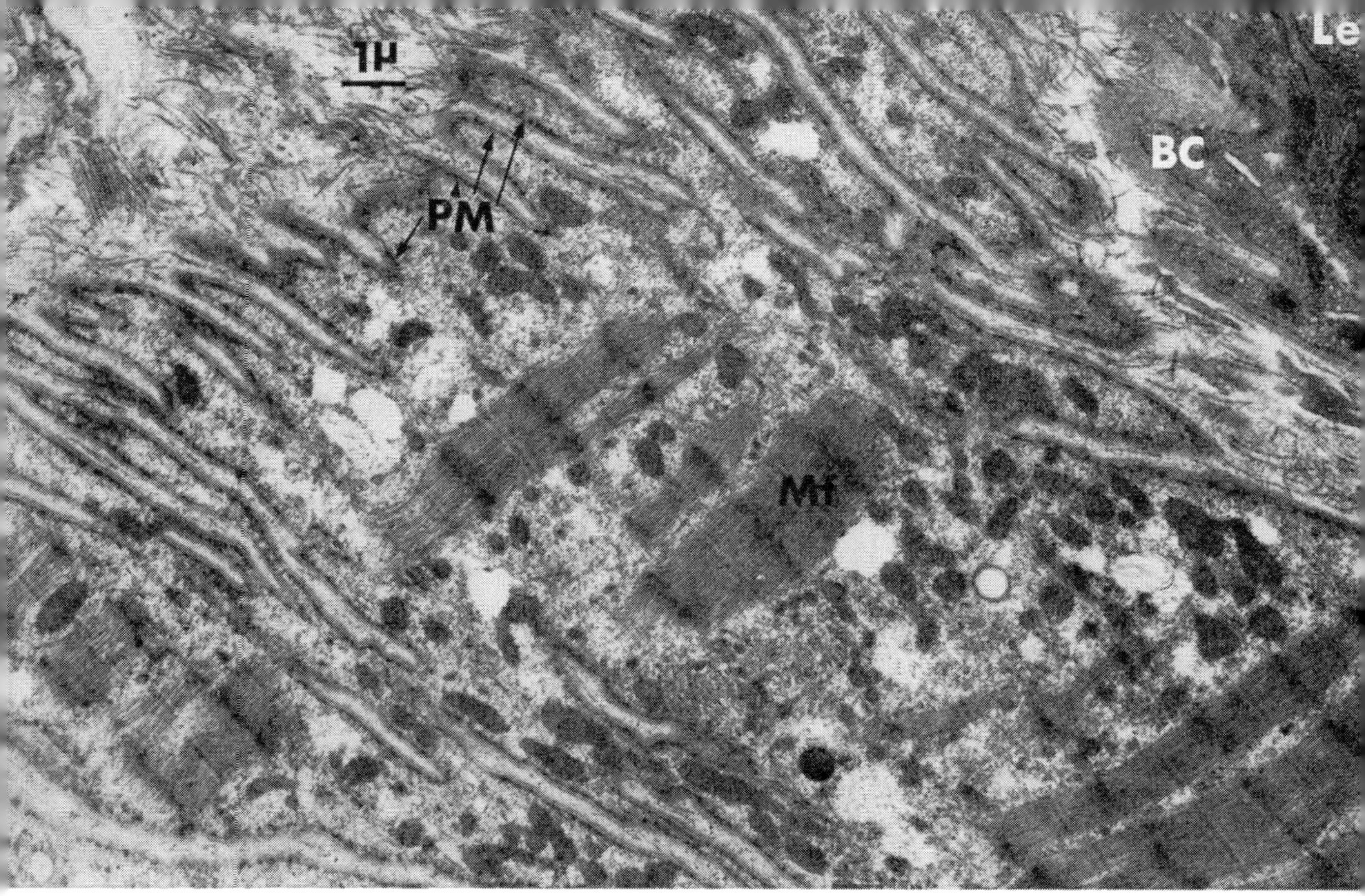

Le
1µ
BC
PM
Mf

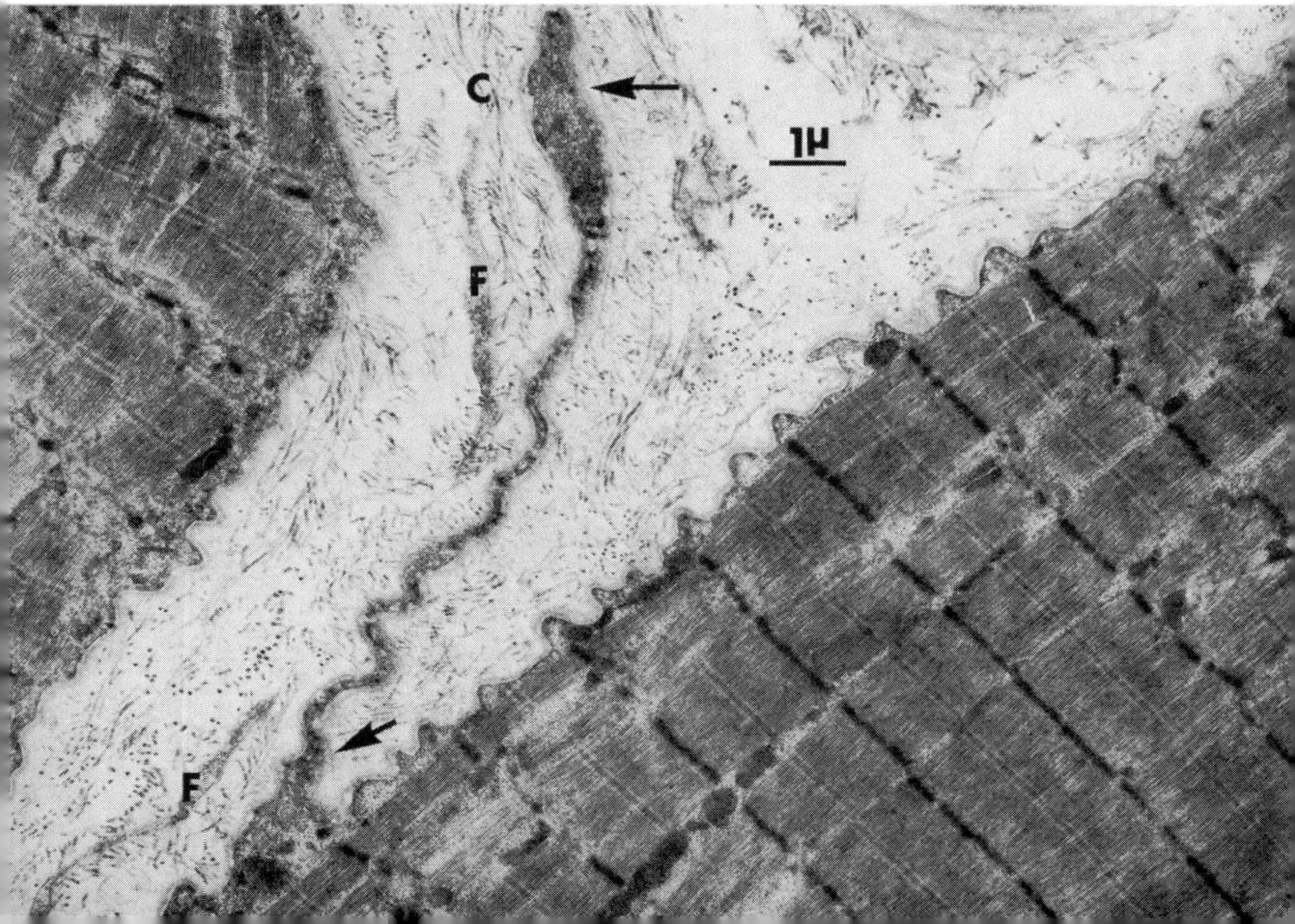

C
1µ
F
F

PLATE 21. MYOFIBRILLARY DEGENERATION

UPPER. Sarcoplasmic Masses.
Loss of myofilaments takes place in several sarcomeres and eventually large parts of the myofibrils disappear. Granular material occupies the regions from which the myofilaments disappear. Many mitochondria accumulate under the surface of the muscle fibre and around the nuclei. The areas from which the myofilaments disappear at the surface of the fibre are termed sarcoplasmic masses. A nucleus, mitochondria and granules lie in the sarcoplasmic mass. Basement membrane covers the beaded plasma membrane of the degenerating muscle fibre. Outside the muscle fibre lie processes of fibroblasts and collagen as well as blood capillaries which in this instance have a thick layer of basement membrane around them. Many vesicles occur in the endothelial cell cytoplasm.

MAGNIFICATION 9,000 ×.

LOWER. Atrophic Muscle Fibre.
The degenerating fibre may become very small with undulating surfaces. The myofilaments and myofibrils have vanished and the fibre is occupied by granular material amongst which occur occasional mitochondria and to the left of the fibre, a nucleus. Dense chromatin lies around the margin of the nucleus. On either side of the atrophied fibre are muscle fibres which contain a large amount of glycogen and this is very evident in the upper fibre.

MAGNIFICATION 7,000 ×.

Both from a patient with muscular dystrophy.

BC	Blood capillary	Gr	Granules
BM	Basement membrane	Mf	Myofibrils
C	Collagen	Mi	Mitochondria
F	Fibroblast	N	Nucleus

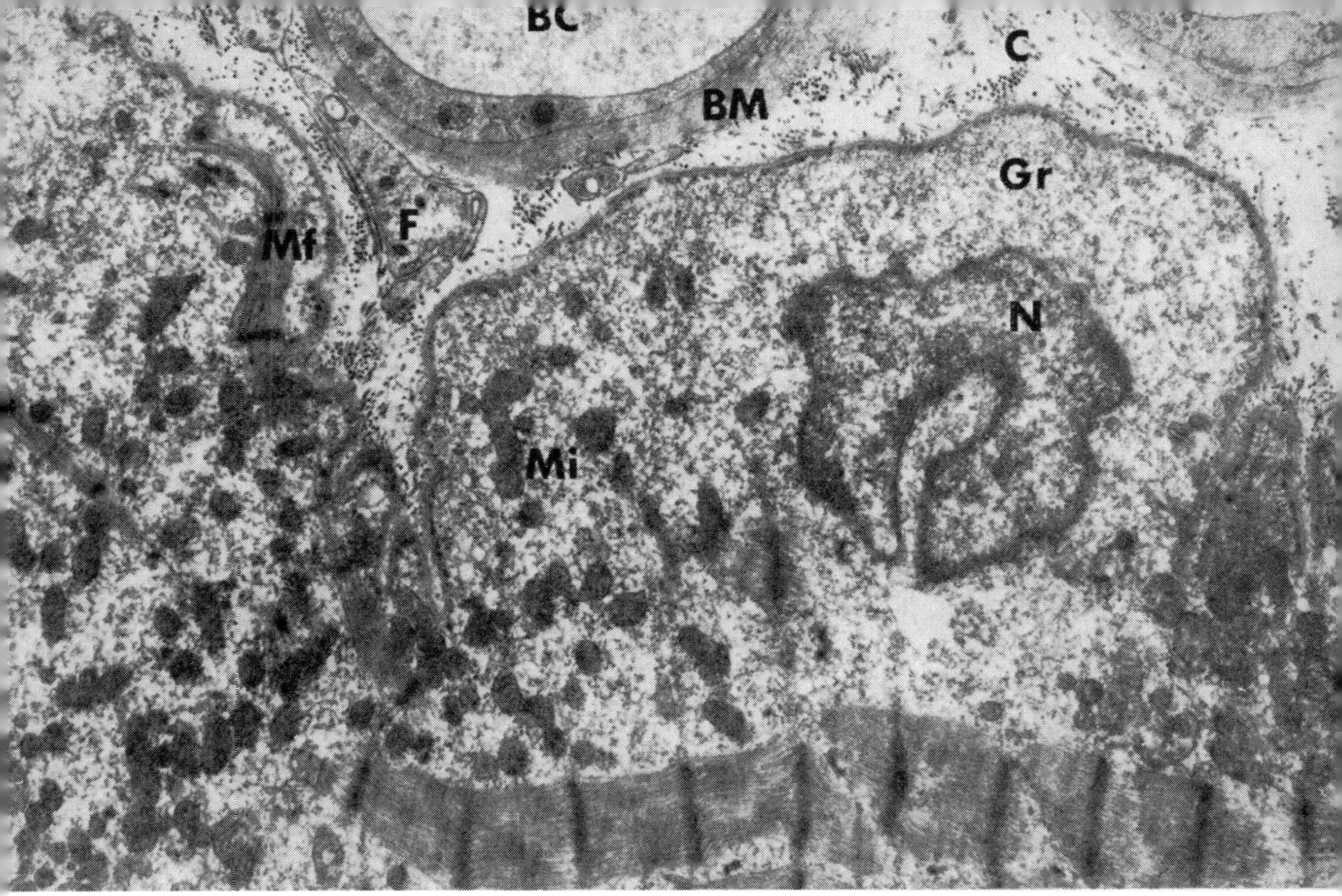
BC
C
BM
Gr
Mf
F
N
Mi

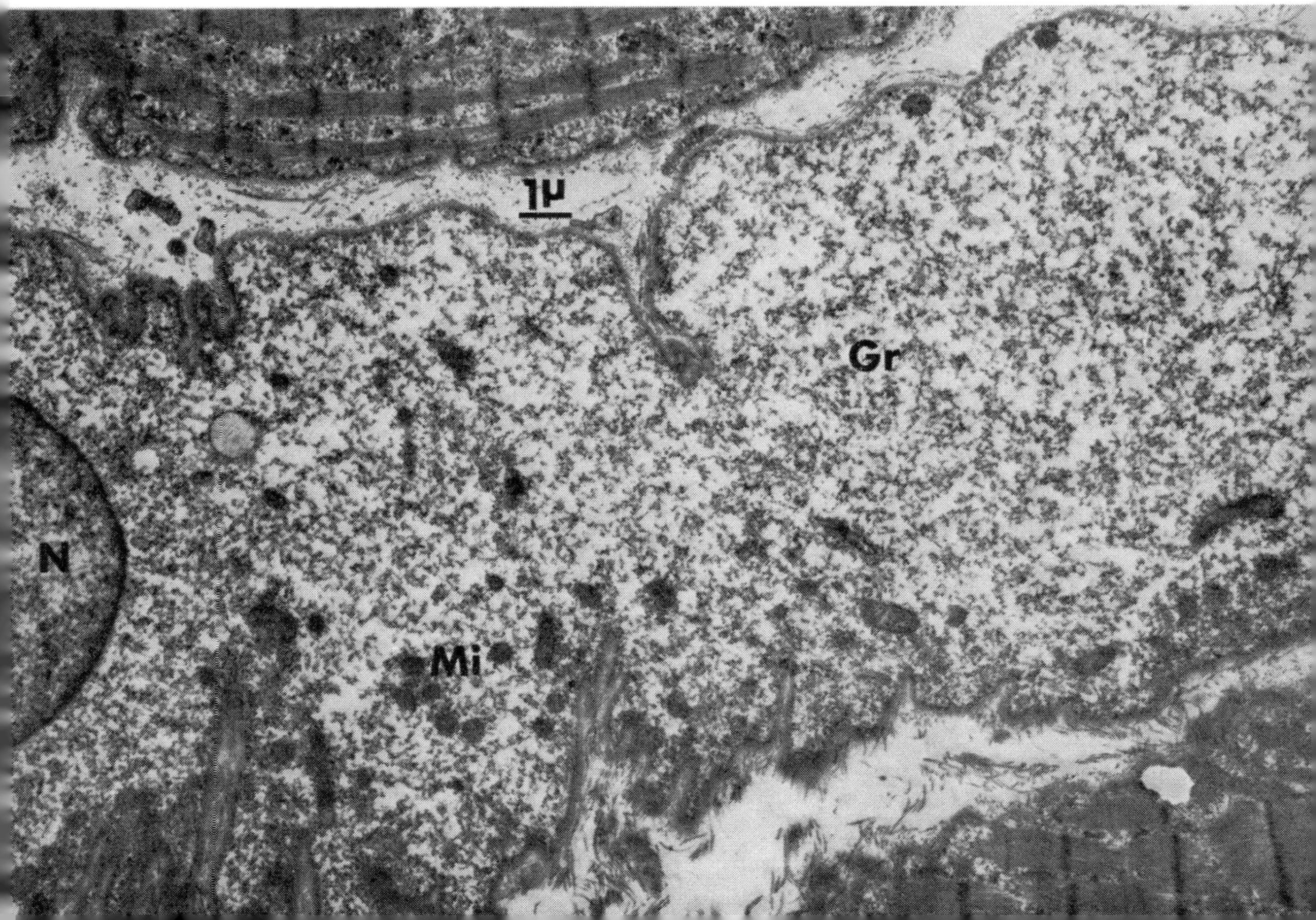
1μ
Gr
N
Mi

PLATE 22. CHANGES IN SHAPE AND SIZE OF DEGENERATE MUSCLE FIBRES

UPPER. A small atrophied muscle fibre shows disorganisation of the myofibrils and the sarcomere pattern. The Z-lines are distorted and thickened and the I-bands have largely disappeared but the A-bands can be identified. Numerous triads and occasional lipid bodies occur in the muscle fibre. The plasma membrane around the top right of the fibre is discontinuous and in parts thickened and very electron dense. Empty folds of basement membrane lie to the right of the fibre and collagen surrounds it.

MAGNIFICATION 10,000 ×.

Temporal muscle from a patient treated with steroids.

LOWER. A rounded atrophied fibre is illustrated: the nucleus lies in the centre of the fibre surrounded by a large amount of glycogen and lipid bodies. The myofibrils around the periphery of the fibre are disorganised: their Z-lines are thickened and distorted, the I-bands cannot be identified but some of the A-bands persist. The plasma membrane shows electron dense beading. Folds of basement membrane lie on either side of the fibre which is surrounded by collagen.

MAGNIFICATION 12,000 ×.

From a patient with motor neurone disease.

BM Basement membrane
C Collagen
G Glycogen
LB Lipid body
Mi Mitochondria
N Nucleus
Tr Triads
Z Z-line

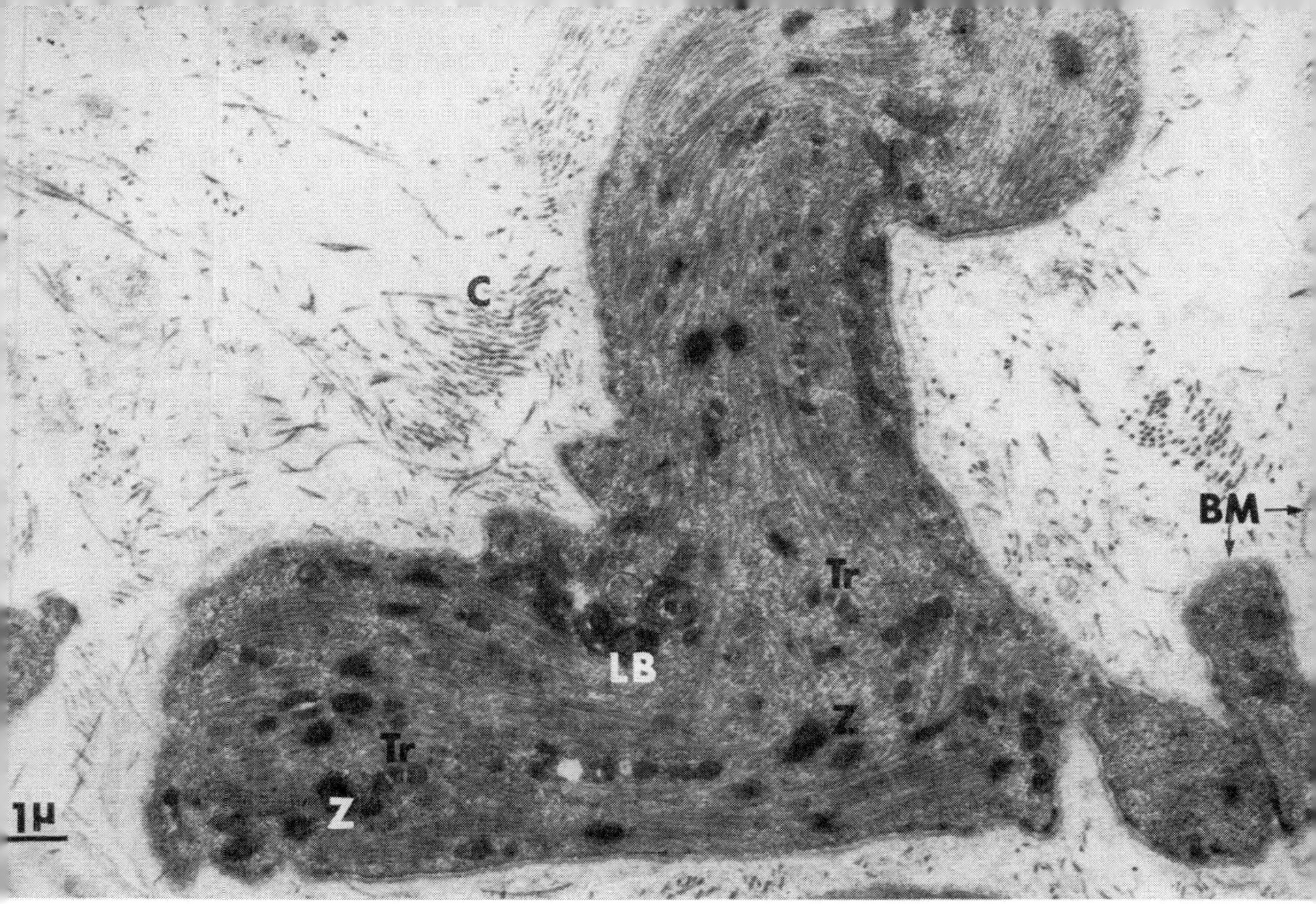
C
BM
Tr
LB
Z
Tr
Z
1μ

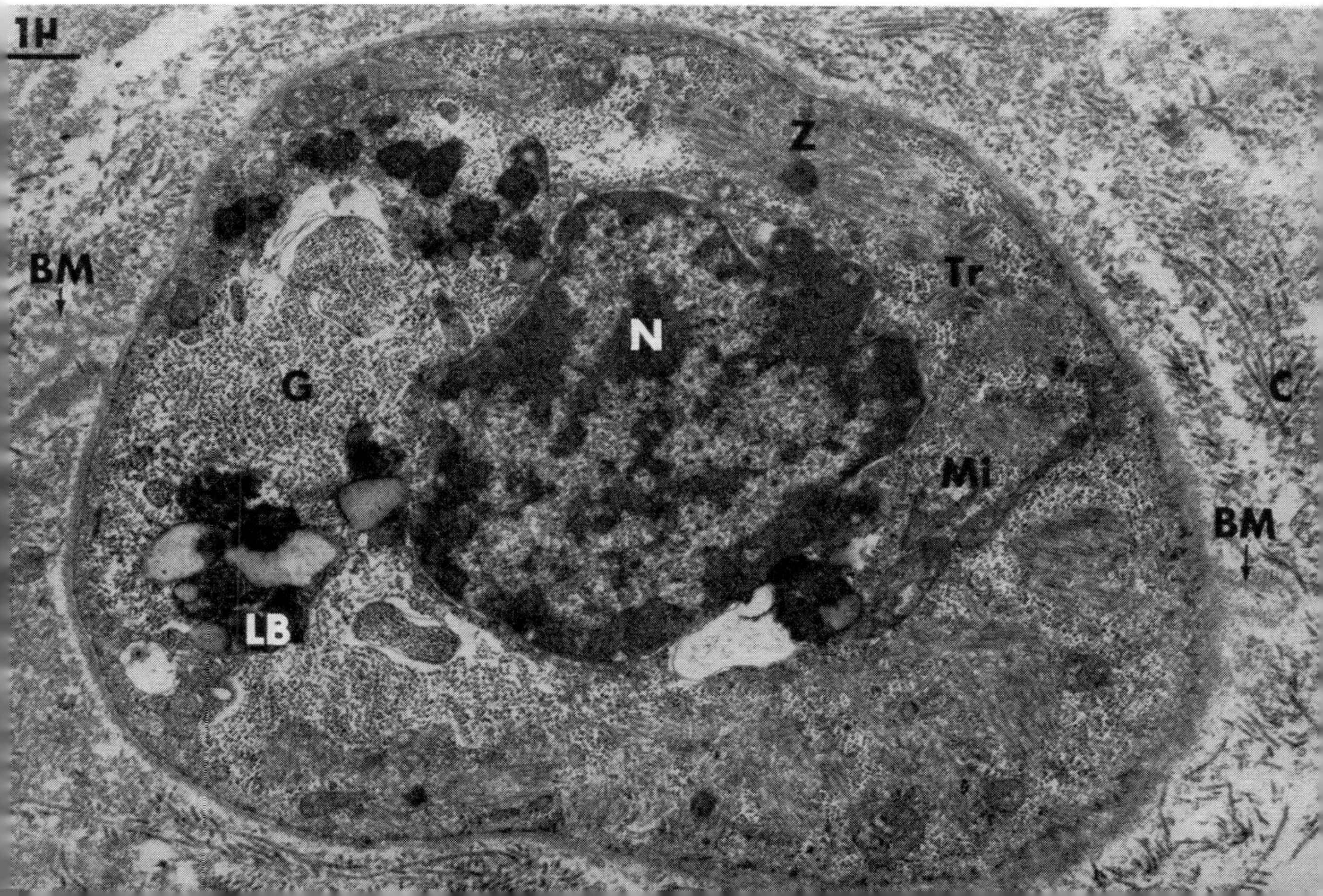
1μ
Z
BM
Tr
N
G
C
Mi
BM
LB

PLATE 23. 'STREAMING' OF THE Z-LINES

All the elements of one or several sarcomeres of a myofibril or adjacent myofibrils may be affected by a change usually referred to as 'streaming' of the Z-line. The Z-line may have a zig-zag appearance or may be replaced by material sometimes slightly less electron dense than the normal Z-line and this material may replace part or all of the I- and A-bands (arrowed). The change is often found at the edge of the muscle fibre.

UPPER LEFT. Consecutive sarcomeres of several adjacent myofibrils are involved by this change (arrowed).

MAGNIFICATION 6,500 ×.

UPPER RIGHT. A sarcomere of adjacent myofibrils is involved by the change. The altered Z-line is arrowed.

MAGNIFICATION 12,000 ×.

Both from a patient with alcoholic myopathy.

LOWER. The change is illustrated at higher magnification. The continuity of the altered material with the Z-line is arrowed.

MAGNIFICATION 25,000 ×.

From a patient with polymyositis.

BC Blood capillary

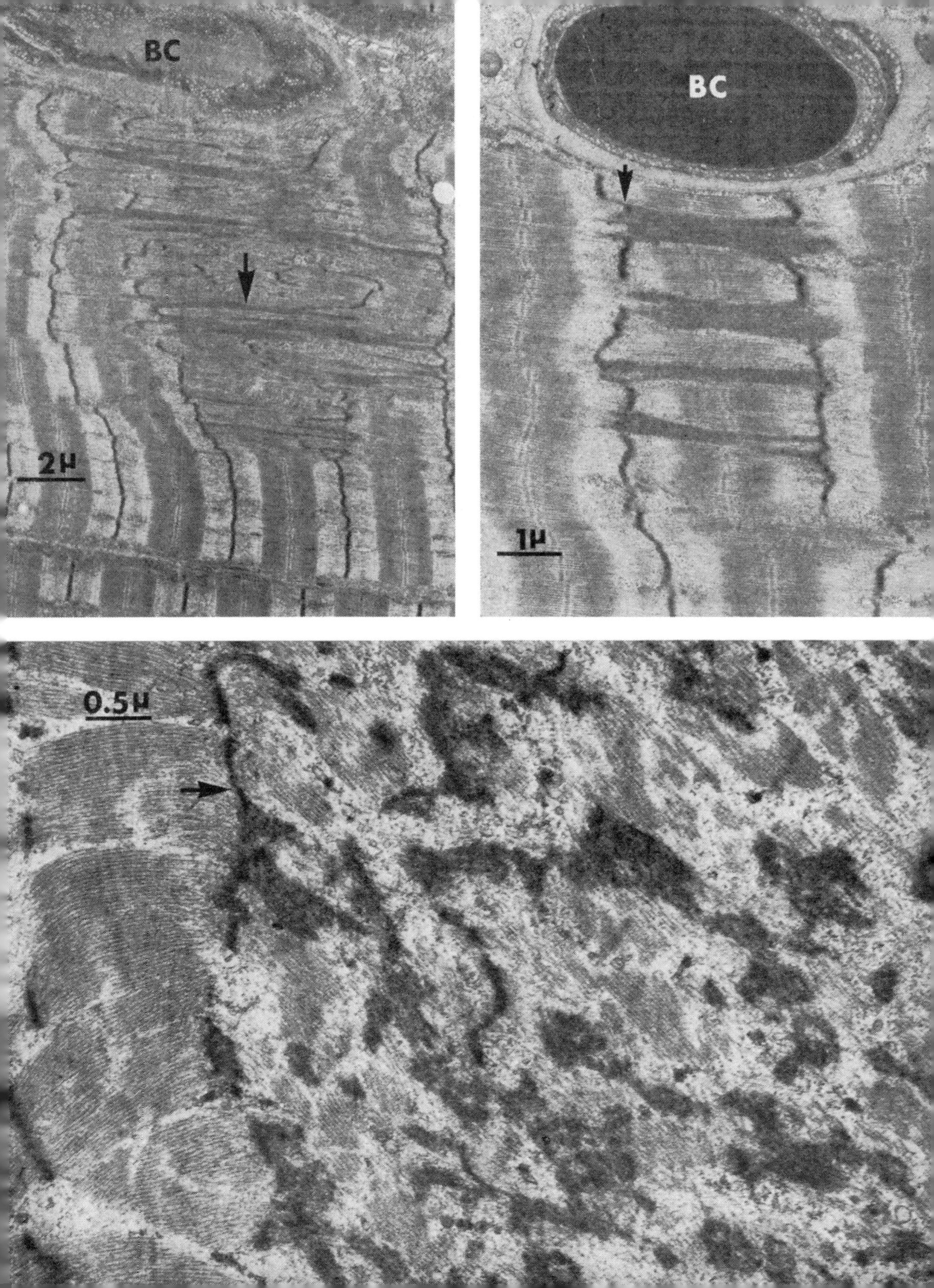
BC
2μ
BC
1μ
0.5μ

PLATE 24. TARGET FIBRES

UPPER LEFT. Target fibres are muscle fibres in which the changes seen between the arrows have occurred. The architecture of several consecutive sarcomeres of several adjacent myofibrils is replaced by electron dense material in which glycogen and mitochondria are not found. Many triads which lie adjacent to one another or in groups are present in the damaged part of the muscle fibre. Between the undamaged and the severely damaged myofibrils, a less damaged region occurs.

MAGNIFICATION 8,500 ×.

UPPER RIGHT. In the lower part of a target fibre sectioned obliquely are collections of irregular shaped electron dense material (arrowed) between which myofilaments can be identified. Numerous triads occur in the muscle around these groups of electron dense material.

MAGNIFICATION 8,000 ×.

Both are from a patient with alcoholic polyneuropathy.

LOWER. The changes in this fibre are less extensive than in the above illustrations. Here, fewer sarcomeres of the involved myofibrils are replaced by the electron dense material (arrowed). Mitochondria and glycogen granules lie close to some of the damaged sarcomeres.

MAGNIFICATION 9,500 ×.

From a patient with dystrophia myotonica.

G Glycogen
Tr Triad

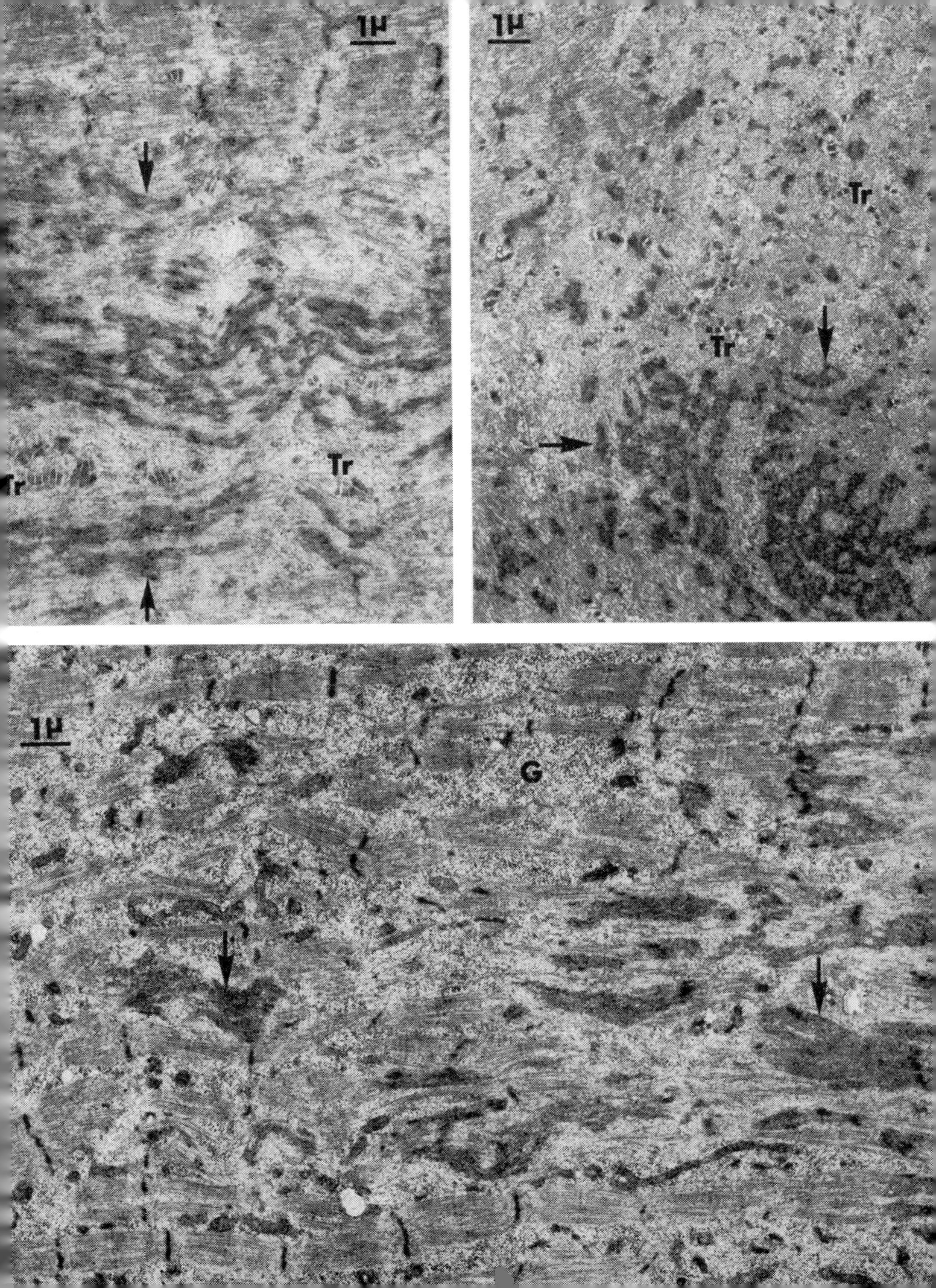
1µ
Tr
Tr
1µ
Tr
Tr
1µ
G

PLATE 25. RODS IN SKELETAL MUSCLE

UPPER. Between the myofibrils of this muscle fibre are roughly parallel rows of rods of similar electron density as the Z-lines which lie in relation to them. The rods have a filamentous structure and merge with the I- and A-bands around them. Some of the Z-lines immediately adjacent to the rods are distorted. The muscle fibre is stretched: in consequence the I-band is long while the A-band remains of constant length.

MAGNIFICATION 14,500 ×.

From a patient with muscular dystrophy.

LOWER. The muscle fibre at the myotendinous junction presents numerous smaller but similar rods as in the upper illustration. The rods occupy the site of the Z-lines. The broadened zone of electron density replacing the thin plasma membrane at the edge of the muscle fibre is also apparent. The mitochondria are ballooned: this is probably due to artefact. The muscle fibre is contracted: the I-band is therefore short.

MAGNIFICATION 15,000 ×.

From the first dorsal interosseous muscle of the foot.

DZ Dense zone
Mf Myofibril
Mi Mitochondria
Ro Rods

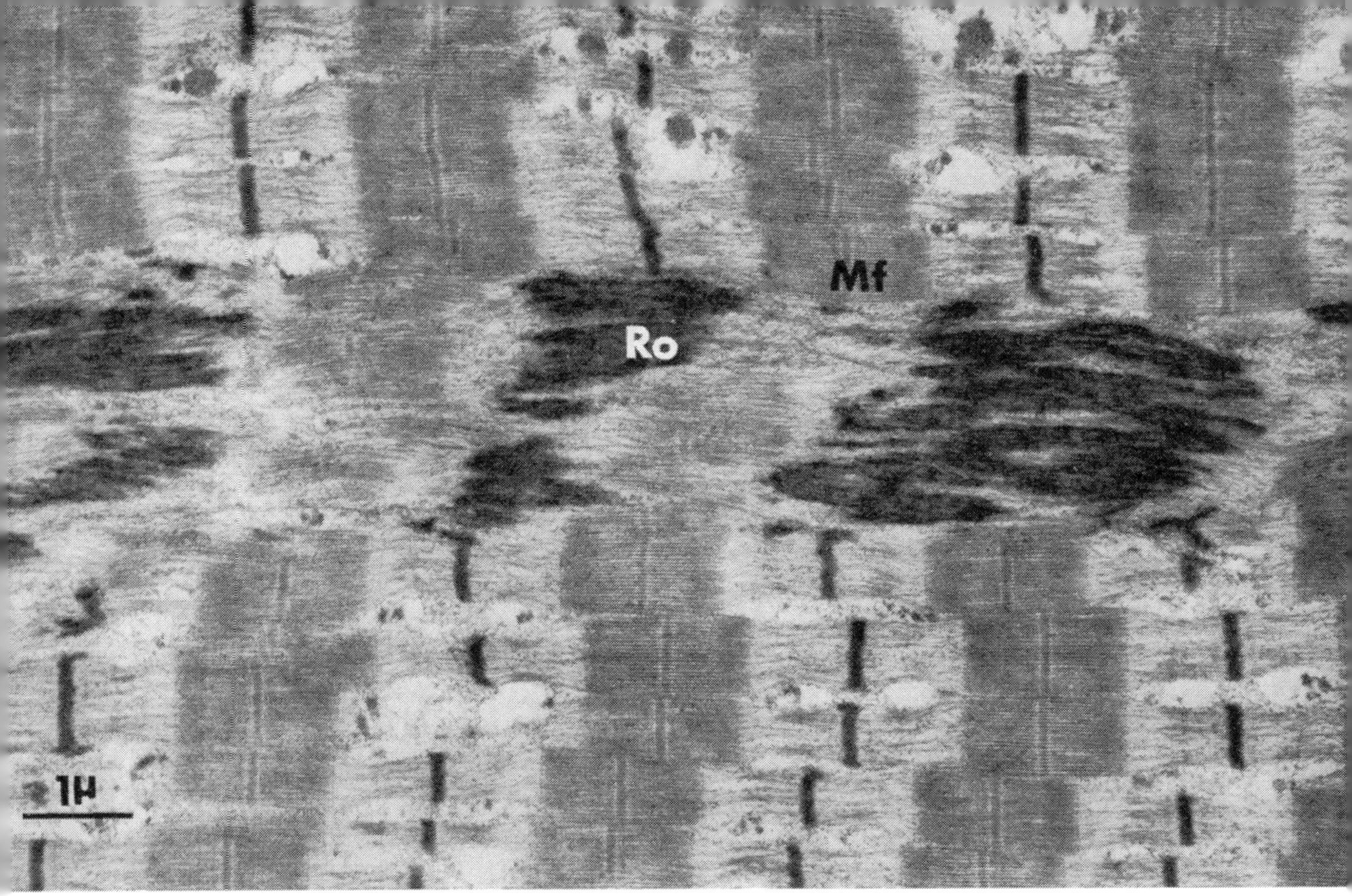
Mf
Ro
1μ

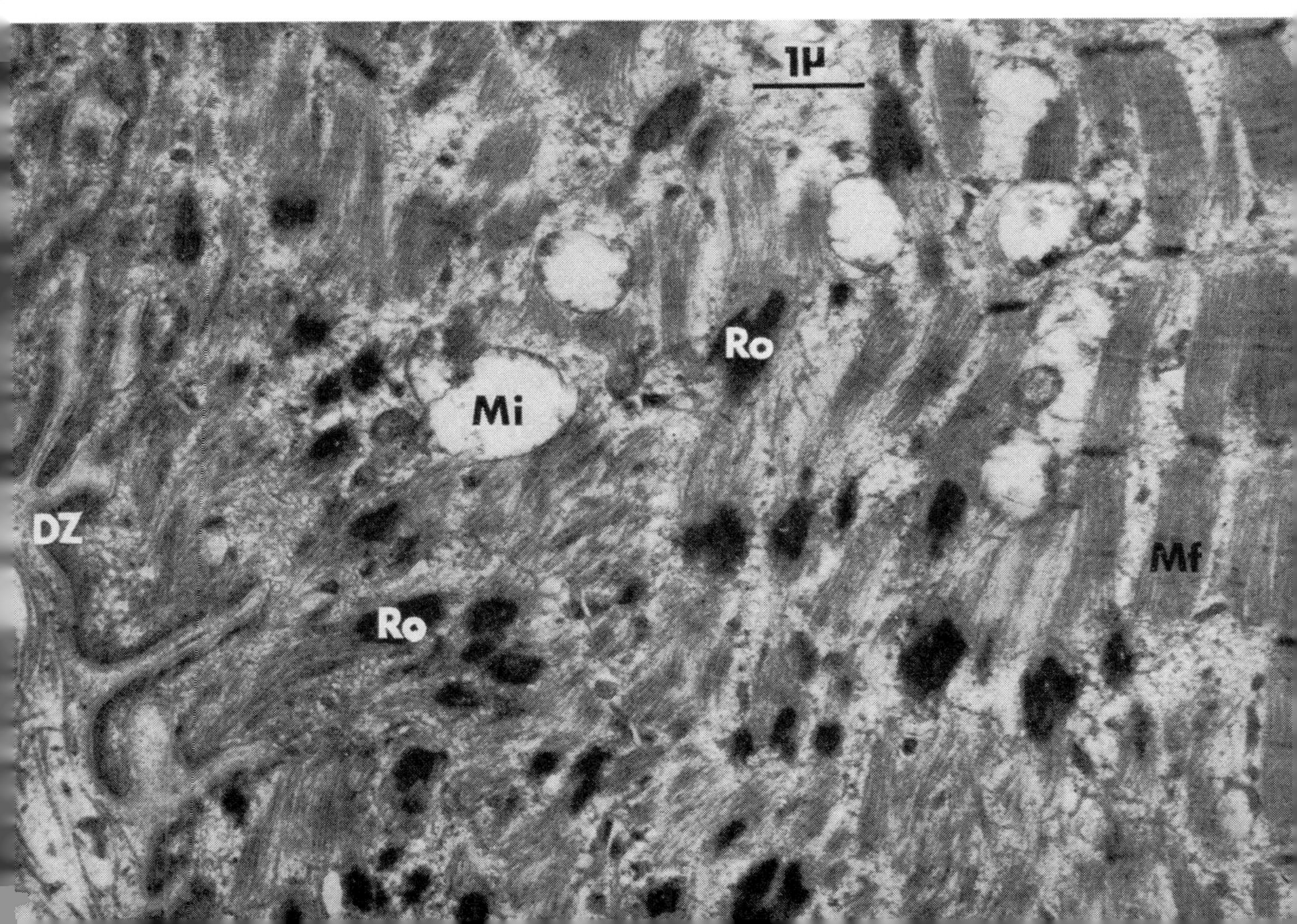
1μ
Ro
Mi
DZ
Ro
Mf

PLATE 26. RODS IN EXTRA-OCULAR MUSCLE

UPPER. In the region of the Z-line in the left half of the muscle fibre are numerous electron dense rods which merge with the surrounding parts of the sarcomeres. These rods which are formed of Z-line material correspond to the rods found in nemaline myopathy. The myofibrils to the left of the fibre are disorganised. In addition the muscle fibre presents large vacuoles near the nucleus and smaller ones between the myofibrils. Numerous mitochondria are present in the fibre.

MAGNIFICATION 9,000 ×.

LOWER. The rods enclosed in the rectangle above are shown here at greater magnification. Their filamentous structure is evident, the filaments continuing with the myofilaments around them (arrowed).

MAGNIFICATION 110,000 ×.

From a patient with diabetes mellitus.

Mi Mitochondria
N Nucleus
Ro Rods
Va Vacuoles

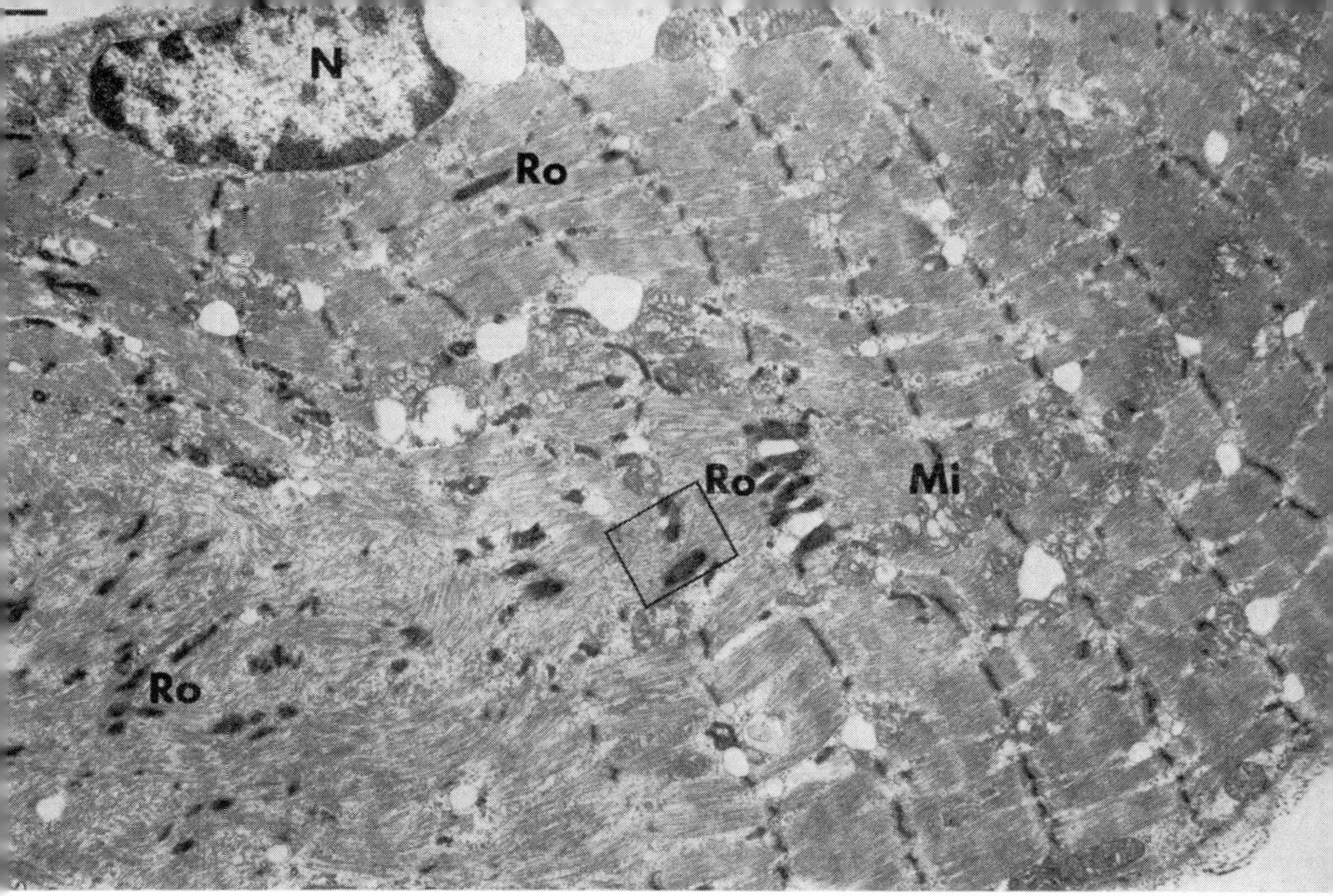
N
Ro
Ro
Mi
Ro

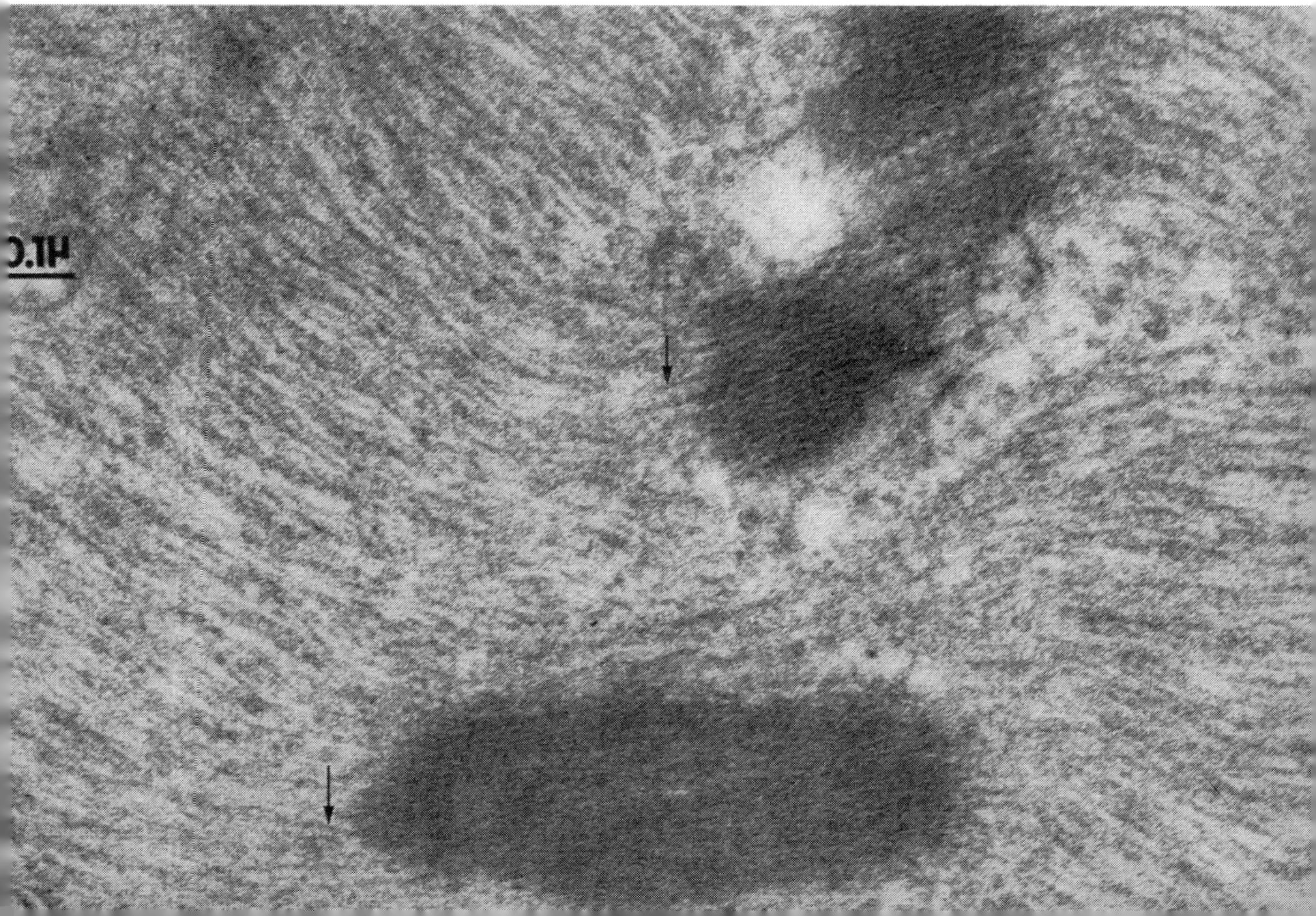

PLATE 27. CYTOPLASMIC BODIES

UPPER. In this degenerating muscle fibre is a very electron dense cytoplasmic body with closely set less electron dense filaments radiating from it. Around the cytoplasmic body are distorted myofibrils with thickened Z-lines. Collections of disorganised filaments are starred at the bottom of the illustration.

MAGNIFICATION 9,500 ×.

From a patient with alcoholic polyneuropathy.

LOWER. A cytoplasmic body which is mushroom shaped and has filaments radiating from it is present in this atrophied fibre. To the left of the cytoplasmic body are some secondary synaptic clefts of a degenerating motor end plate. The myofibrils are disorganised. Collections of glycogen granules are abundant in the muscle fibre: to the left is a nucleus and around it some mitochondria. Collagen and processes of fibroblasts lie around the muscle fibre.

MAGNIFICATION 10,000 ×.

From a patient with muscular dystrophy.

C Collagen
CB Cytoplasmic body
F Fibroblast
Fi Filaments
G Glycogen
N Nucleus
SSC Secondary synaptic clefts

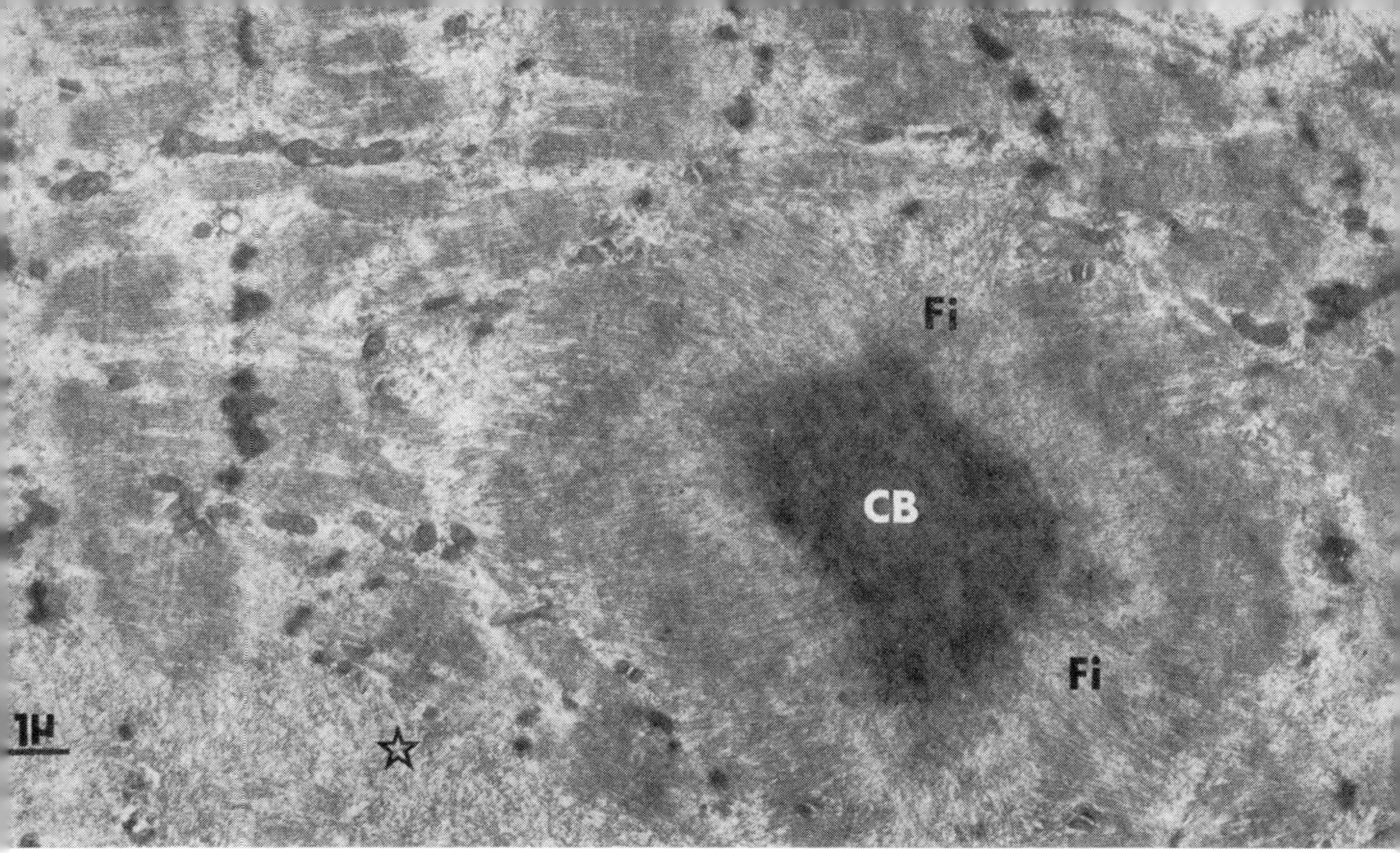

Fi
CB
Fi
1μ

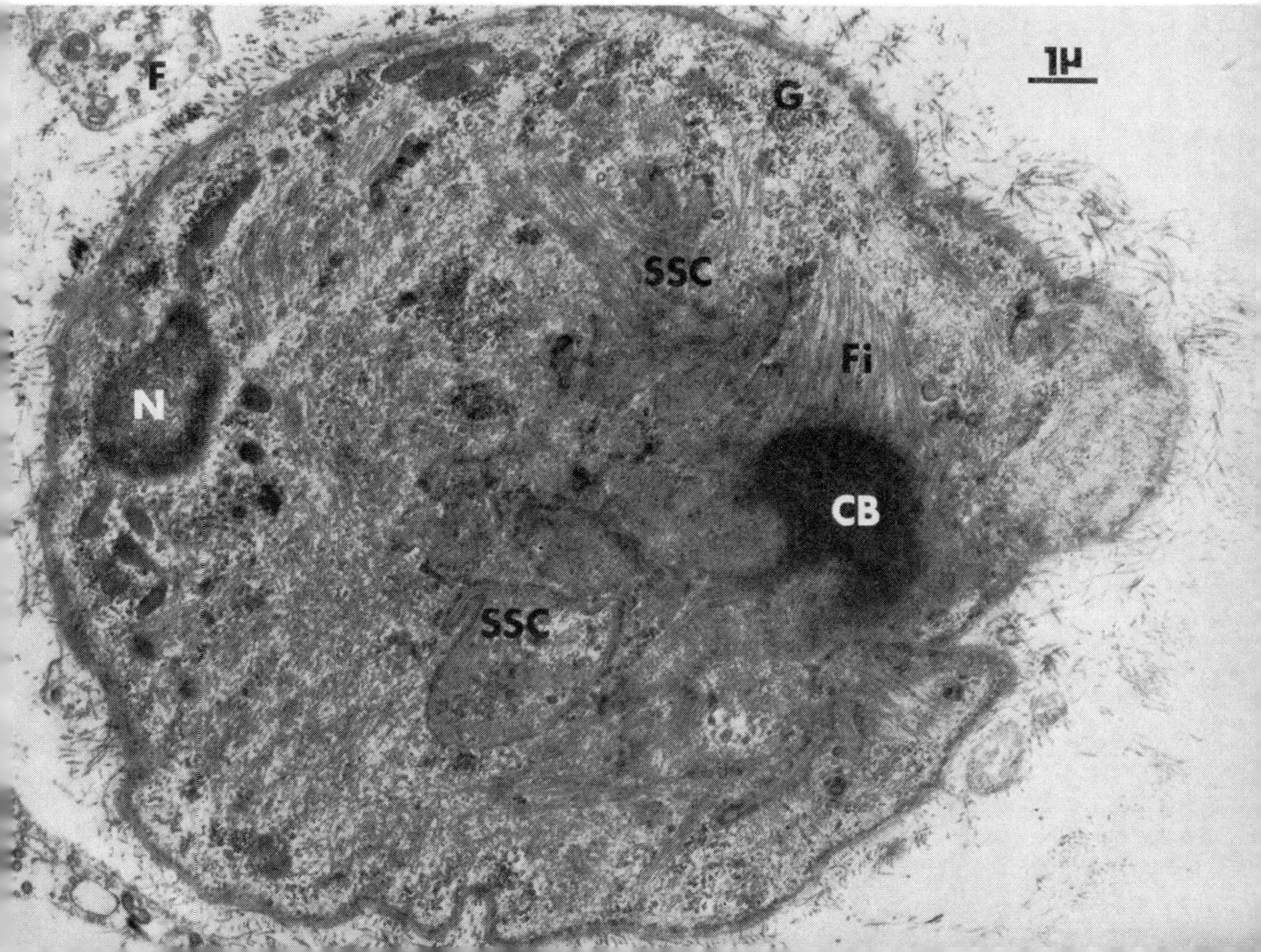

F
G
1μ
SSC
N
Fi
CB
SSC

PLATE 28. FILAMENTOUS BODIES

UPPER. Filamentous bodies may occur in the muscle fibres in very different conditions. Amongst the myofilaments between the surface and the nuclei of this atrophying muscle fibre is a collection of closely packed filaments which do not form myofibrils. Glycogen granules, polysomes and a collection of tubules forming a honeycomb structure also occur. On the right is a greatly thickened Z-line.

MAGNIFICATION 24,000 ×.

From a patient with polyneuropathy.

LOWER. A similar collection of filaments is present in a sarcoplasmic mass of an atrophying muscle fibre. Numerous granules and mitochondria occur in the sarcoplasm and to the left of the filamentous body are lipid bodies.

MAGNIFICATION 16,000 ×.

From a patient with muscular dystrophy.

G	Glycogen	My	Myofilaments
HC	Honeycomb structure	N	Nucleus
LB	Lipid bodies	Po	Polysomes
Mf	Myofibrils	Z	Z-line
Mi	Mitochondria		

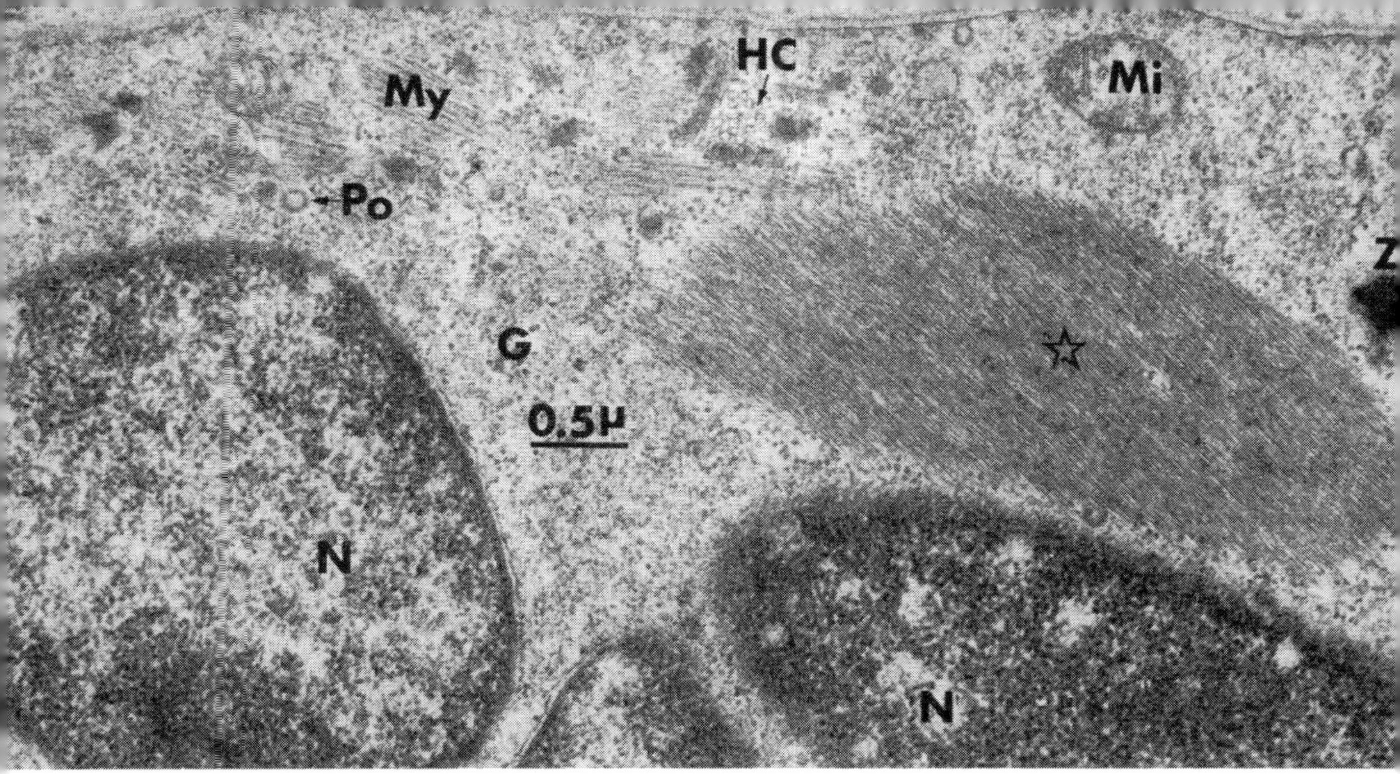
My
HC
Mi
Po
Z
G
☆
0.5μ
N
N

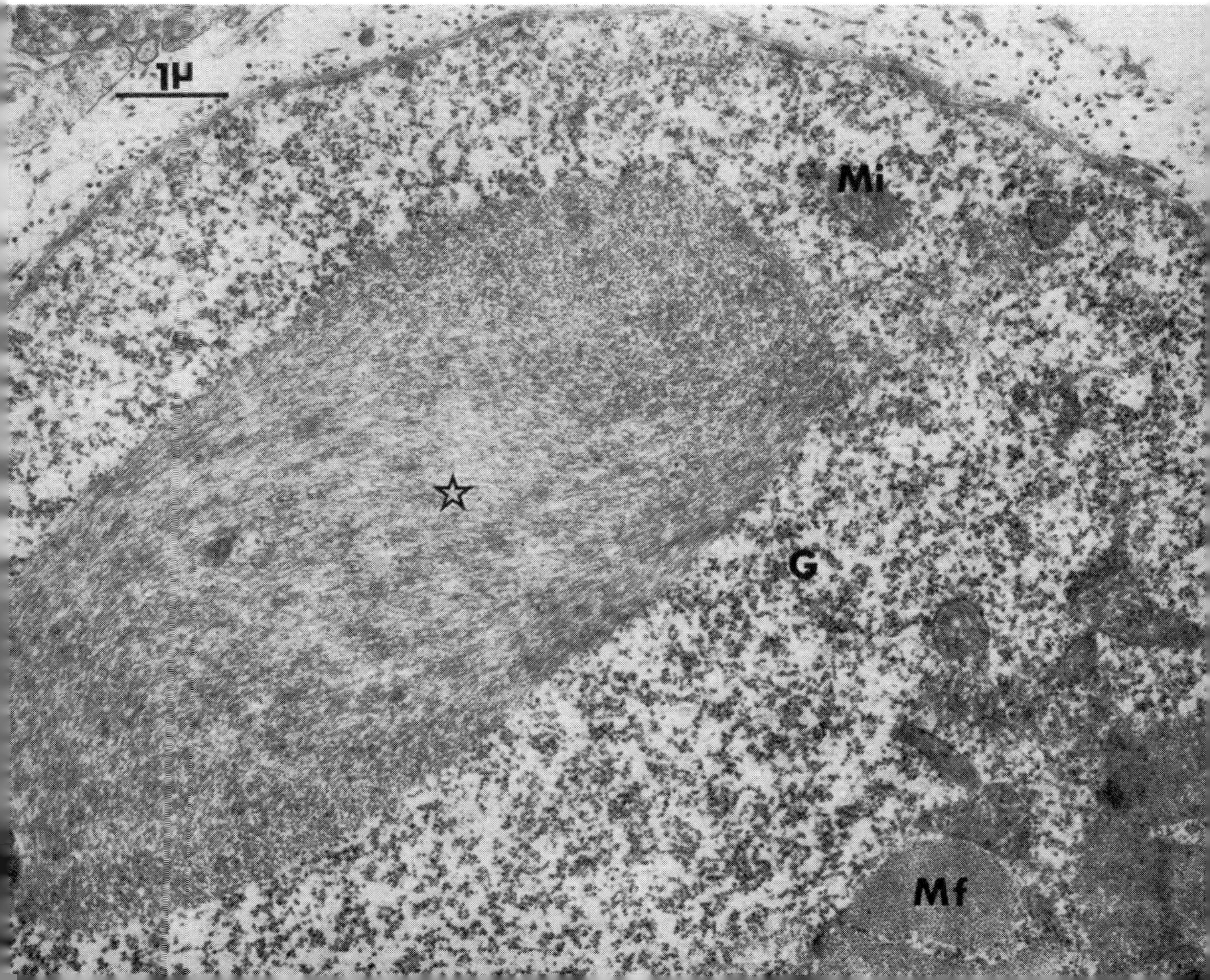
1μ
Mi
☆
G
Mf

PLATE 29. CENTRAL NUCLEI IN MUSCLE FIBRES

UPPER. A transversely cut muscle fibre shows a central nucleus which is granular with a rim of electron dense chromatin at the periphery. The myofibrils show the Z-line and the I- and A-bands distinctly. In the middle of the A-band lies the H-zone with the M-line in its centre. The myofibrils are well preserved.

MAGNIFICATION 10,000 ×.

From a patient with vitamin E deficiency.

LOWER. The nucleus lies in the centre of the muscle fibre. The inner and the outer nuclear membranes are distinct. Around the nucleus lie the A- and I-bands and the Z-lines which are cut transversely. Collections of glycogen granules lie between the myofibrils and at the poles of the nucleus. Triads occur between the myofibrils.

MAGNIFICATION 15,000 ×.

From a patient with dystrophia myotonica.

A	A-band	M	M-line
H	H-zone	N	Nucleus
G	Glycogen	Tr	Triad
I	I-band	Z	Z-lines

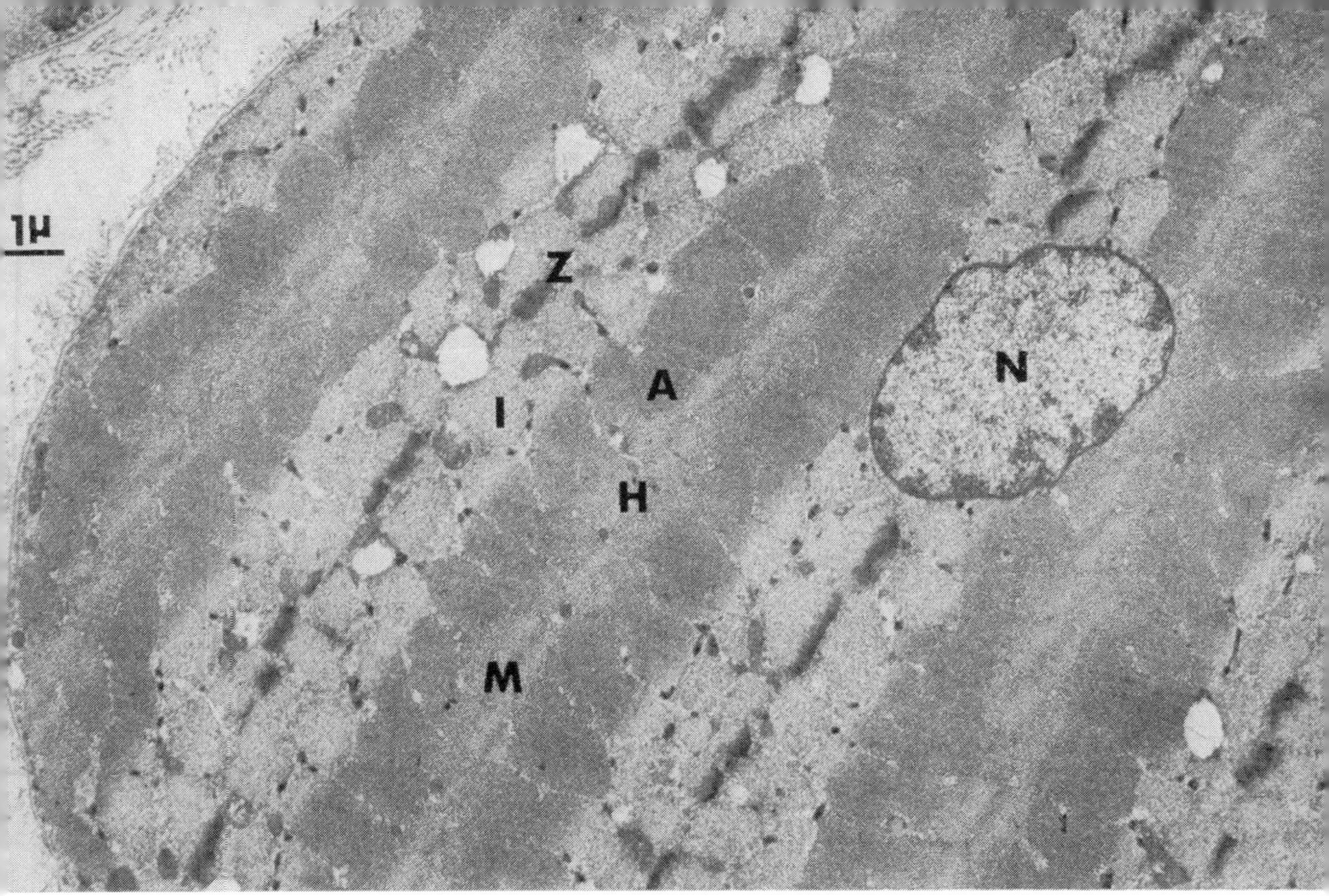
1μ
Z
N
A
I
H
M

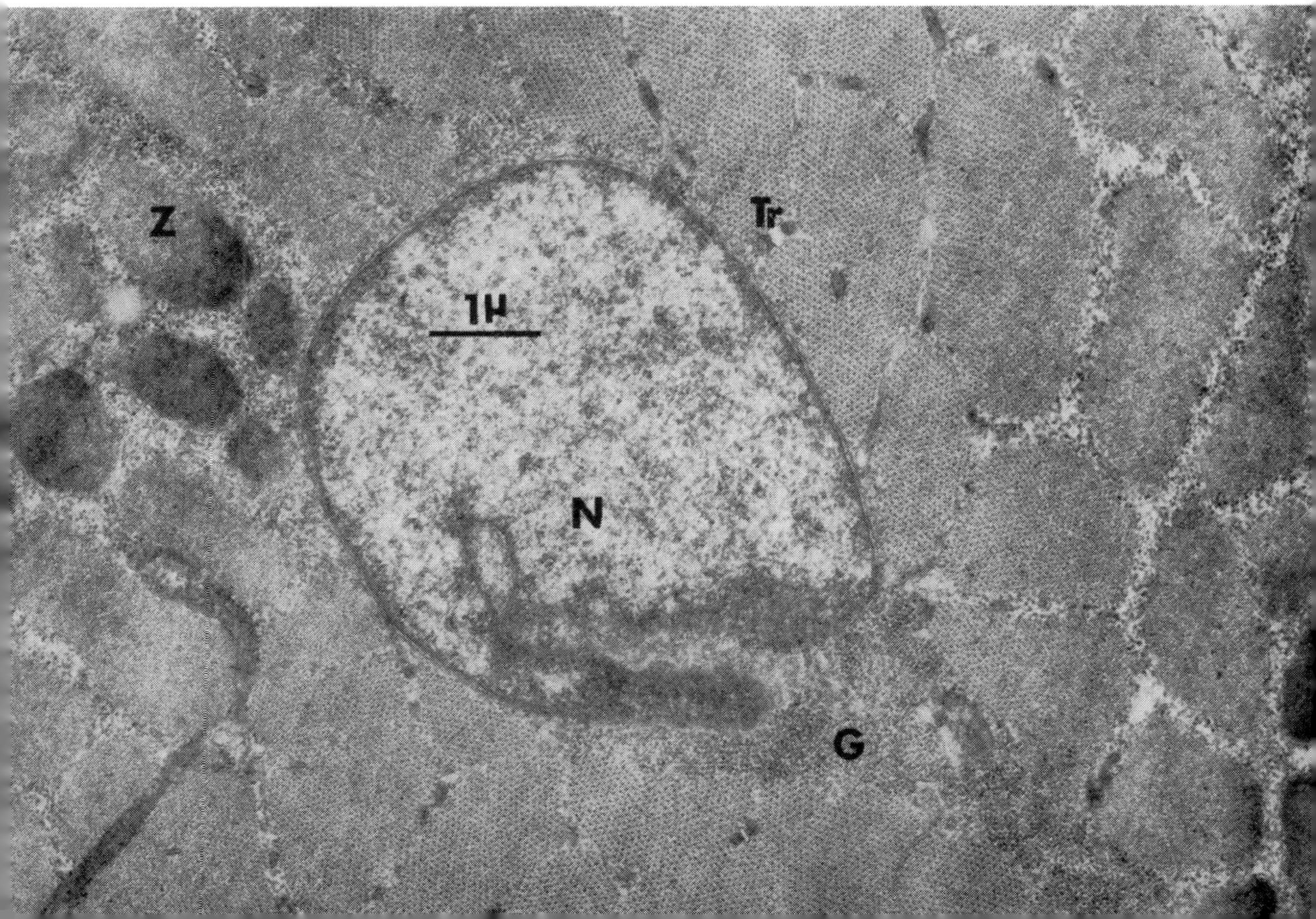
Z
Tr
1μ
N
G

PLATE 30. MITOCHONDRIAL ABNORMALITIES

UPPER. Mitochondria are prominent between the myofibrils. The upper central mitochondrion is swollen but the cristae around its periphery are readily identifiable. Within the mitochondrion are portions of cristae and a collection of glycogen granules. The mitochondrion to the left also contains glycogen granules associated with membranes. Some small electron dense bodies lie in the mitochondria between the lower myofibrils.

MAGNIFICATION 24,000 ×.

LOWER. The mitochondria are distended and most of the cristae have disappeared. Within a membranous body in one of them are collections of glycogen granules. Vacuoles are found near the mitochondria.

MAGNIFICATION 30,000 ×.

From a patient with muscular dystrophy of the Duchenne type.

Cr Cristae
DB Dense bodies
G Glycogen
Va Vacuole

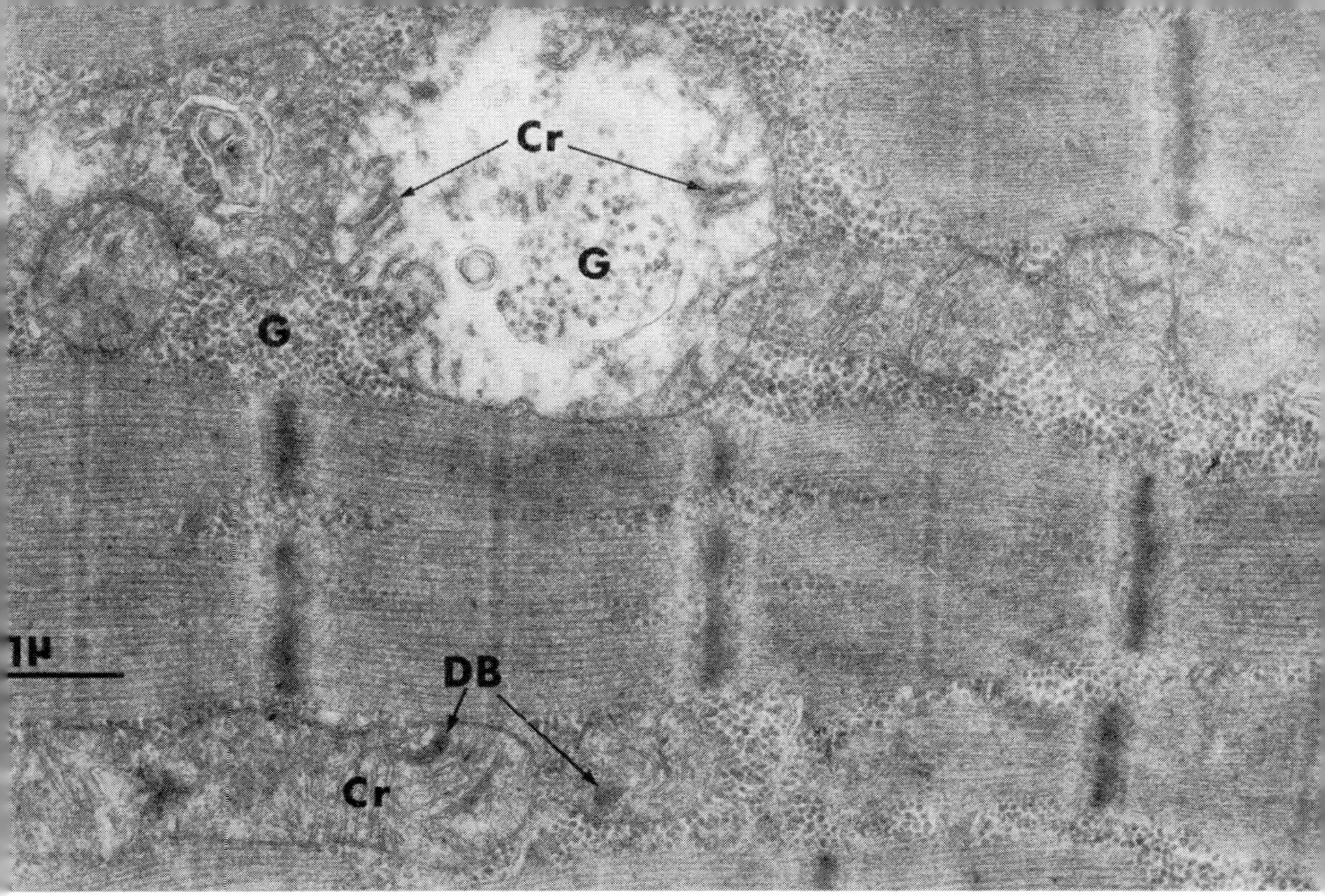
Cr
G
G
1μ
DB
Cr

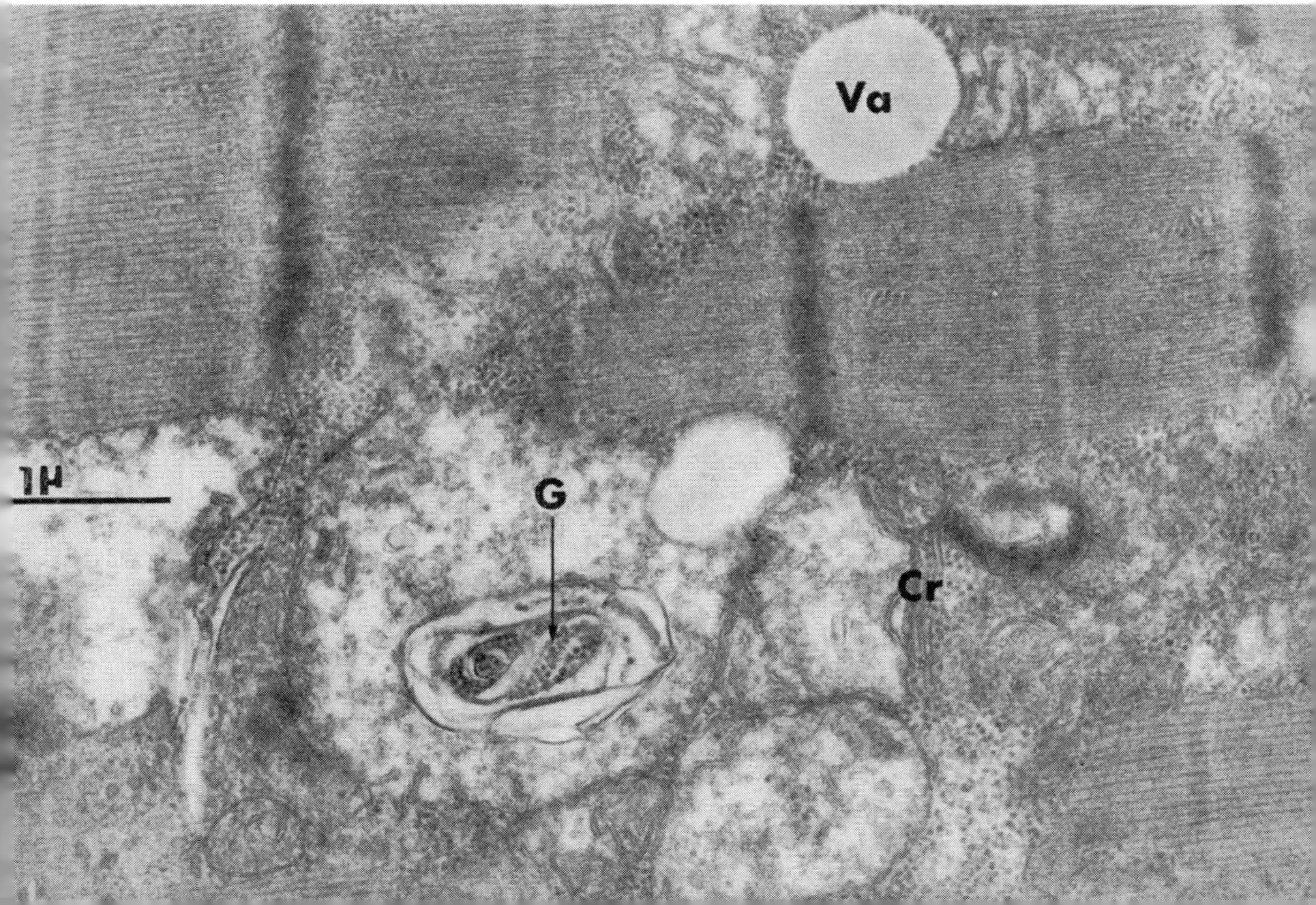
Va
1μ
G
Cr

PLATE 31. MITOCHONDRIAL ABNORMALITIES

UPPER. The mitochondria exhibit distensions some of which are large and contain membranous bodies of varying size and structure (arrowed). Some membranous bodies are bound by a double membrane and contain tubules; others are formed of multiple membranes like myelin bodies. Numerous glycogen granules surround the mitochondria.

MAGNIFICATION 26,000 ×.

From a patient treated with vincristine sulphate for malignant disease.

LOWER. The mitochondria are distended and their cristae broken down: within or near them are membranous and myelin bodies. One of the mitochondria (arrowed) contains collections of electron dense bodies of varying size and shape.

MAGNIFICATION 21,000 ×.

From a patient with polymyositis.

Cr	Cristae	MeB	Membranous bodies
Fi	Filaments	MB	Myelin bodies
G	Glycogen	Tu	Tubules
Mi	Mitochondria	Z	Z-line

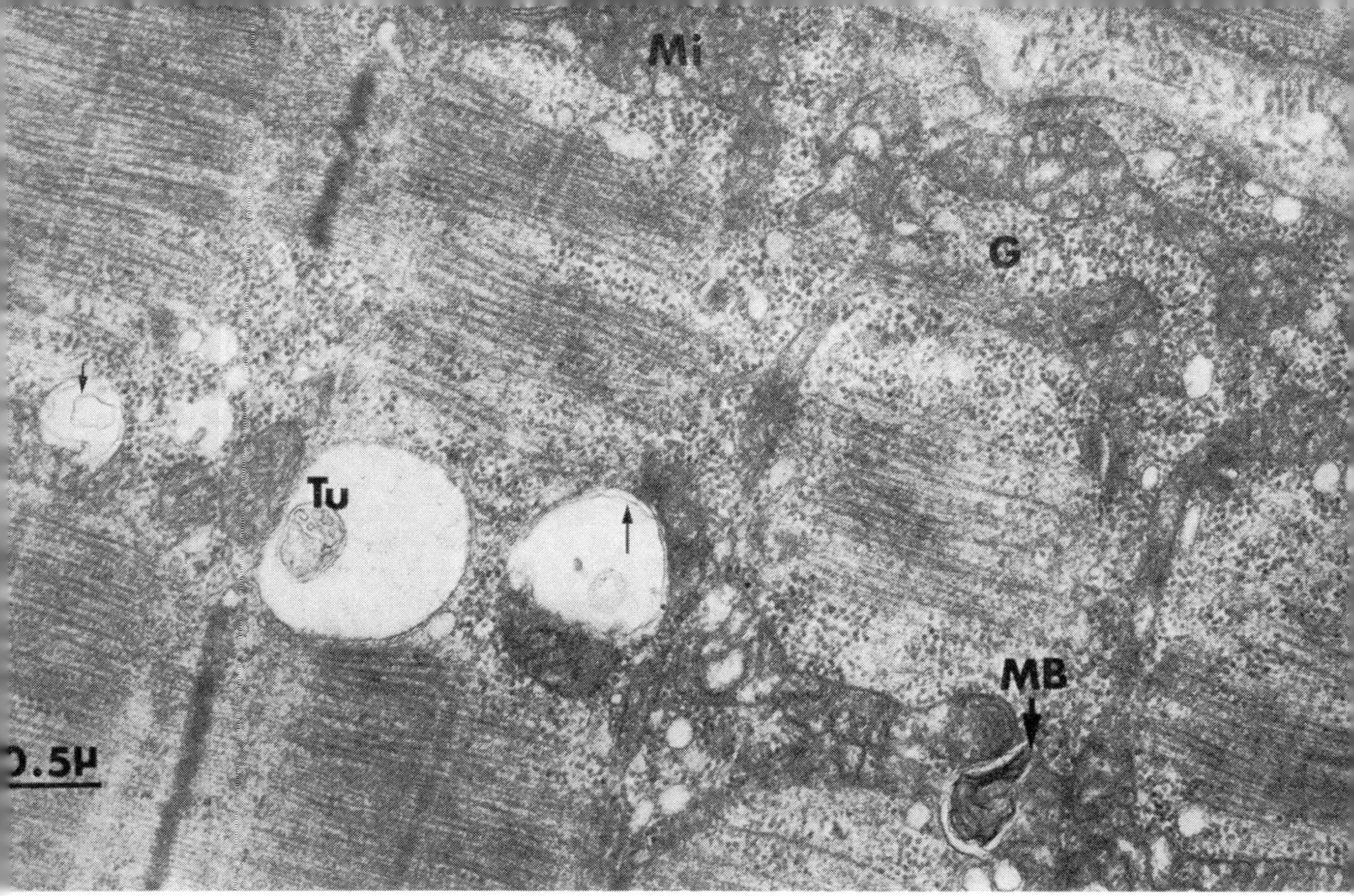
Mi
G
Tu
MB
0.5μ

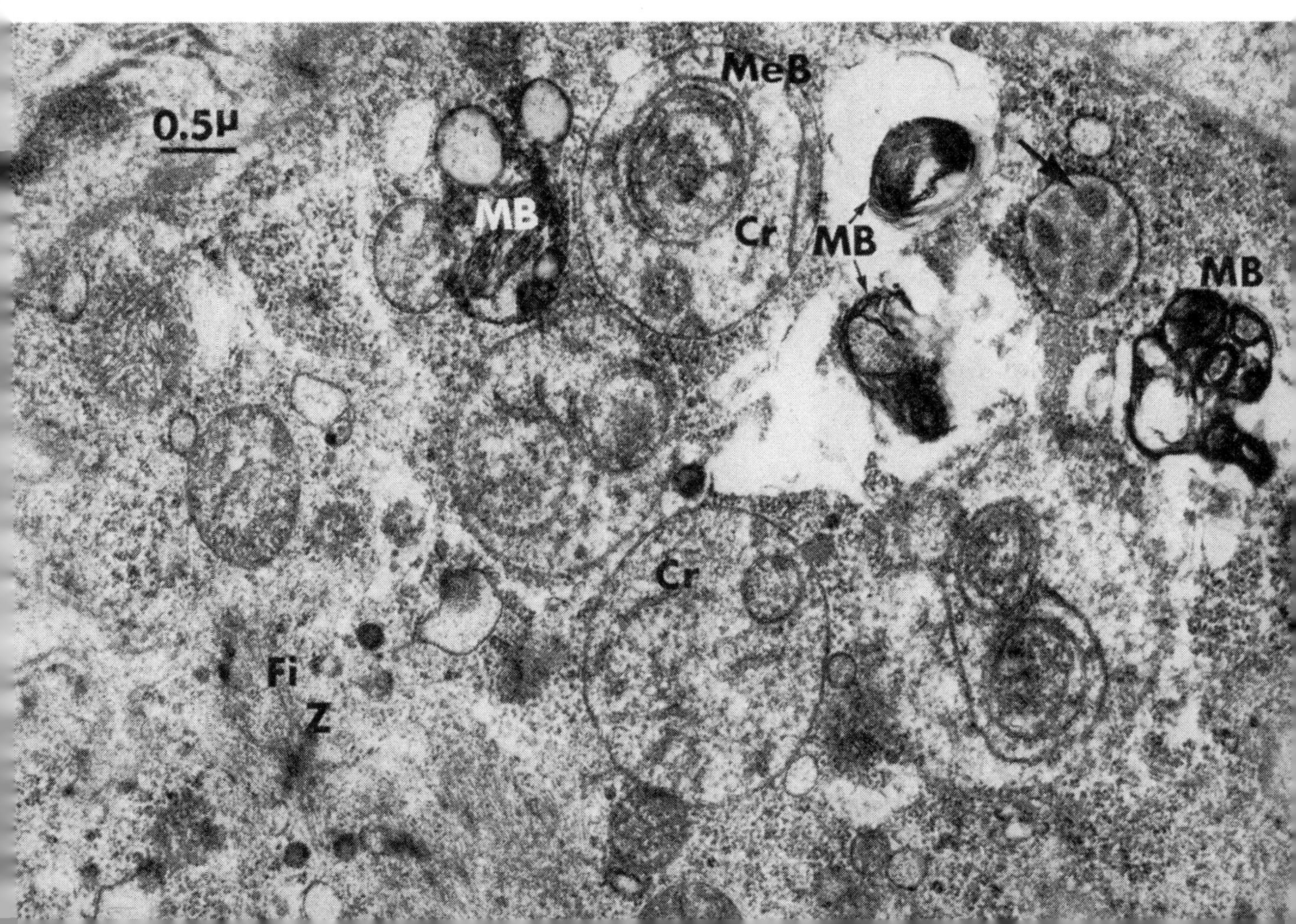
MeB
0.5μ
MB
Cr
MB
MB
Cr
Fi
Z

PLATE 32. MITOCHONDRIAL ABNORMALITIES

Crystalline inclusions are illustrated in the mitochondria between the myofibrils, in serial sections of a muscle fibre. The inclusions are laminated and quadrilateral in shape but of varying size. Their lamellae are about 100 Å thick and 35 Å apart. The numbers and shape of the inclusions in the same mitochondria of the two sections vary considerably. Small electron dense granules are also present in them (arrowed). Numerous glycogen granules occur between the myofibrils. A lipid body lies at the bottom of the sections.

MAGNIFICATION 41,000 ×.

From a patient with limb girdle muscular dystrophy.

In Inclusions
LB Lipid body

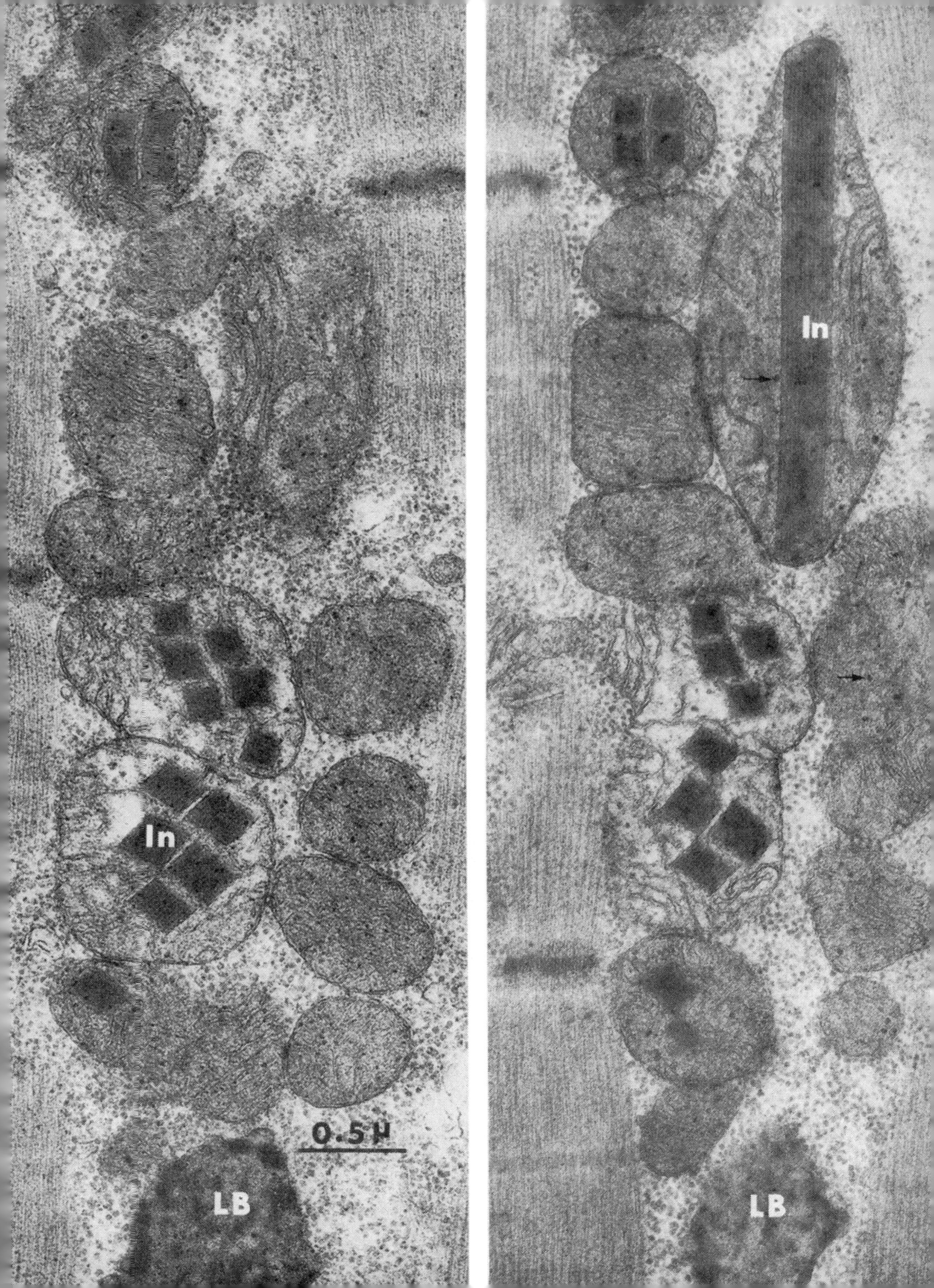

In
0.5μ
LB
In
LB

PLATE 33. GLYCOGEN IN INCREASED AMOUNT

UPPER. In this muscle fibre there is a great increase in glycogen both under the plasma membrane and between the myofibrils. Discontinuity of the myofibrils may be due to their displacement by the glycogen. Empty folds of basement membrane are very prominent overlying the muscle fibre.

MAGNIFICATION 18,000 ×.

LOWER. Accumulations of glycogen may occur free or within double membranes (arrowed) between the myofibrils. Mitochondria and membranous bodies also occur amongst the glycogen.

MAGNIFICATION 38,000 ×.

From patients with muscular dystrophy.

BM Basement membrane
G Glycogen
Mf Myofibrils
Mi Mitochondria
MeB Membranous body

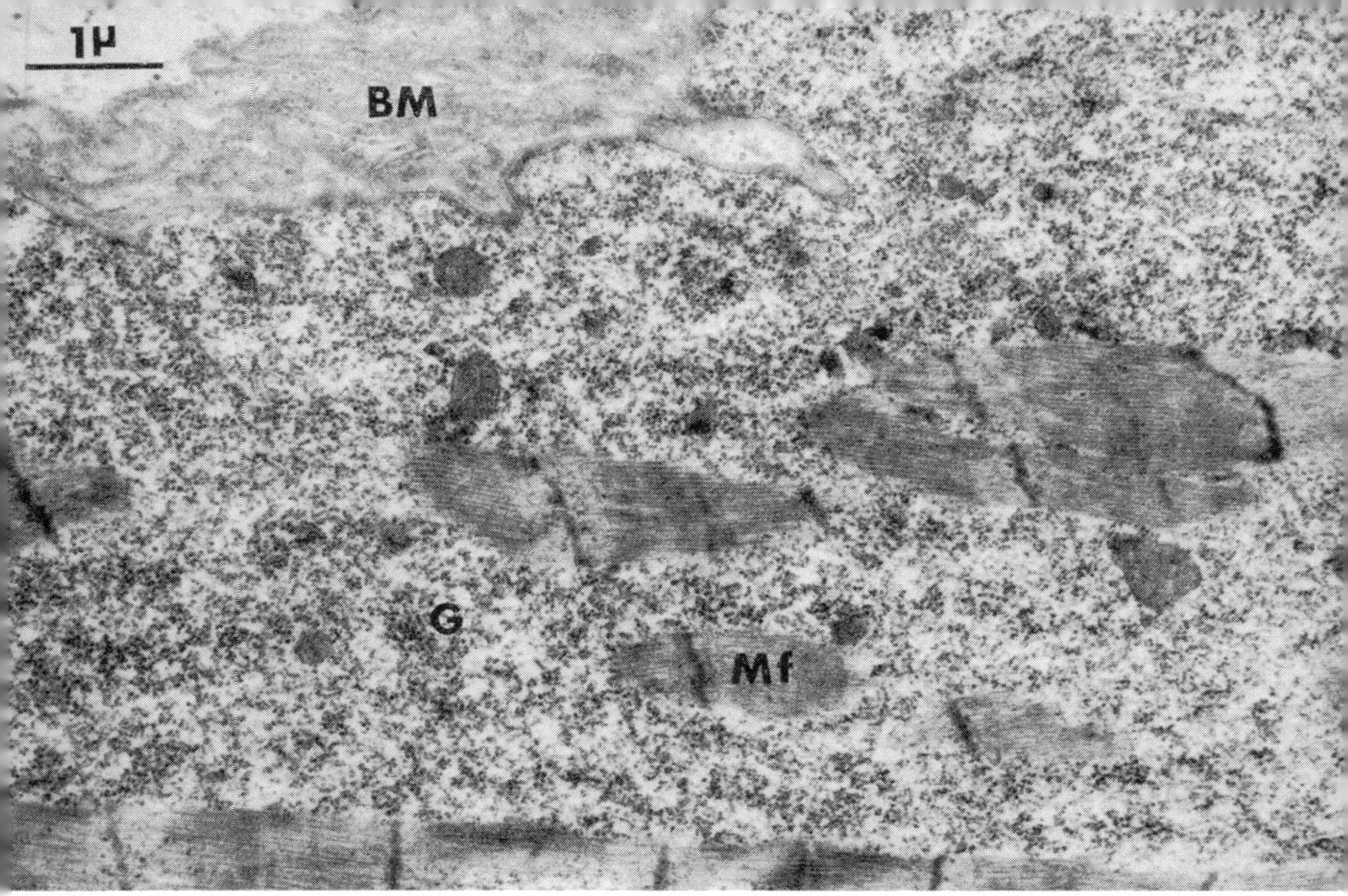
1μ
BM
G
Mf

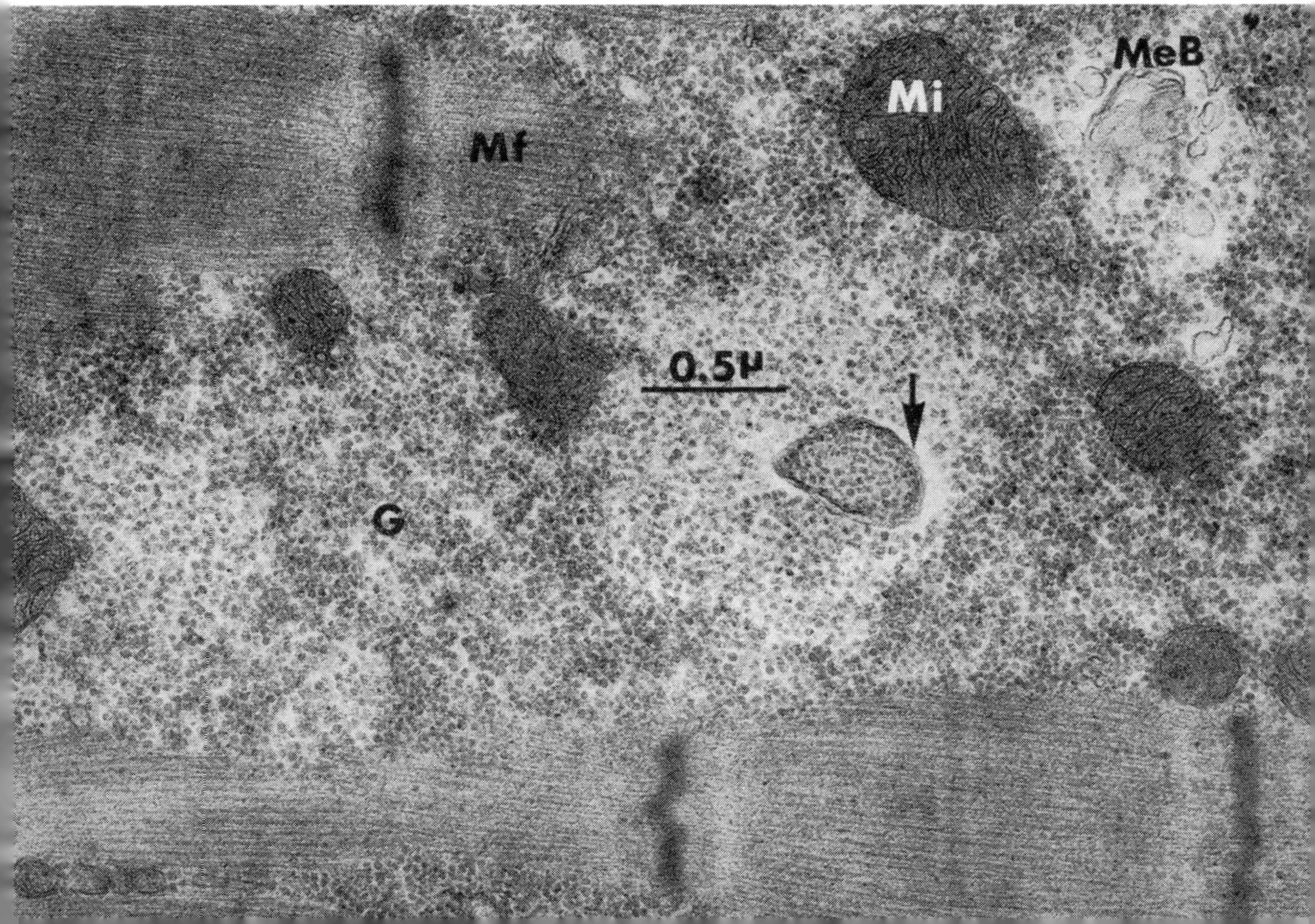
MeB
Mi
Mf
0.5μ
G

PLATE 34. LIPID BODIES IN DEGENERATING MUSCLE FIBRES

UPPER. Here are two degenerating muscle fibres separated by fibroblasts and collagen. The fibre on the left presents a nucleus and around it degenerating myofilaments, mitochondria, lipid material and a readily identifiable triad. The fibre on the right shows parts of two nuclei one of which has a nucleolus. Around the nuclei are very prominent conglomerates of lipid, some lying free amongst the myofibrils and some enclosed in large autophagic vacuoles. Parts of the lipid are electron dense and parts are clear. Membranous material also occurs in the vacuoles as well as the early stages of a myelin body.

MAGNIFICATION 7,000 ×.

LOWER. Four adjacent muscle fibres are separated by fibroblast processes and bundles of collagen. Both central muscle fibres are atrophied but contain some myofilaments and a prominent nucleus. Part of a Golgi apparatus lies at the pole of the nucleus of the upper fibre and lipid bodies, vacuoles, vesicles and glycogen granules at the poles of the nucleus of the lower fibre. Significant structural changes are not apparent in the lowermost fibre.

MAGNIFICATION 13,000 ×.

Both are from a patient with alcoholic polyneuropathy.

C	Collagen	My	Myofilaments
F	Fibroblast	MB	Myelin body
G	Glycogen	N	Nucleus
LB	Lipid body	Tr	Triad
Mf	Myofibril	Va	Vacuole
Mi	Mitochondria	Z	Z-line

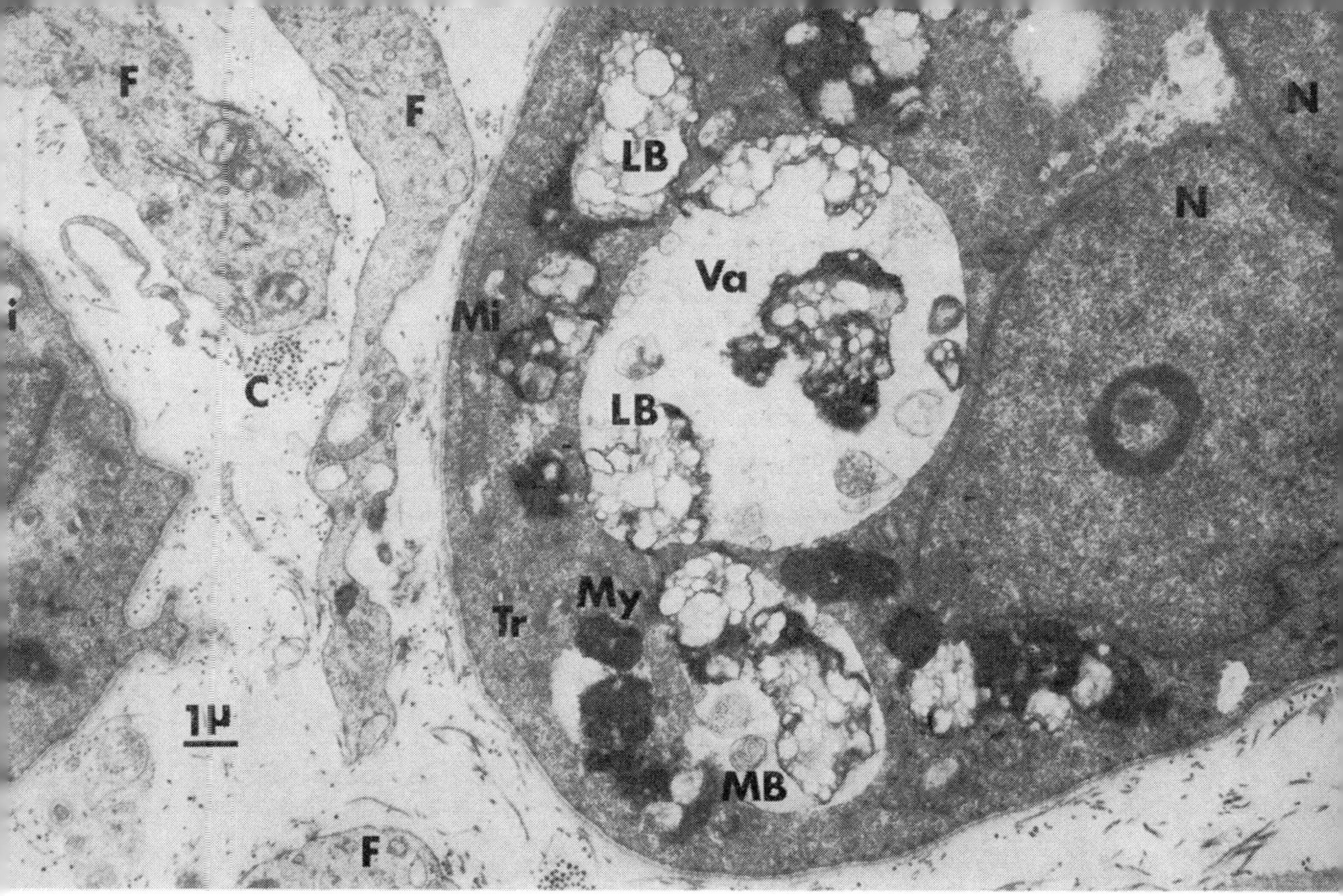
F
F
N
N
LB
Va
Mi
C
LB
Tr
My
1μ
MB
F

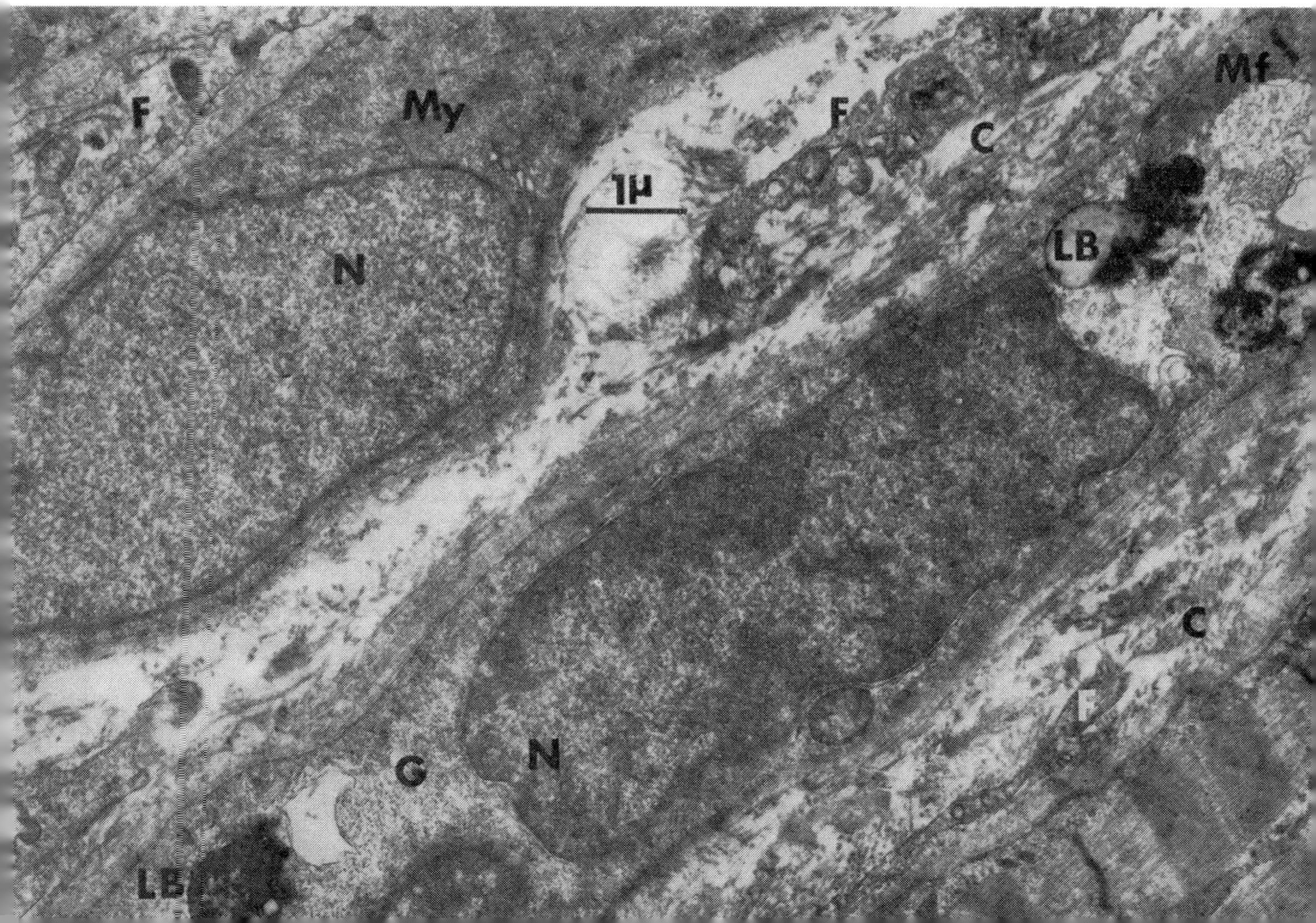
F
My
F
C
Mf
1μ
N
LB
C
F
G
N
LB

PLATE 35. TRIADS IN DEGENERATING MUSCLE FIBRES

UPPER. The degenerating muscle fibre presents thickened Z-lines and numerous triads formed by a central tubule (the T-system) and the electron dense lateral sacs of the sarcoplasmic reticulum. Some T-systems can be followed over a long course. Mitochondria and glycogen granules occur in the fibre.

MAGNIFICATION 45,000 ×.

LOWER. This fibre shows in addition to the altered distribution of the myofibrils, some of which are cut longitudinally and others transversely, an apparent increase in the number of triads. Some of the T-systems are very long: they are bounded by the very obvious electron dense zones of the lateral sacs of the sarcoplasmic reticulum. Numerous glycogen granules and occasional mitochondria occur in the sarcoplasm. Some Z-lines are broadened and occasional rods occur.

MAGNIFICATION 36,000 ×.

Both are from a patient with polymyositis.

G Glycogen
LS Longitudinal section
Mi Mitochondria
Ro Rod
SR Sarcoplasmic reticulum
T T-system
TS Transverse section
Z Z-line

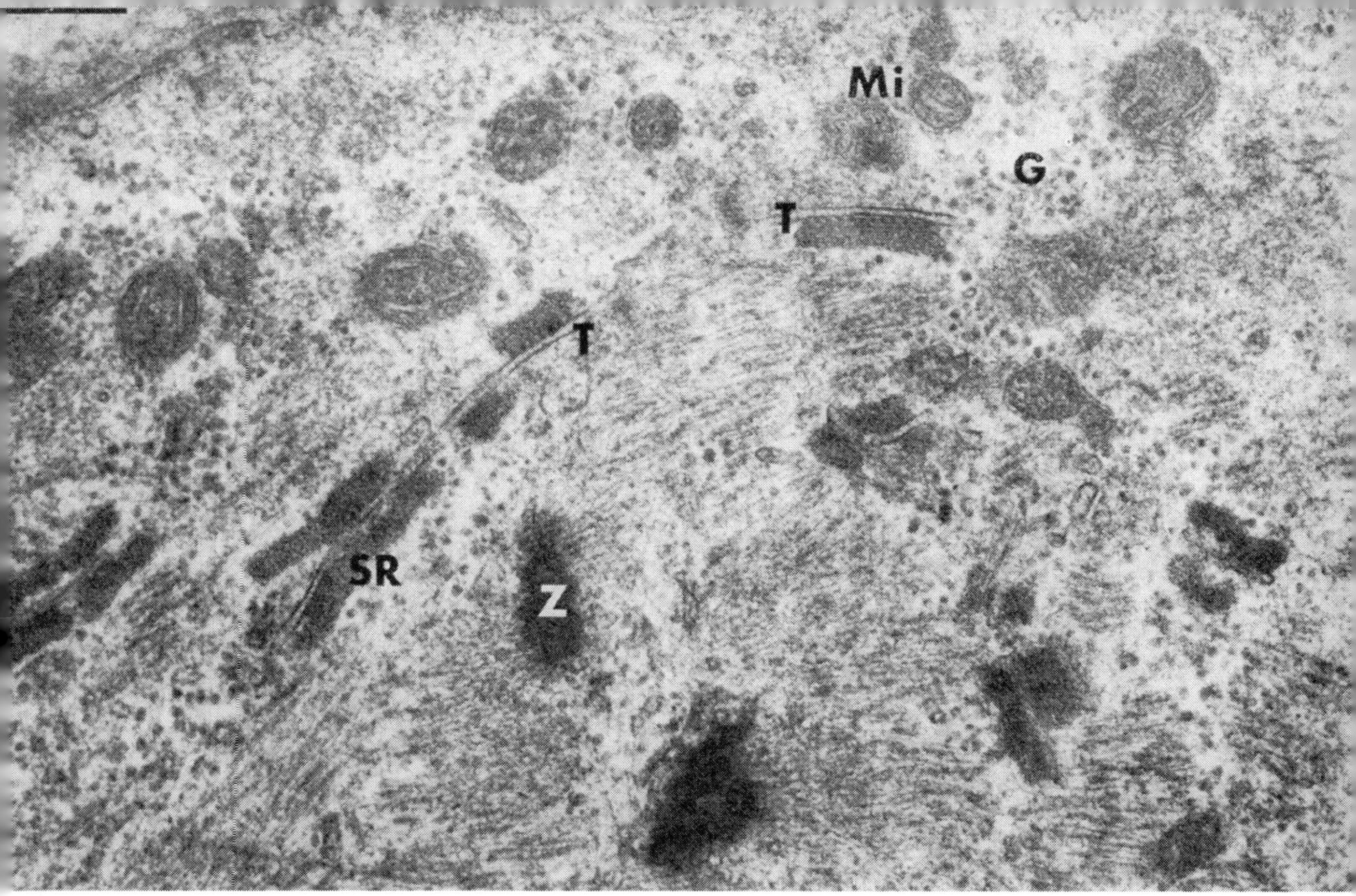
Mi
G
T
T
SR
Z

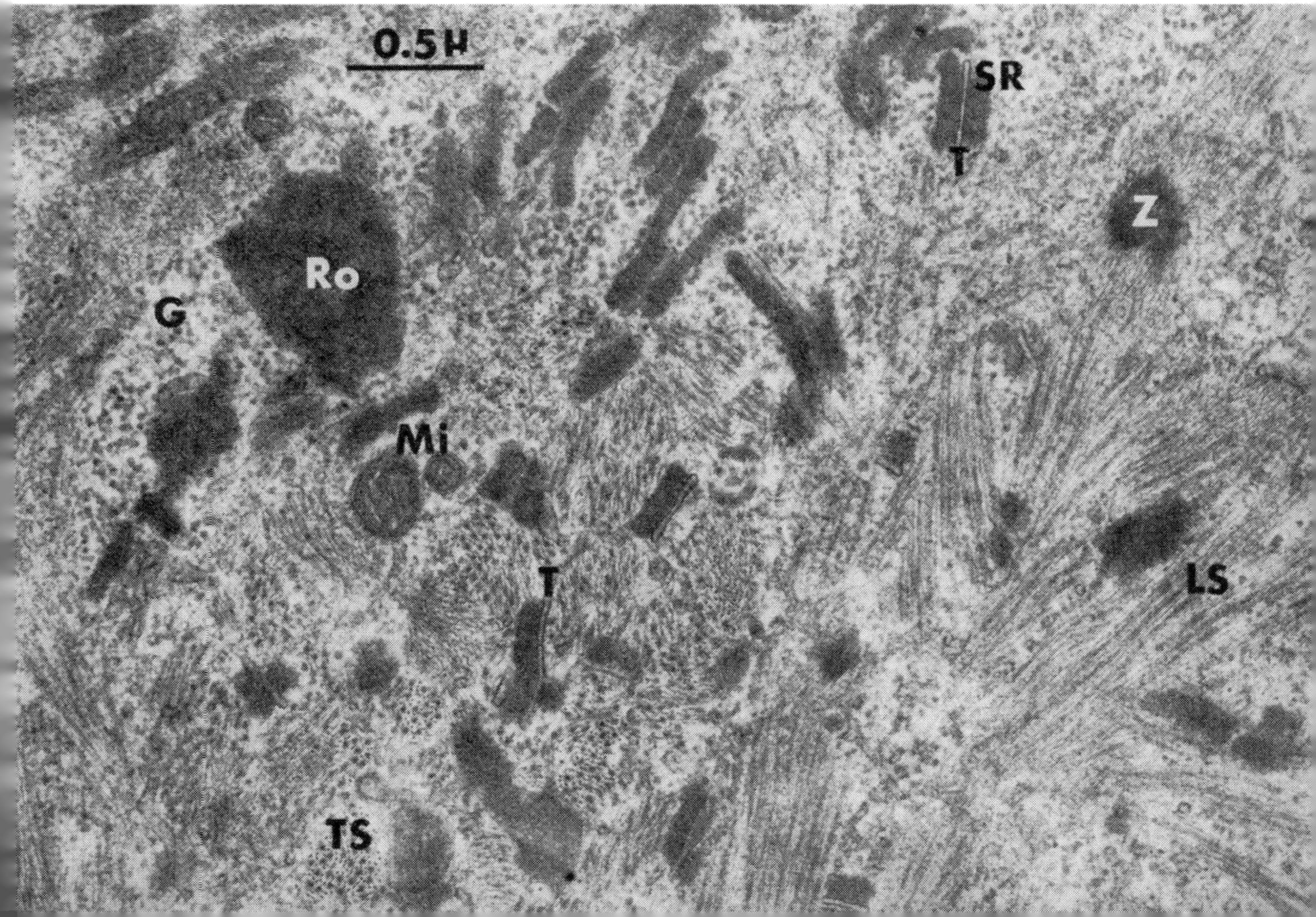
0.5μ
SR
T
Z
Ro
G
Mi
T
LS
TS

PLATE 36. COLLECTIONS OF TRIADS

UPPER. In a target fibre rows of triads lie close together. They have a clear central tubule, the T-system (arrowed), on either side of which are the electron dense ellipsoid lateral sacs of the sarcoplasmic reticulum. Some T-tubules are distended. Vacuoles, some containing membranous material, occur amongst the degenerate myofibrils.

MAGNIFICATION 16,000 ×.

LOWER. At higher magnification, the triads show granularity of the electron dense lateral sacs of the sarcoplasmic reticulum (arrowed). The parallel electron dense membranes bounding the T-system are distinct: a less electron dense space separates the T-system from the sarcoplasmic reticulum, the membranes of which are also distinct. Some T-systems are distended and contain membranous material.

MAGNIFICATION 35,000 ×.

From a case of alcoholic neuropathy.

T T-system
Tr Triads
Va Vacuoles

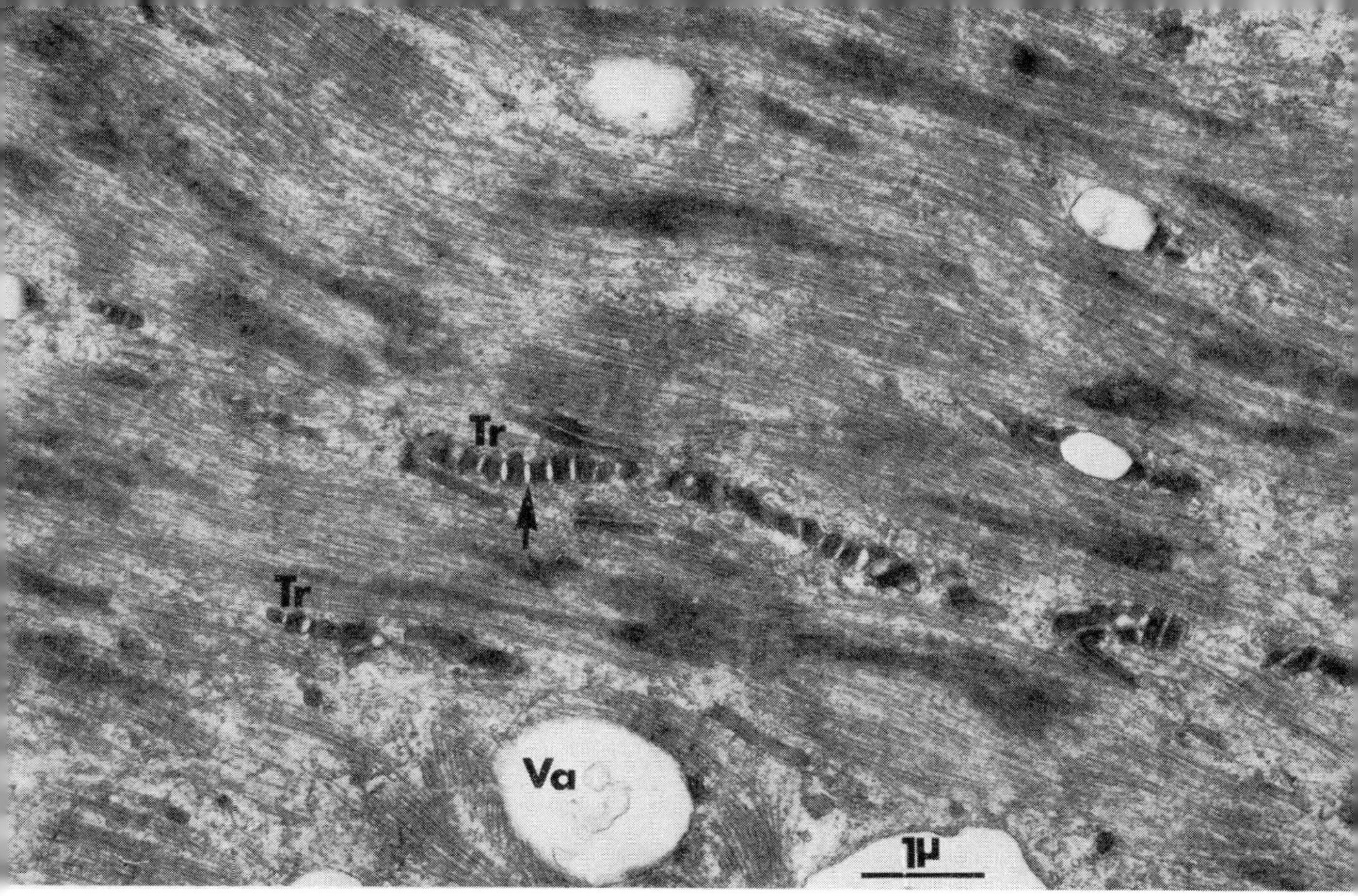
Tr
Tr
Va
1μ

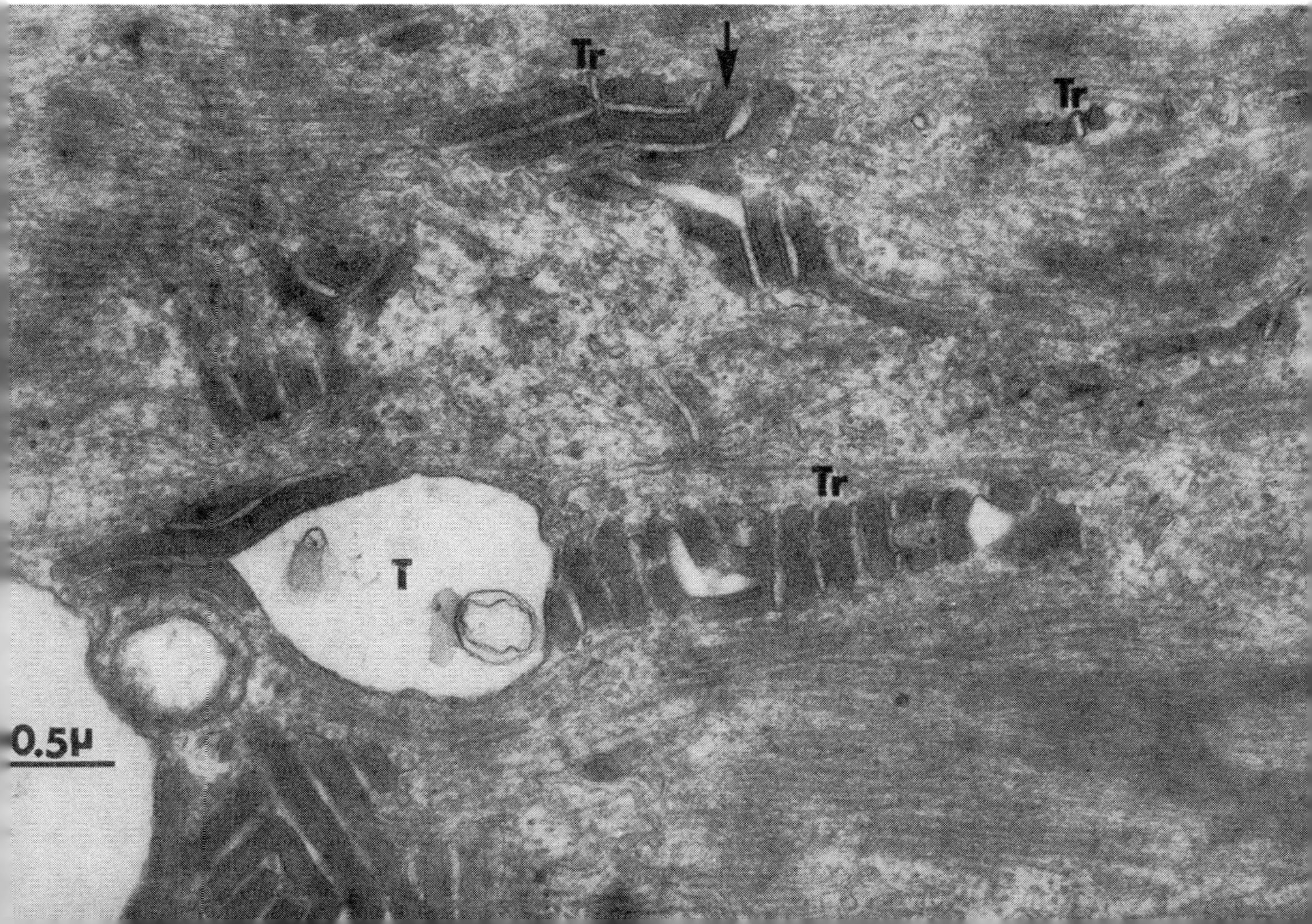
Tr
Tr
Tr
T
0.5μ

PLATE 37. DISTENSION OF THE SARCOPLASMIC RETICULUM

UPPER LEFT. The sarcomere pattern of this degenerating muscle fibre is deranged. The triads are more numerous than normal and lie haphazardly throughout the fibre: some are in close apposition to one another. Many glycogen granules are present in the sarcoplasm. Vacuoles occur next to the electron dense lateral sacs of the sarcoplasmic reticulum.

MAGNIFICATION 25,000 ×.

UPPER RIGHT. The *upper part* shows a triad at higher magnification. A less electron dense zone lies between the more electron dense boundaries of the T-system and the dilated lateral sacs of the sarcoplasmic reticulum. A vacuole and numerous glycogen granules lie around the triad.

MAGNIFICATION 80,000 ×.

The *lower part* shows granular material in the distended sarcoplasmic reticulum with an electron dense zone between it and the T-system.

MAGNIFICATION 45,000 ×.

LOWER. The distended sarcoplasmic reticulum contains a large amount of granular material. Vacuoles occur in some of the distensions. A T-system can be identified between the sarcoplasmic reticulum and the myofibrils to the right of the illustration. Glycogen granules are present between some of the sacs of the sarcoplasmic reticulum. The myofibrils are disorganised, some being cut transversely and others longitudinally.

MAGNIFICATION 27,000 ×.

All from a patient with amyotrophic lateral sclerosis.

G Glycogen
LS Longitudinal section
My Myofilaments
SR Sarcoplasmic reticulum
T T-system
Tr Triads
TS Transverse section
Va Vacuoles
Z Z-line

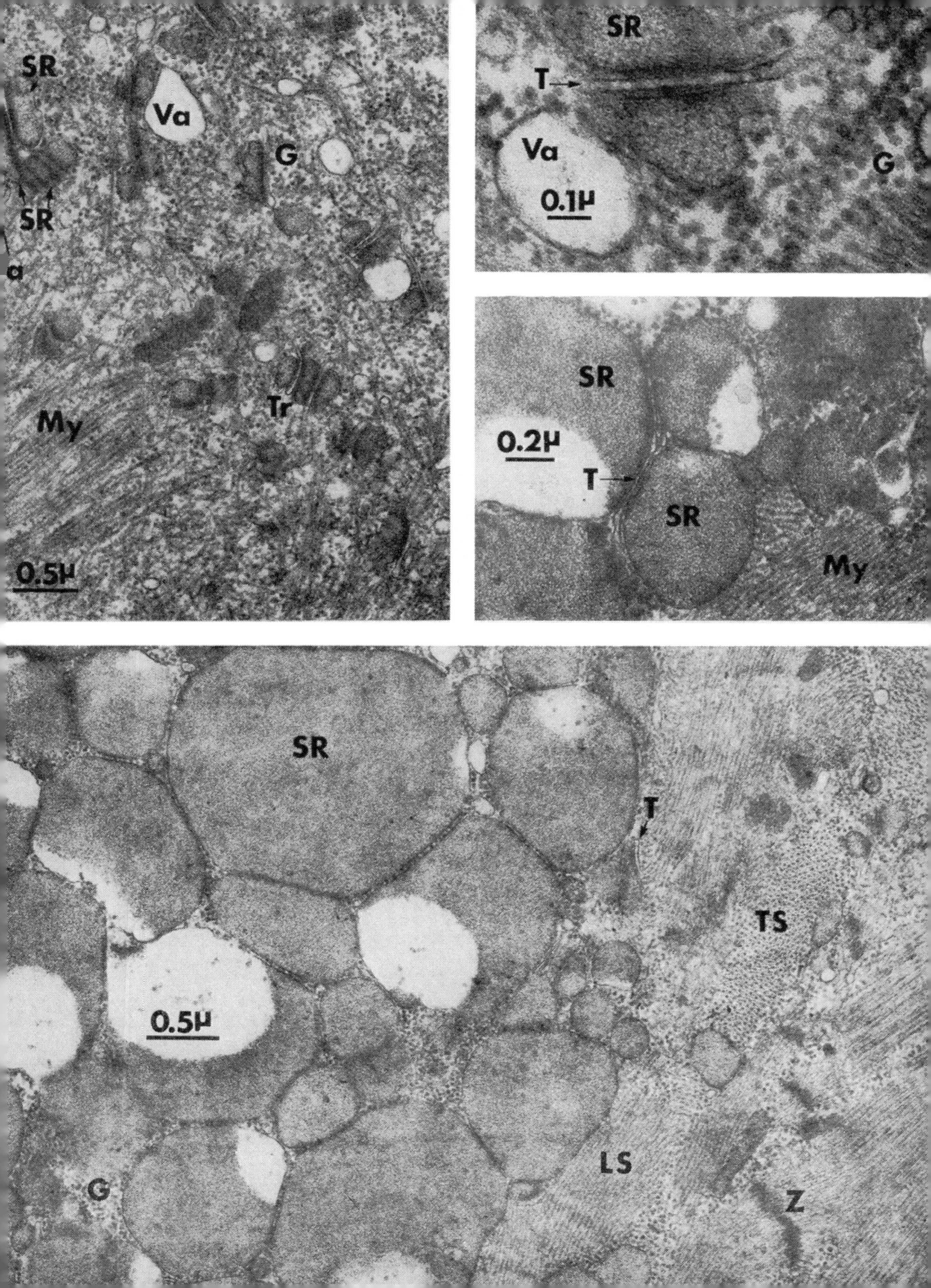

SR
SR
a
Va
G
Tr
My
0.5μ
SR
T
Va
0.1μ
G
SR
0.2μ
T
SR
My
SR
T
TS
0.5μ
G
LS
Z

PLATE 38. HONEYCOMB STRUCTURES

Honeycomb structures may appear in the muscle in various clinical conditions such as denervation, polymyositis and in various intoxications.

UPPER. A honeycomb structure lies between the A-band of the myofibril and the altered mitochondria in which occur glycogen granules. Some tubular structures are present at the bottom of the illustration.

MAGNIFICATION 72,000 ×.

From a patient with alcoholic neuropathy.

LOWER LEFT. Here similar honeycomb structures are present between the plasma membrane and the nucleus of the muscle fibre.

MAGNIFICATION 64,000 ×.

From a patient with polymyositis.

LOWER RIGHT. A less elaborate honeycomb is seen in relation to the T-system from the proliferation of which the honeycomb structures are said to be derived. A distended sac of the sarcoplasmic reticulum lies adjacent to the T-system. Vacuoles and glycogen granules also occur between the myofibrils.

MAGNIFICATION 72,000 ×.

From a patient with amyotrophic lateral sclerosis.

A A-band
G Glycogen
HC Honeycomb structures
Mi Mitochondria
N Nucleus
SR Sarcoplasmic reticulum
T T-system
Tu Tubules
Va Vacuoles

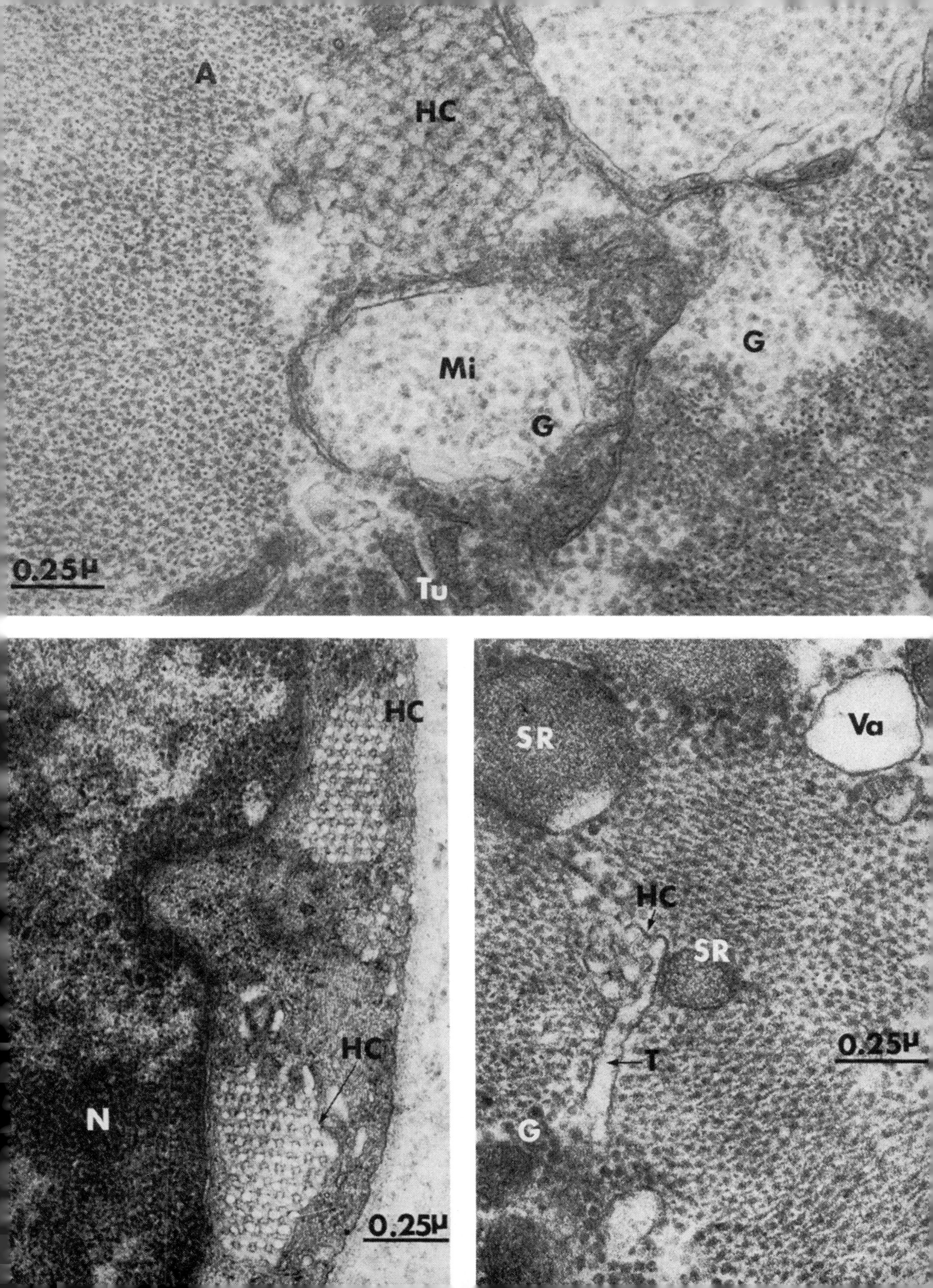
A
HC
Mi
G
G
0.25µ
Tu
HC
HC
N
0.25µ
SR
Va
HC
SR
0.25µ
T
G

PLATE 39. AUTOPHAGIC VACUOLES

UPPER. In some disorders of muscle there appear within the muscle fibre, and also in the basement membrane covering it, varying sized collections of bodies of irregular shape and different electron density. These are autophagic vacuoles. Within the muscle they are surrounded by a membrane.

MAGNIFICATION 6,000 ×.

LOWER. Higher magnification of the autophagic vacuole on the right of the muscle fibre of the upper illustration shows numerous vesicles immediately around its membrane as well as various outpouchings (arrowed) of the membrane bounding it. Amongst the various contents of the vacuole are glycogen granules and membrane bound bodies.

MAGNIFICATION 52,000 ×.

From a patient with dystrophia myotonica.

AV Autophagic vacuole
BM Basement membrane
G Glycogen
V Vesicles

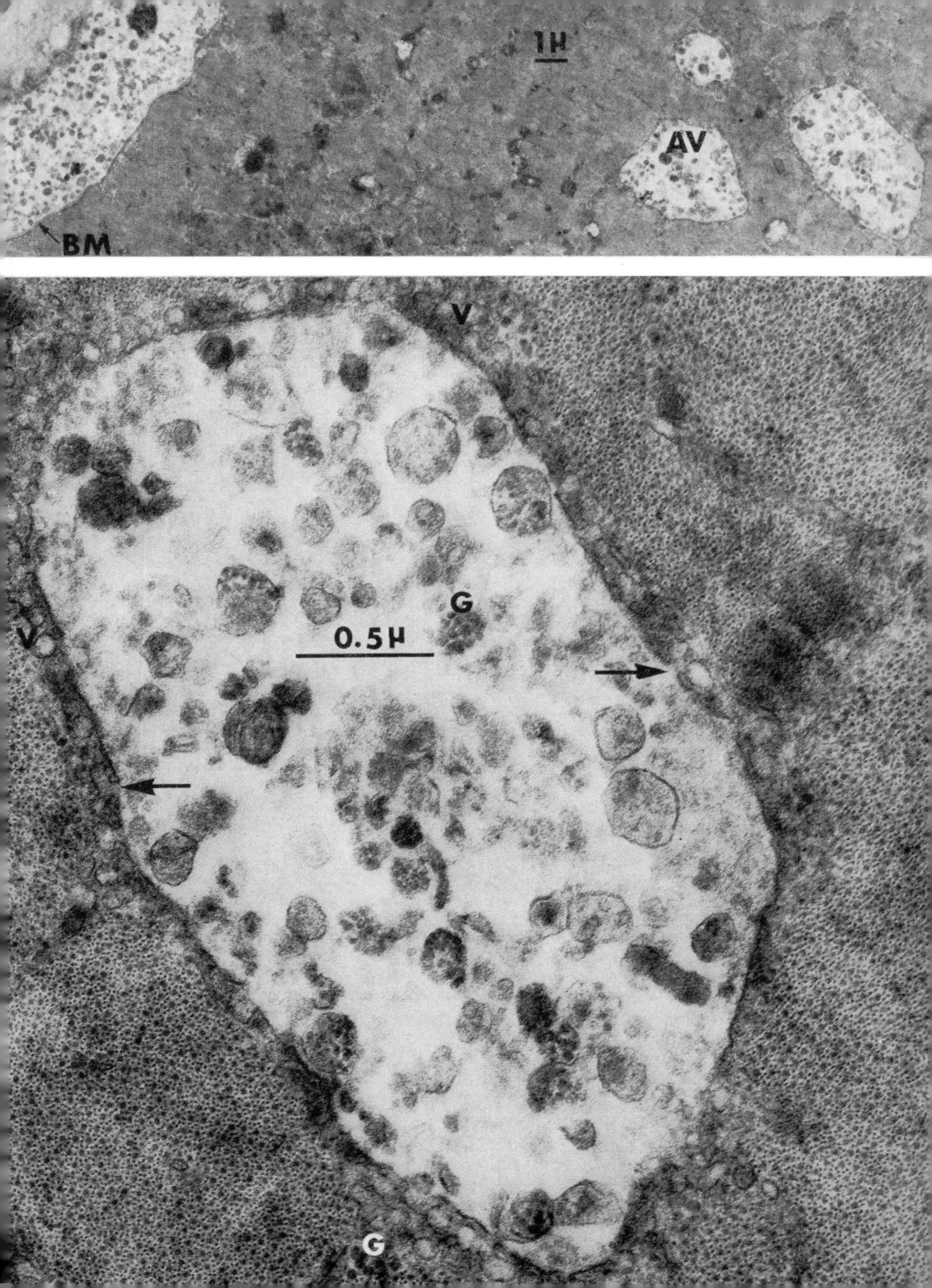
1μ
AV
BM
V
V
G
0.5μ
G

PLATE 40. EXTRUSION OF THE AUTOPHAGIC VACUOLE CONTENTS INTO THE BASEMENT MEMBRANE

UPPER. Spaces of varying size are numerous in the basement membrane of this muscle fibre which shows numerous sarcoplasmic projections containing vesicles and granules. The spaces contain collections of granular material of varying size, shape and electron density. The plasma membrane of the muscle fibre shows electron dense beading: a myelin body surrounded by glycogen granules lies on the right and on the left a nucleus. Collagen and layers of basement membrane lie outside the fibre.

Similar material is demonstrated in the basement membrane and autophagic vacuoles within the muscle fibre in Plate 39. The material in the autophagic vacuoles is presumably extruded from the muscle fibre via the basement membrane.

MAGNIFICATION 15,500 ×.

LOWER. A prominent laminated myelin body is surrounded by the basement membrane of the muscle fibre. Collagen is abundant alongside the basement membrane.

MAGNIFICATION 20,000 ×.

Both are from a patient with dystrophia myotonica.

BM Basement membrane
C Collagen
MB Myelin body
MF Muscle fibre
N Nucleus

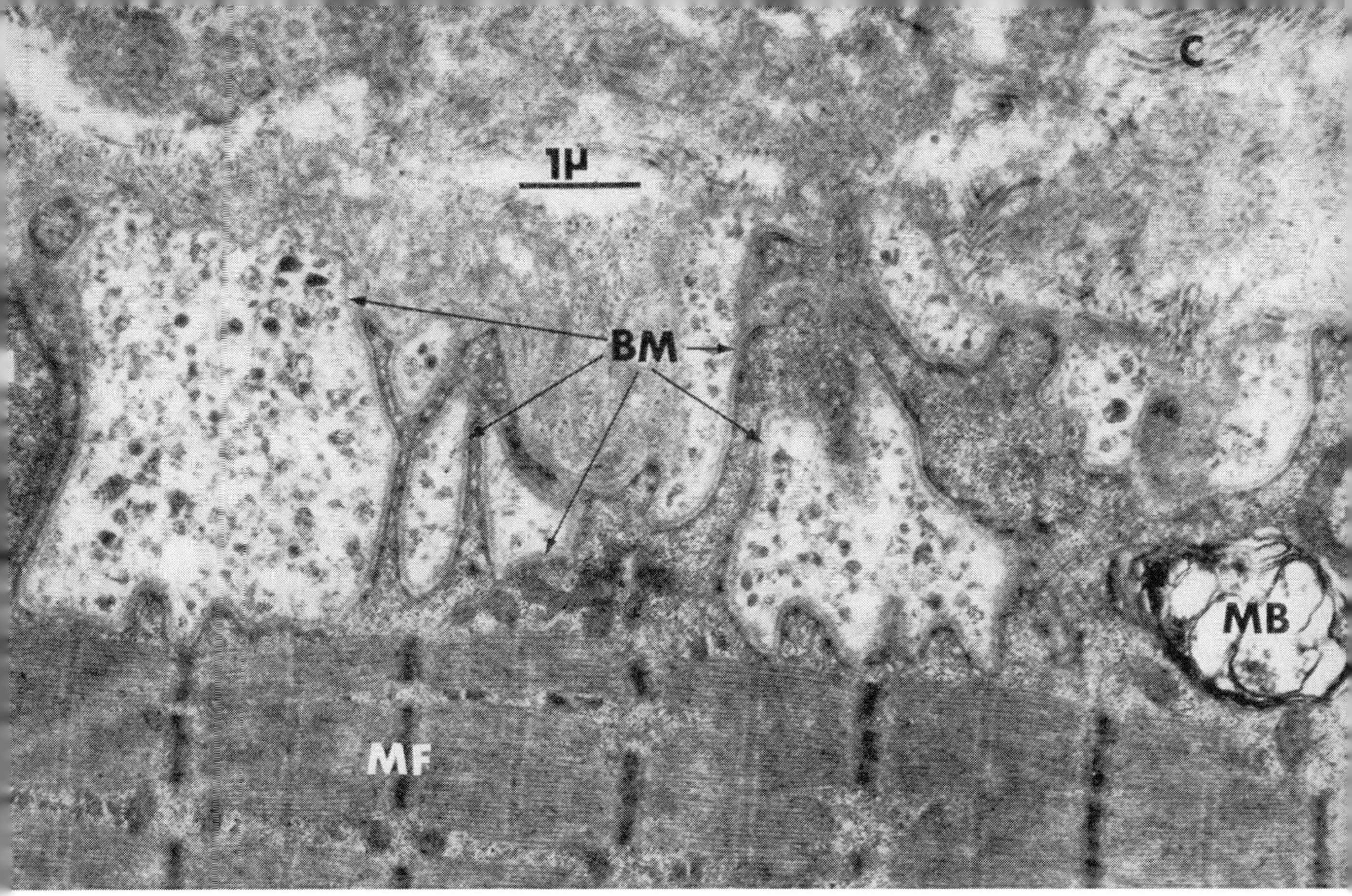
C
1μ
BM
MB
MF

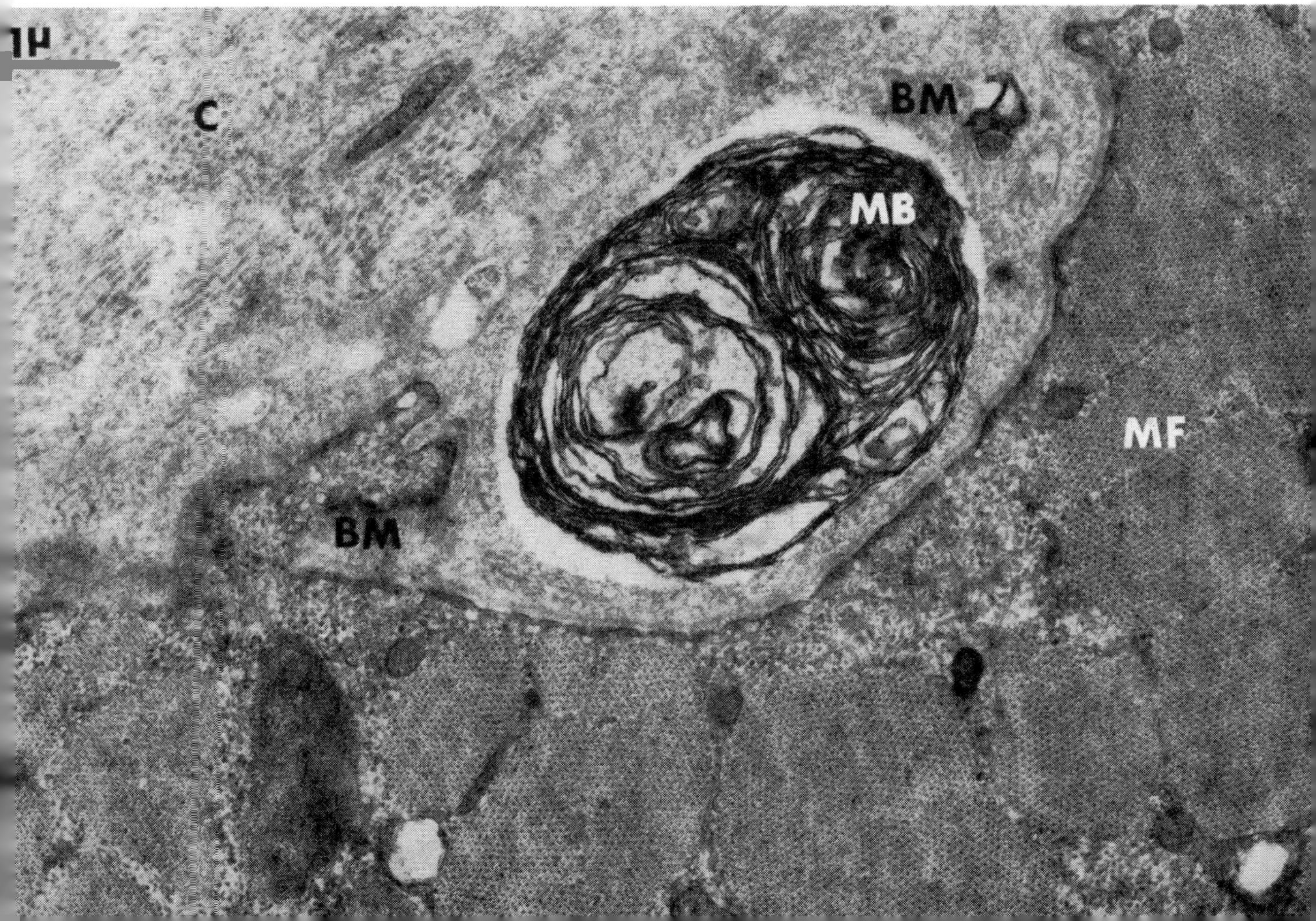
1μ
C
BM
MB
BM
MF

PLATE 41. MYELIN BODIES IN DEGENERATING MUSCLE FIBRES

UPPER. The architecture of the muscle fibre is completely deranged. The myofibrils have been destroyed but remnants of thickened Z-lines with filaments extending from them can still be identified. These have the same features as nemaline rods. In addition, numerous myelin bodies of irregular shape and size are present in the altered muscle fibre as well as vesicles and degenerating mitochondria.

MAGNIFICATION 10,000 ×.

From a patient with periarteritis nodosa.

LOWER. This muscle fibre is less severely damaged. The nucleus, some myofibrils and related mitochondria remain intact. Between them and the surface of the fibre which is crenated lie numerous filaments and granular material, amongst which are vacuoles of varying size containing myelin bodies. A fibroblast and collagen lie to the top left.

MAGNIFICATION 17,500 ×.

From a patient with polymyositis.

F Fibroblast
Fi Filaments
Mf Myofibrils
Mi Mitochondria
MB Myelin body
N Nucleus
Ro Rods

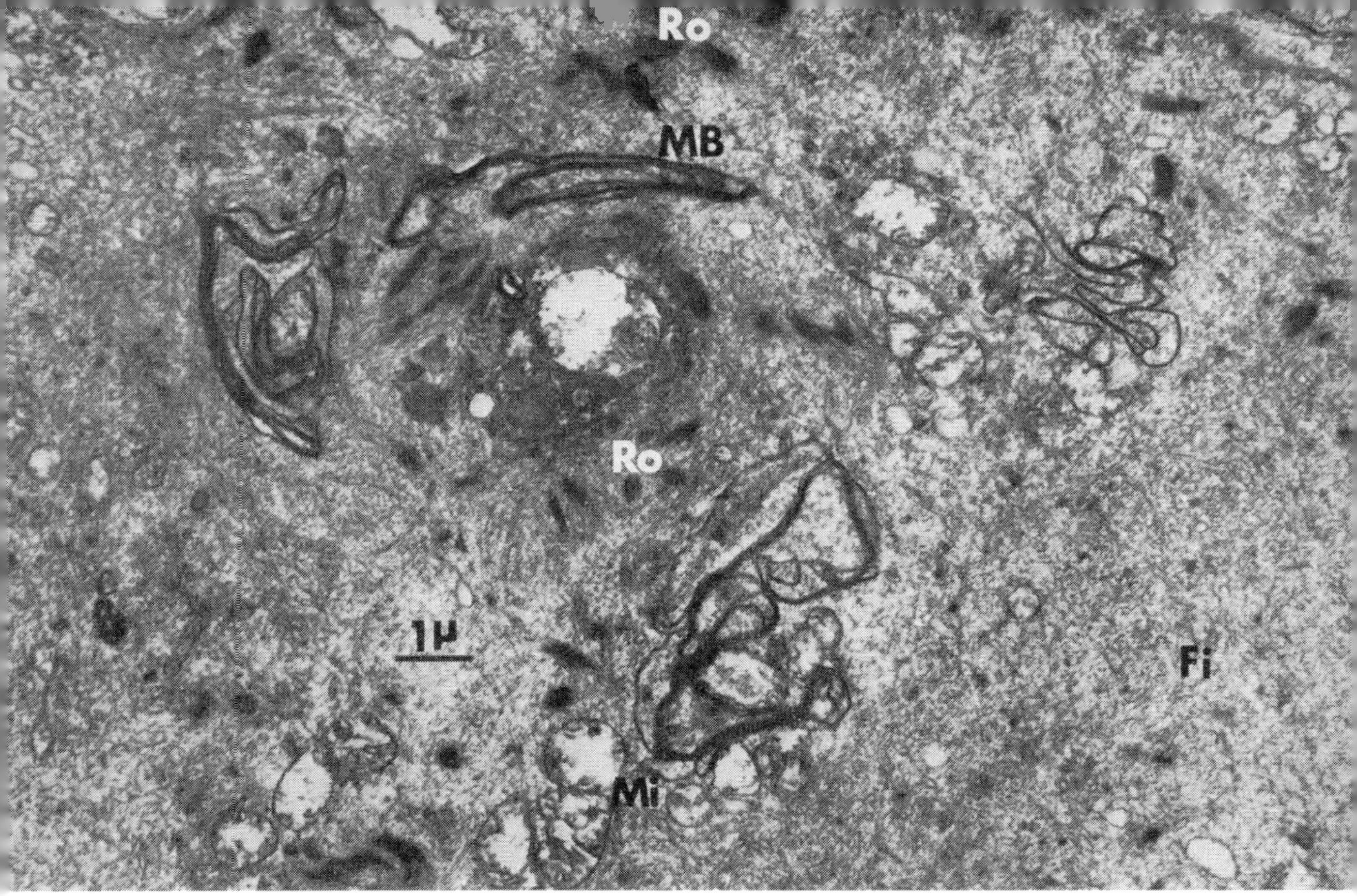
Ro
MB
Ro
1µ
Fi
Mi

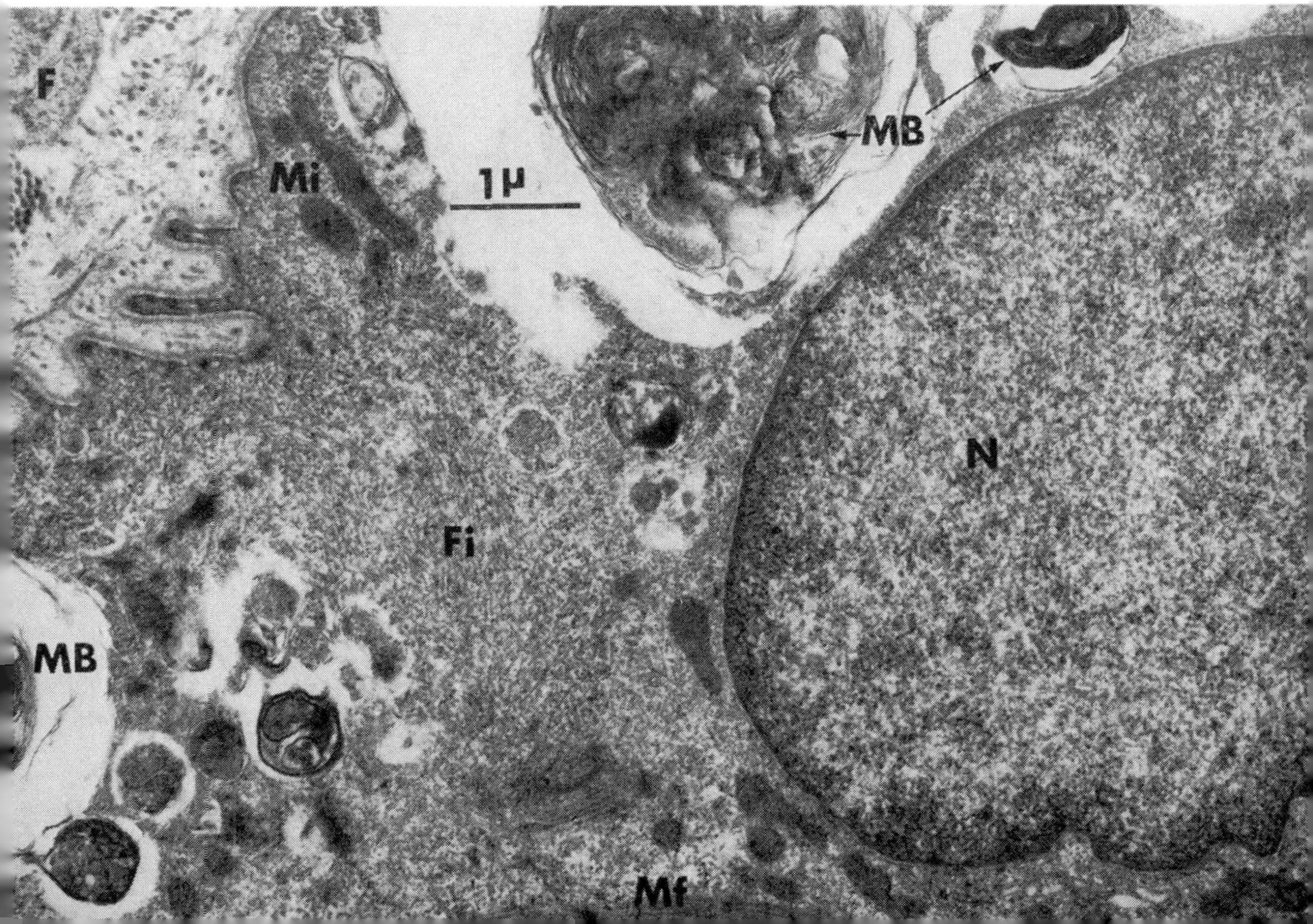
F
Mi
1µ
MB
N
Fi
MB
Mf

PLATE 42. MEMBRANOUS BODIES IN SKELETAL MUSCLE

UPPER. Laminated membranous bodies lie under the surface and between the nuclei of a degenerating muscle fibre showing thickening of the Z-lines and alteration of the myofibrils. A triad is prominent near the membranous body next to the nucleus. Glycogen granules and mitochondria also occur in the fibre.

MAGNIFICATION 20,000 ×.

From a patient with polyneuropathy.

LOWER LEFT. A concentric laminar body with a granular central zone lies to the left of the nucleus. Mitochondria and altered myofilaments also occur in the fibre.

MAGNIFICATION 30,000 ×.

From a patient with polyneuropathy.

LOWER RIGHT. Concentric membranous bodies lie near the nucleus of the fibre. One of them appears to be within a mitochondrion with broken cristae.

MAGNIFICATION 35,000 ×.

From a patient with muscular dystrophy.

G	Glycogen	My	Myofilaments
MeB	Membranous body	N	Nucleus
Mf	Myofibril	Tr	Triad
Mi	Mitochondria	Z	Z-line

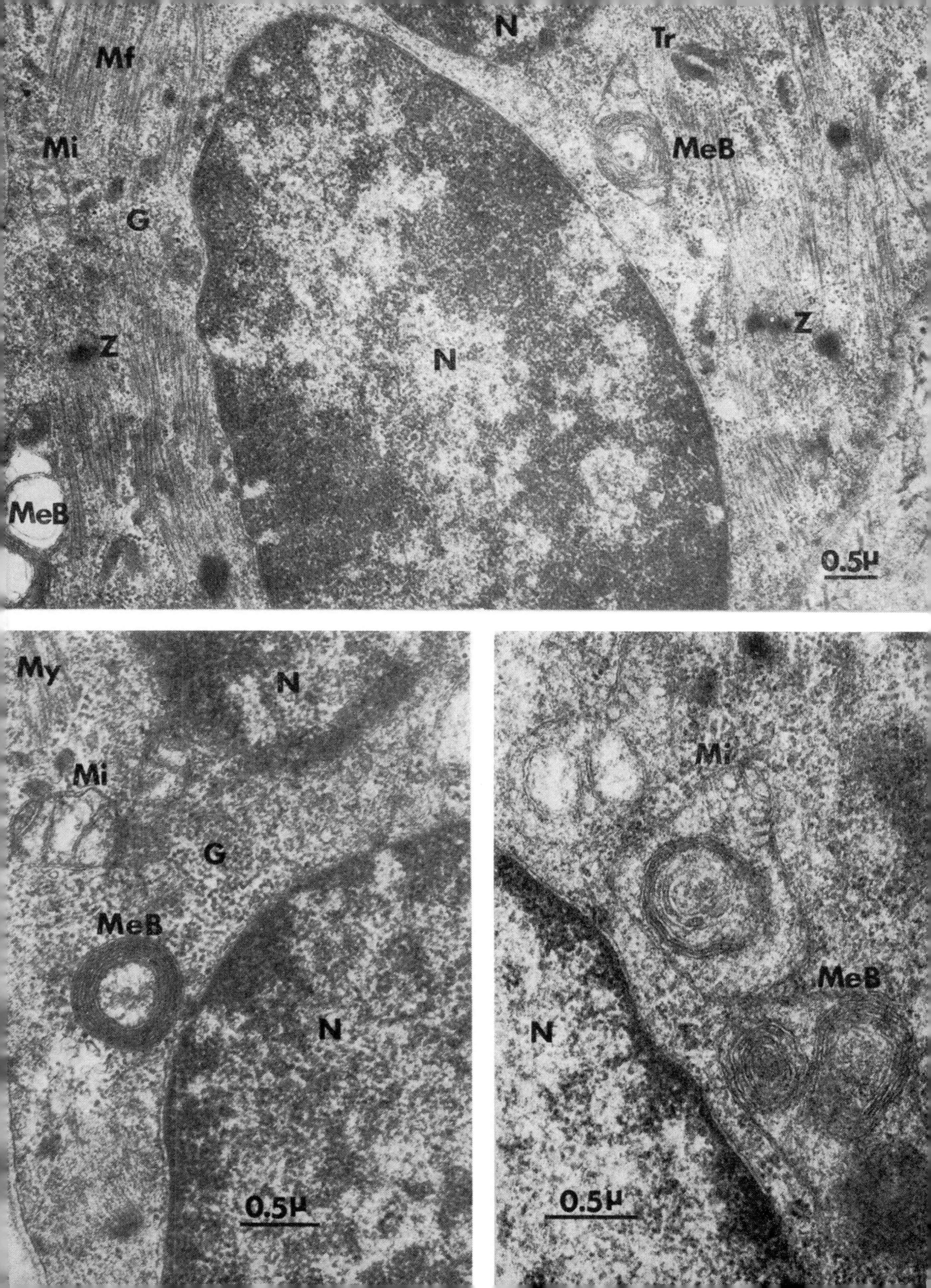

N
Tr
Mf
Mi
MeB
G
Z
N
Z
MeB
0.5μ
My
N
Mi
G
MeB
N
0.5μ
Mi
MeB
N
0.5μ

PLATE 43. MEMBRANOUS BODIES IN EXTRA-OCULAR MUSCLE

UPPER. This muscle fibre contains, besides the zebra body on the left, several peculiar inclusions. They consist of collections of concentric tubules and large vacuoles containing membranous material and smaller vacuoles filled with electron dense material. Glycogen granules are scattered between these various structures and around the mitochondria between the myofibrils in the lower half of the muscle fibre.

MAGNIFICATION 9,000 ×.

LOWER. A higher magnification of the upper right part of the same muscle fibre shows, in addition to the various tubules and electron dense material, collections of mitochondria around the secondary synaptic clefts of a motor end plate.

MAGNIFICATION 15,000 ×.

G	Glycogen
MeB	Membranous bodies
Mi	Mitochondria
SSC	Secondary synaptic clefts
Va	Vacuoles
ZB	Zebra body

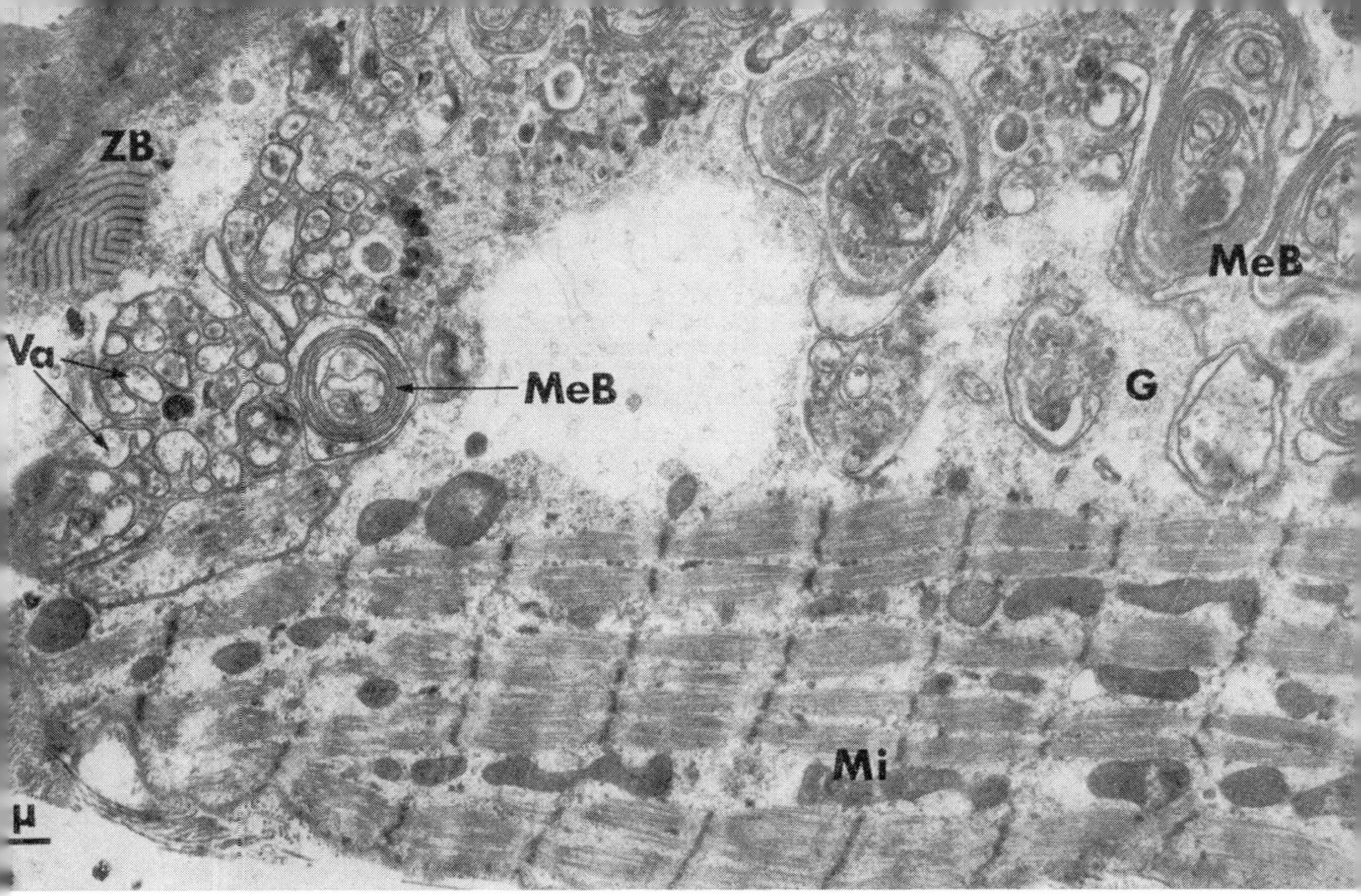
ZB
Va
MeB
MeB
G
Mi
μ

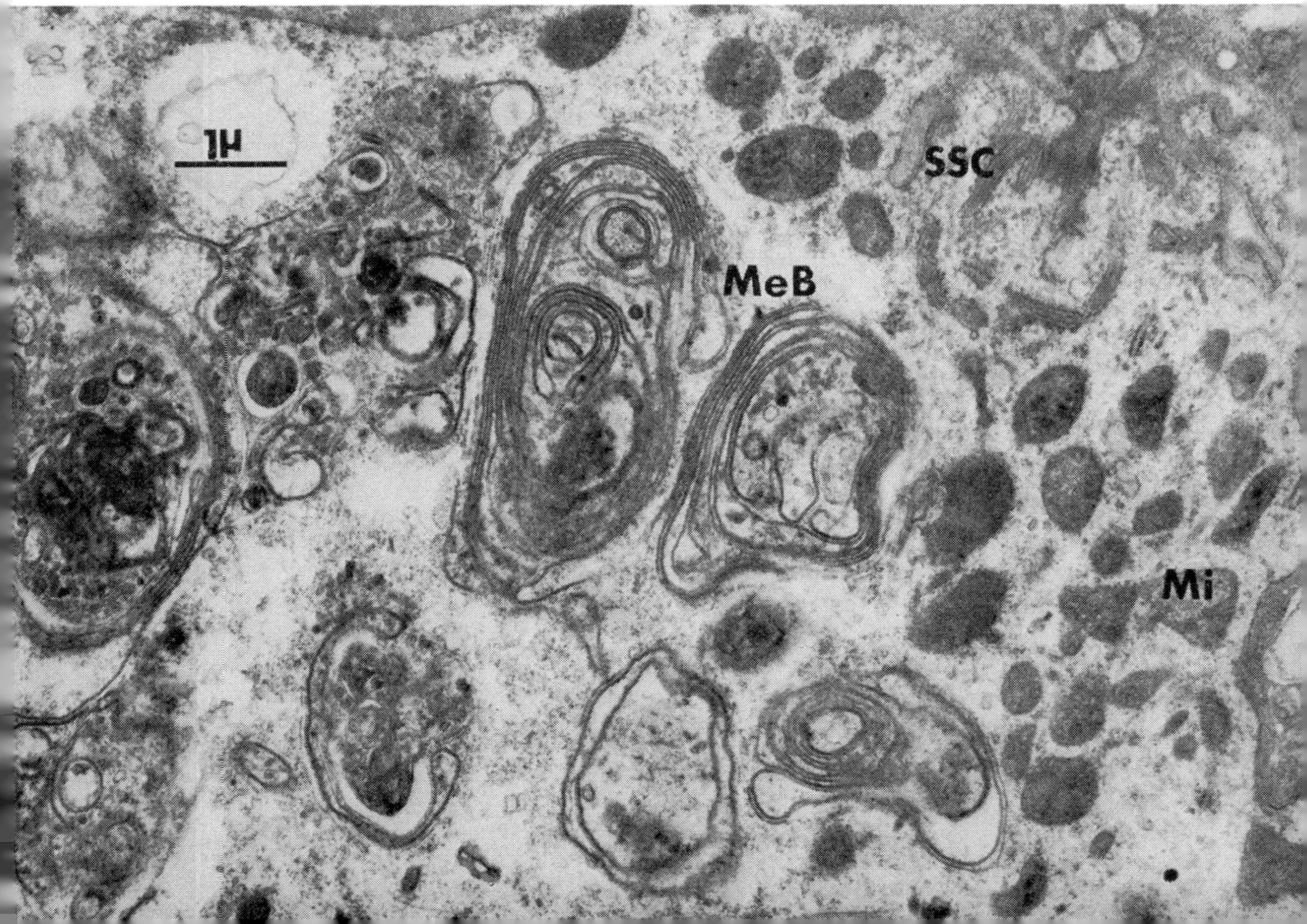
1μ
SSC
MeB
Mi

PLATE 44. CONCENTRIC LAMINATED BODIES IN DEGENERATING MUSCLE FIBRES

UPPER. In a very atrophied muscle fibre with undulating sarcoplasmic projections are numerous concentrically laminated bodies of varying diameter, the largest being about 0·7 μ. Around these bodies and in their centre are numerous granules some of which are glycogen granules. Strands of collagen and processes of fibroblasts lie between the atrophied muscle fibre and another muscle fibre which contains a satellite cell.

MAGNIFICATION 11,000 ×.

INSET. Higher magnification of the concentric bodies within the rectangle shows details of their structure. They are formed of lamellae of about 70 Å thick. In part of one on the left, the lamellae are interrupted.

MAGNIFICATION 60,000 ×.

From a patient with alcoholic polyneuropathy.

LOWER. Similar concentric laminated bodies cut obliquely and longitudinally are seen at greater magnification. They are formed of interrupted lamellae: granules lie around them and in their centres. Some of the granules are glycogen. Myofibrils lie on the left of the illustration.

MAGNIFICATION 31,000 ×.

From a patient with polyneuropathy of unknown aetiology.

C	Collagen	Mi	Mitochondria
DMF	Degenerating muscle fibre	My	Myofilaments
F	Fibroblast	OS	Oblique section
LS	Longitudinal section	S	Satellite cell

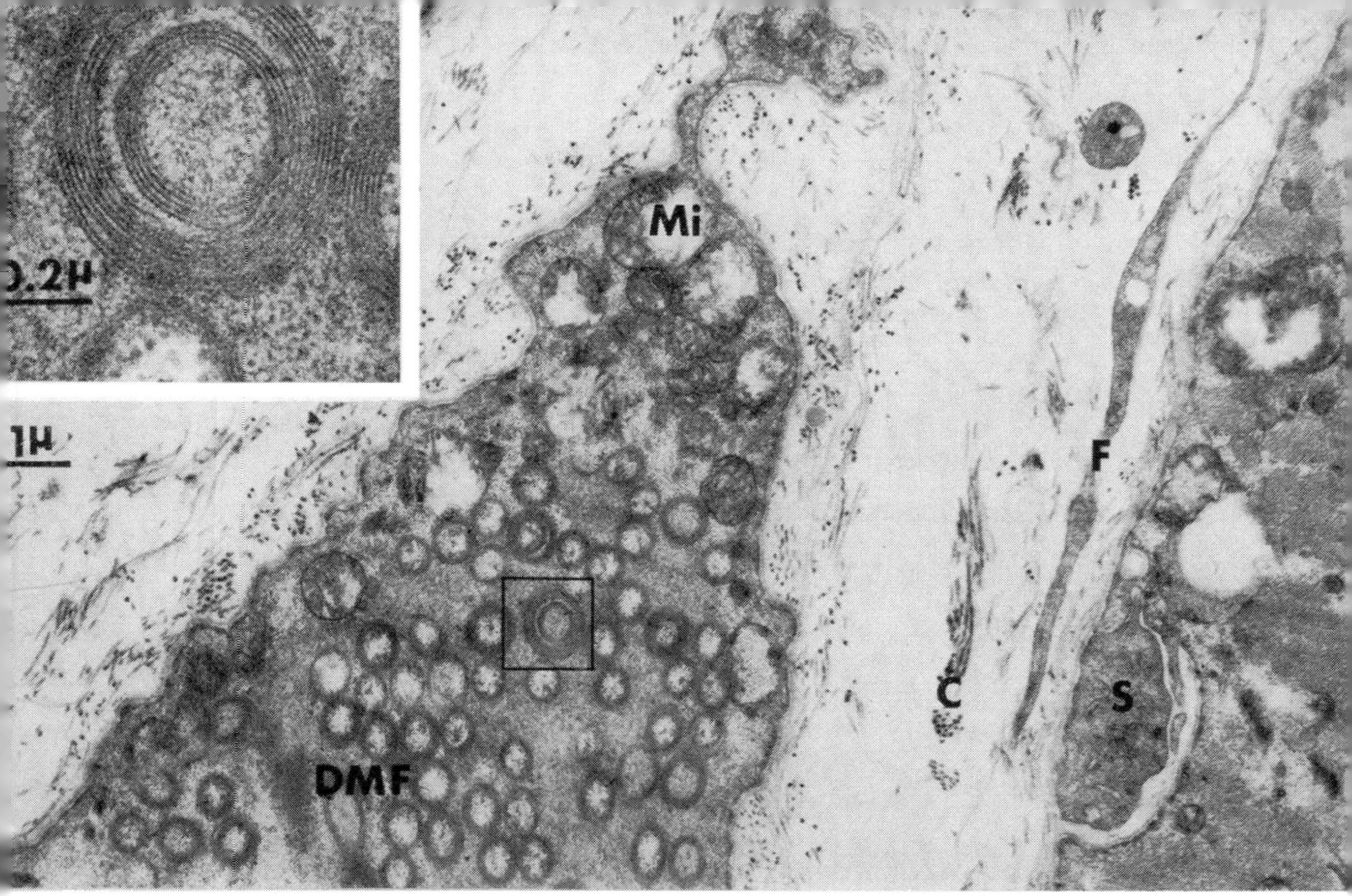
0.2μ
1μ
Mi
F
C
S
DMF
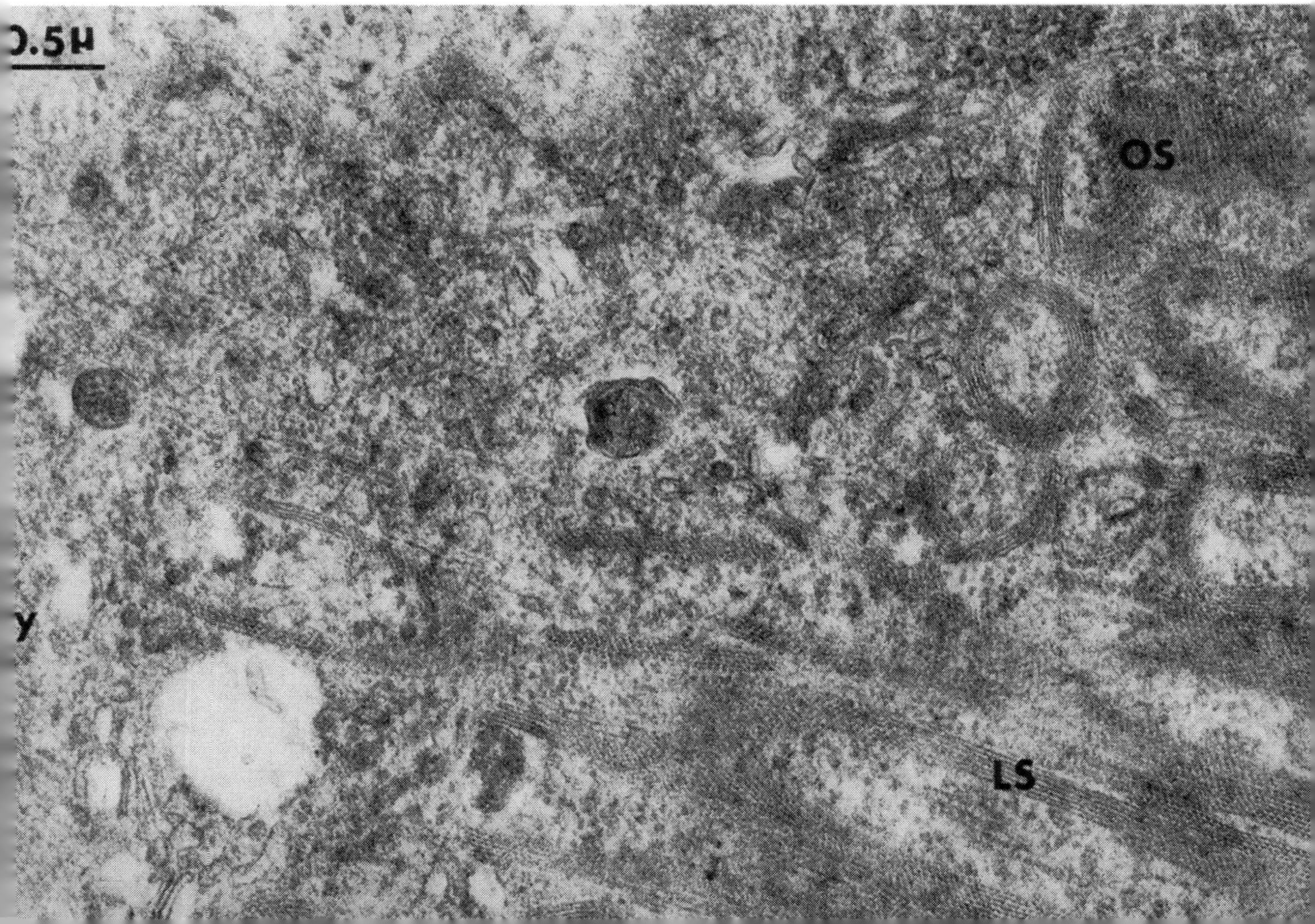
0.5μ
OS
LS

PLATE 45. CONCENTRIC AND PARALLEL TUBULES IN MUSCLE FIBRES

This muscle fibre shows concentric and parallel arrays of up to 19 tubules between the plasma membrane and the myofibrils. The tubules are 40–80 mμ wide and are separated from each other by a space of 40–70 mμ containing glycogen granules. In the sarcoplasm to the left are longitudinal and cross sections of myofilaments while around the tubules are lipid bodies, mitochondria, triads, vesicles and glycogen granules. Basement membrane covers the muscle fibre and outside it lies collagen.

MAGNIFICATION 42,000 ×.

From a patient with alcoholic neuropathy.

BM Basement membrane
C Collagen
G Glycogen
LB Lipid bodies
Mf Myofibrils
Mi Mitochondria
My Myofilaments
PM Plasma membrane
Tr Triads
Tu Tubules
V Vesicles

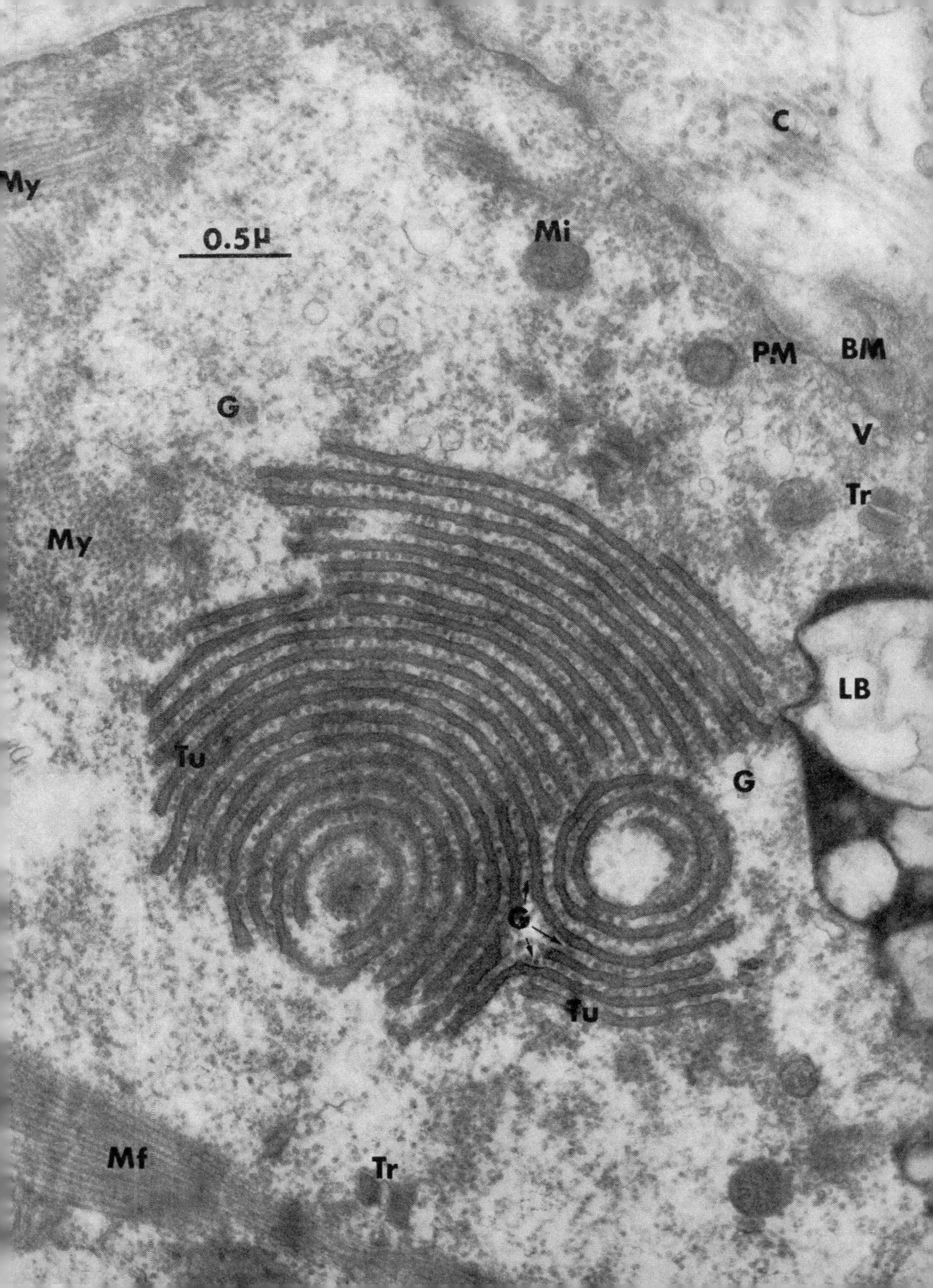

My
C
0.5µ
Mi
PM
BM
G
V
Tr
My
LB
Tu
G
G
Tu
Mf
Tr

PLATE 46. TUBULAR AGGREGATES IN MUSCLE FIBRES

Aggregates of tubules are present in the muscle fibres. Some are present under the plasma membrane or around the nuclei and less frequently in the centre of the fibre. The tubules are 400–500 Å in diameter with a central mass 250–300 Å in diameter and a clear zone 70–120 Å wide separating the central mass from the outer wall which is about 80 Å thick. The tubules lie in hexagonal array. They may be cut transversely, longitudinally or obliquely in the same section of the muscle. In addition occasional honeycomb structures are present near the tubules (upper right). Glycogen granules separate the myofibrils. A prominent T-system is demonstrated amongst the tubules and a triad lies to the right in the lower left illustration. The tubules are sometimes associated with large vacuoles.

MAGNIFICATION	*Upper* Left	27,000 ×.	Right	28,000 ×.
	Lower Left	43,000 ×.	Right	40,000 ×.

From a patient with myopathy.

F	Fibroblast	OS	Oblique section
G	Glycogen	T	T-system
HC	Honeycomb structure	Tr	Triad
LS	Longitudinal section	Tu	Tubule
Mf	Myofibril	TS	Transverse section
N	Nucleus	Va	Vacuole

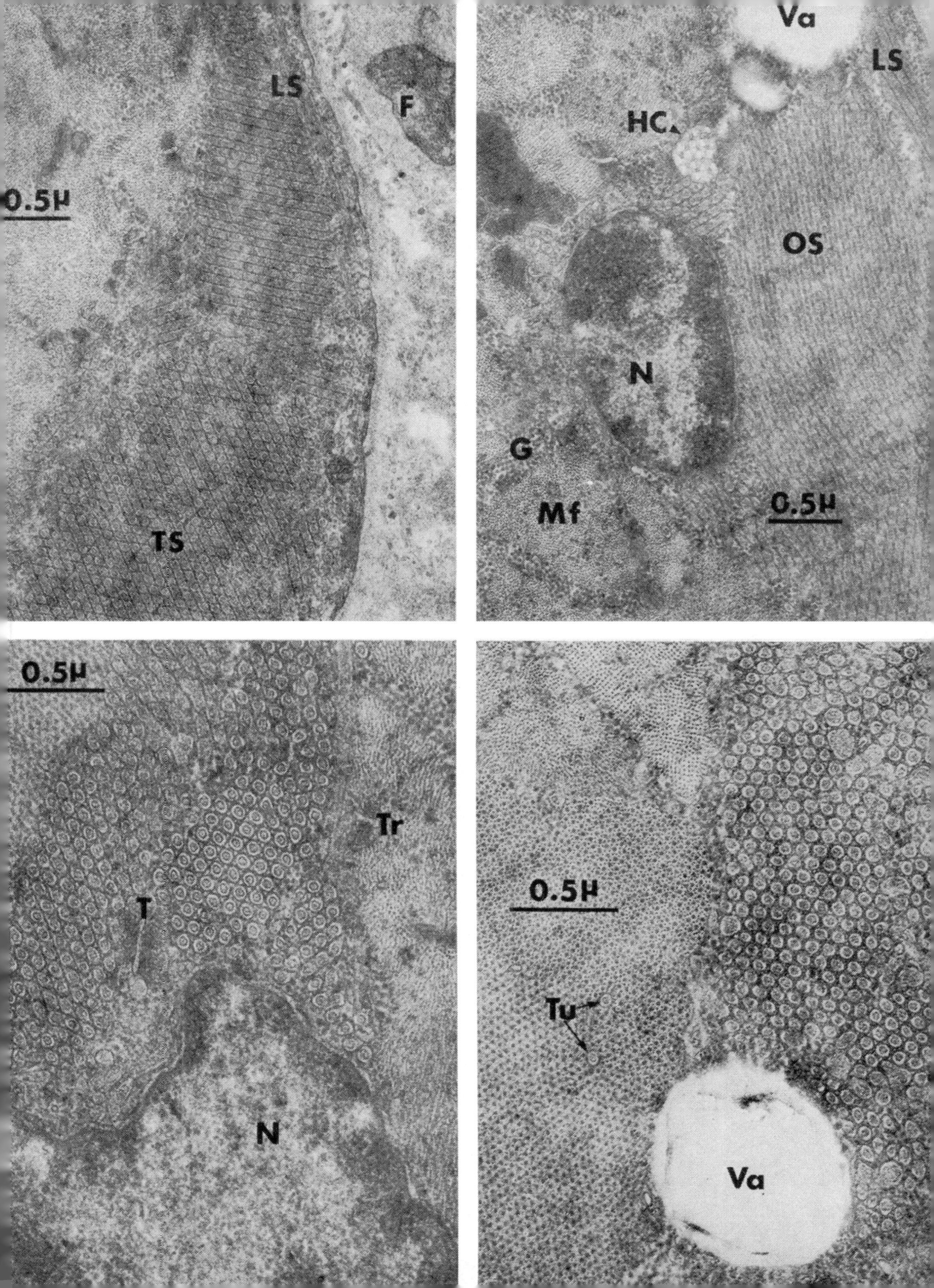

LS
F
0.5μ
TS
Va
LS
HC
OS
N
G
Mf
0.5μ
0.5μ
Tr
T
N
0.5μ
Tu
Va

PLATE 47. TUBULAR AGGREGATES IN MUSCLE FIBRES

The muscle fibres contain tubules which are bounded by electron dense margins and contain less electron dense granular material. Their diameters vary considerably, some being up to 900 Å in diameter.

UPPER HALF. The *upper part* shows tubules (arrowed) running longitudinally between the myofibrils. Vacuoles and numerous glycogen granules are present near the tubules.

MAGNIFICATION 26,000 ×.

In the *lower part* the tubules lie between the plasma membrane and the myofibrils. Some tubules are cut transversely and others longitudinally. A vacuole lies near them.

MAGNIFICATION 50,000 ×.

LOWER HALF. On the left the tubules (arrowed) run obliquely across the myofibrils.

MAGNIFICATION 40,000 ×.

On the right the *upper part* shows the tubules cut transversely. They are between the myofibrils.

MAGNIFICATION 41,000 ×.

On the right the *lower part* shows tubules (arrowed) cut transversely, obliquely and longitudinally.

MAGNIFICATION 48,000 ×.

From a patient with muscular dystrophy.

G	Glycogen	PM	Plasma membrane
LS	Longitudinal section	TS	Transverse section
Mf	Myofibril	Va	Vacuole

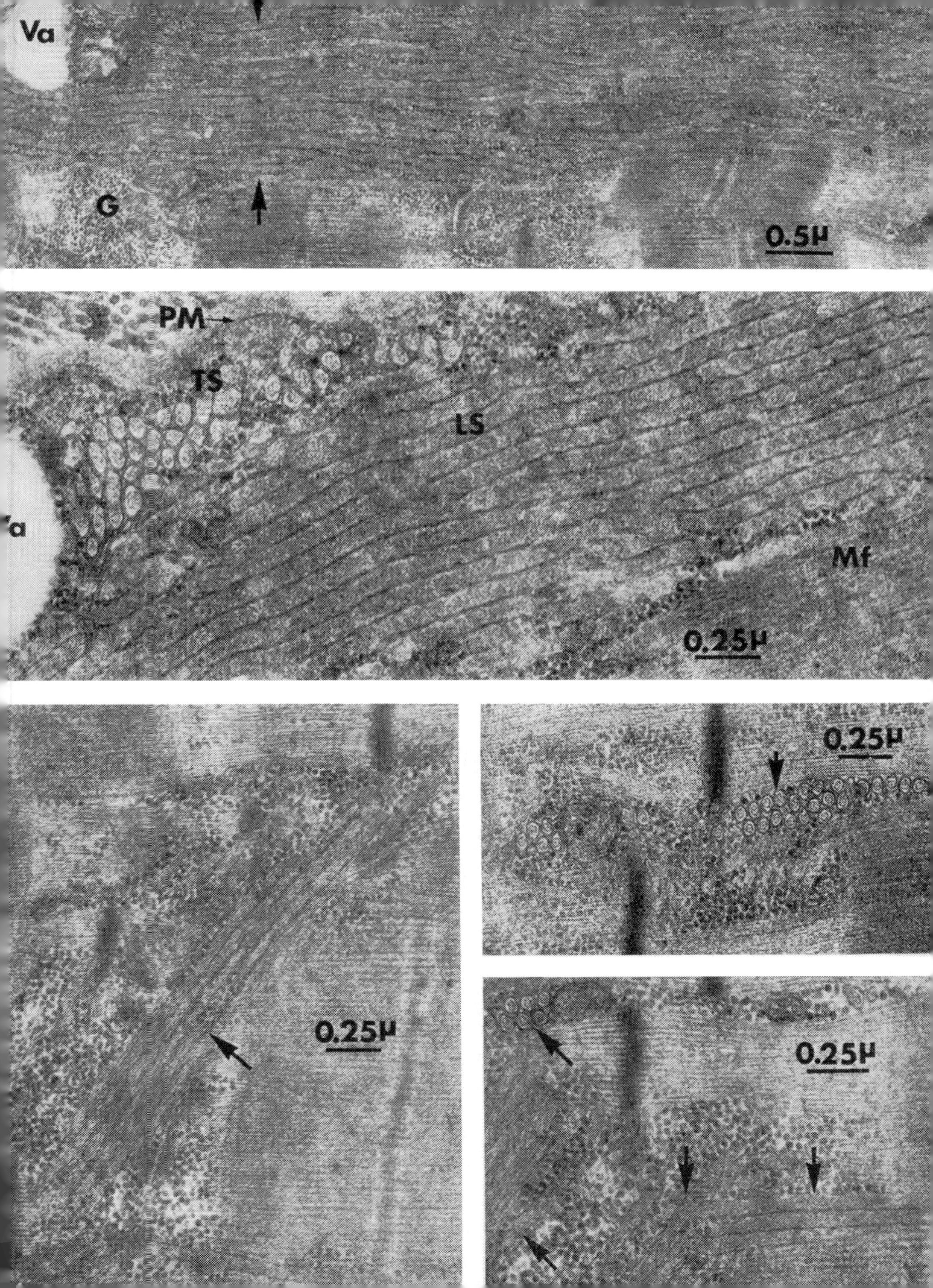
Va
G
0.5μ
PM
TS
LS
Mf
0.25μ
0.25μ
0.25μ
0.25μ

PLATE 48. TUBULAR AGGREGATES IN MUSCLE FIBRES

UPPER. Here are collections of tubules with electron dense margins and less electron dense content (arrowed). They lie between the nucleus and a myofibril and adjacent mitochondria, one of which is vacuolated. Collagen separates the two muscle fibres, the lower of which appears normal.

MAGNIFICATION 31,000 ×.

From a patient with alcoholic myopathy.

LOWER. Under the surface of the muscle fibre are tubules lying amongst some obliquely cut filaments. The tubules have an electron dense membrane and a central electron dense mass separated from one another by a clear space. The tubules are 500–600 Å in diameter. Close to the tubules are mitochondria and large vacuoles one of which contains membranous material.

MAGNIFICATION 45,000 ×.

From a patient with rheumatoid arthritis treated with steroids.

C	Collagen	Mi	Mitochondria
Fi	Filaments	N	Nucleus
Mf	Myofibril	Va	Vacuole

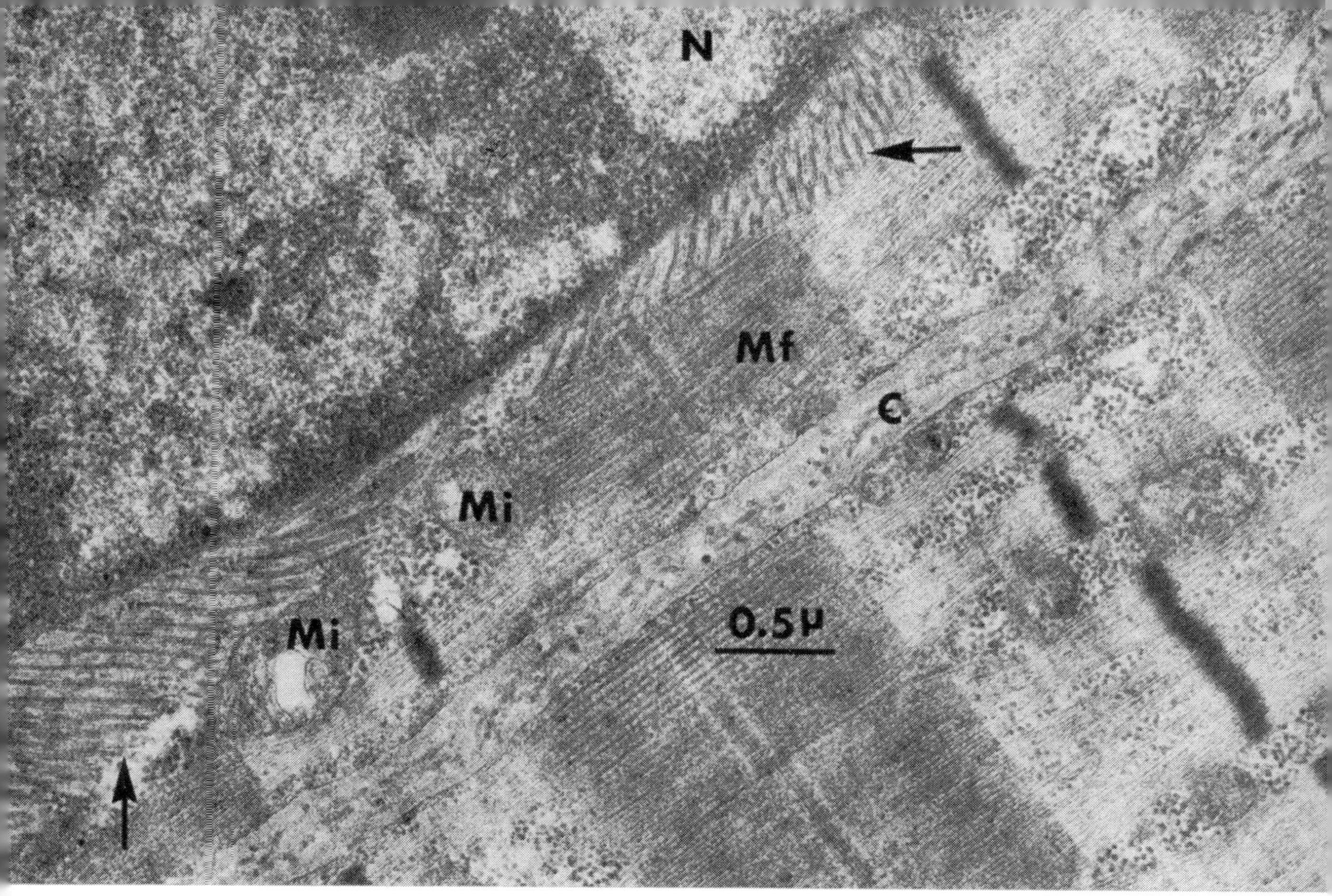
N
Mf
C
Mi
Mi
0.5μ

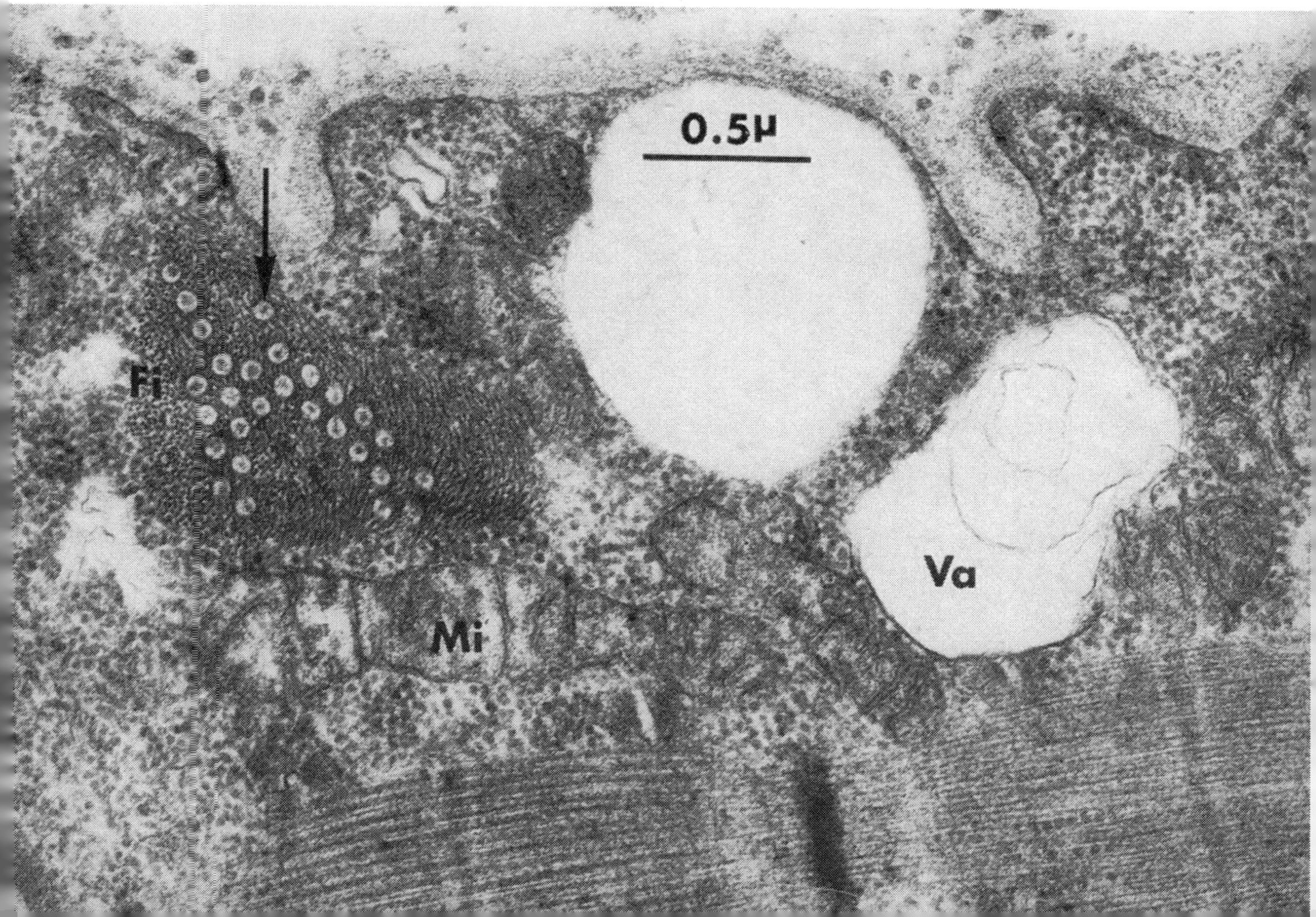
0.5μ
Fi
Va
Mi

PLATE 49. PLASMA AND BASEMENT MEMBRANES IN DEGENERATING MUSCLE FIBRES

UPPER. Blood capillaries, strands of collagen and granular material lie between two degenerating muscle fibres. The upper fibre shows more advanced signs of degeneration. The myofibrils and the plasma membrane have disappeared. Filaments are scattered in a profusion of granules and a group of altered mitochondria lie at the top. The basement membrane of the muscle fibre remains. The lower fibre shows separation of the basement membrane from the plasma membrane and myelin bodies lie between them. Degenerating myofilaments, vesicles and some mitochondria can be seen in the fibre.

MAGNIFICATION 8,000 ×.

LOWER. Two adjacent degenerating muscle fibres are separated by collagen, amorphous material and the process of a fibroblast. Degeneration is much more advanced in the lower fibre where myofibrils cannot be identified. The sarcoplasm is filled with granular material, a few filaments and some vesicles. The plasma membrane is fine and shows interruptions in its continuity: it lies close to the basement membrane. In the upper fibre degeneration of the myofilaments is seen in its lower part.

MAGNIFICATION 15,000 ×.

Both are from a patient with polyneuropathy.

BC	Blood capillary	Mi	Mitochondria
BM	Basement membrane	My	Myofilaments
C	Collagen	MB	Myelin body
F	Fibroblast	MF	Muscle fibre
Fi	Filaments	PM	Plasma membrane

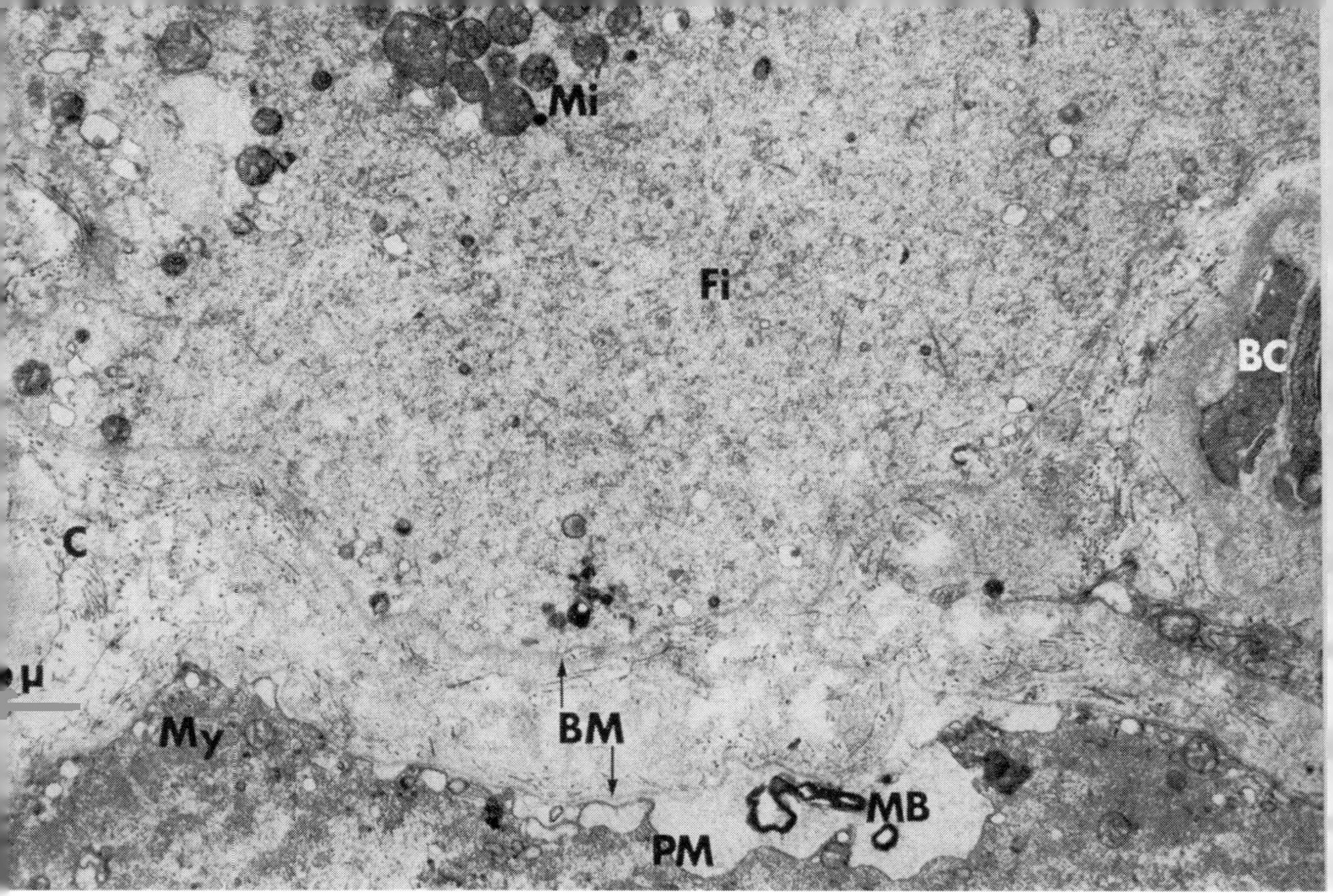
Mi
Fi
BC
C
μ
My
BM
BM
MB
PM

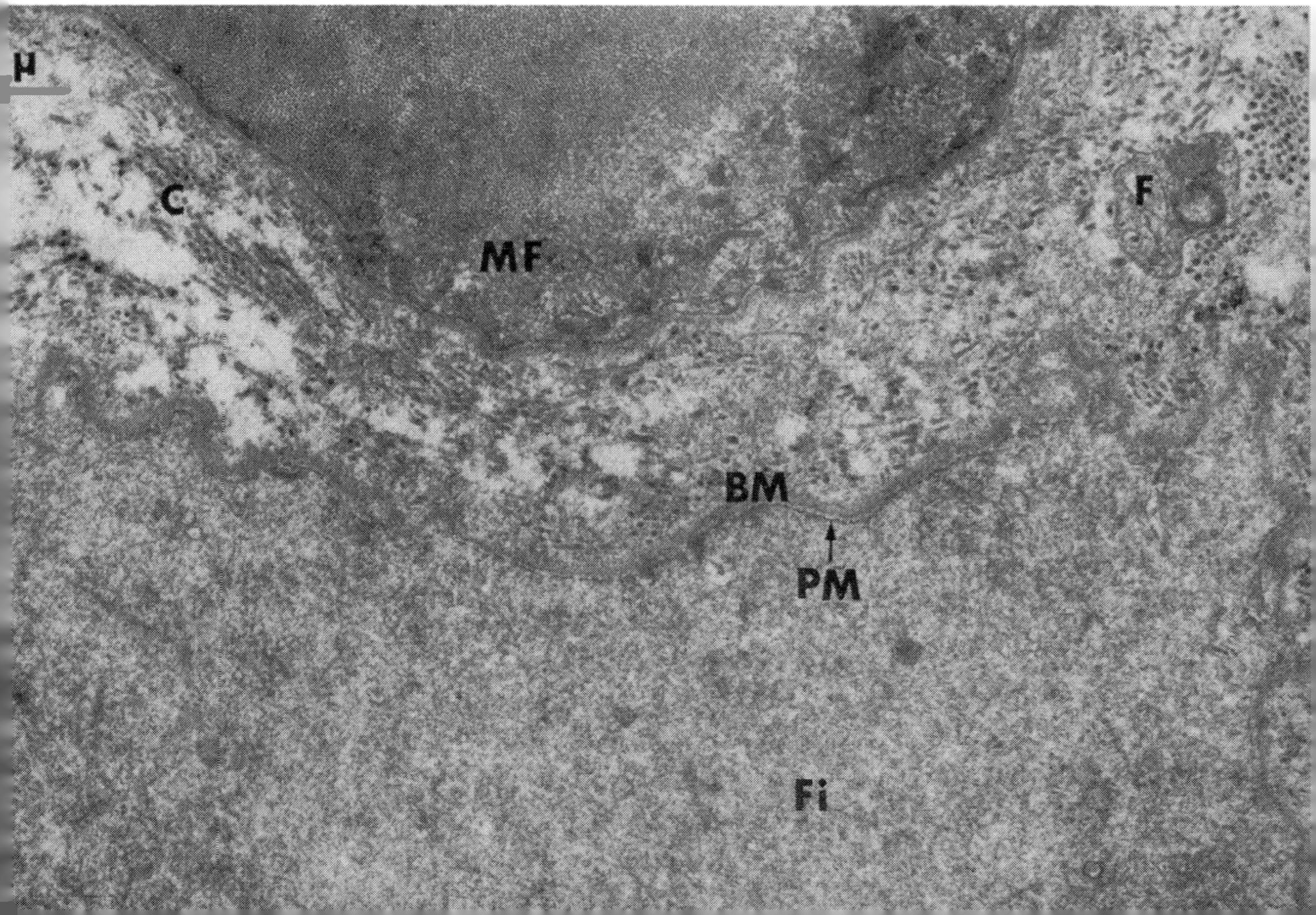
μ
C
MF
F
BM
PM
Fi

PLATE 50. BASEMENT MEMBRANE PROJECTIONS FROM AN ATROPHYING MUSCLE FIBRE

Undulating folds of basement membrane protrude from a degenerating muscle fibre exhibiting distorted Z-lines, disorganised myofibrils and collections of glycogen granules. Most of the folds are completely devoid of any sarcoplasm: strands of collagen surround them. A process of a fibroblast lies to the right of the illustration.

MAGNIFICATION 14,500 ×.

From a patient with muscular dystrophy.

BM Basement membrane
C Collagen
DMF Degenerating muscle fibre
F Fibroblast

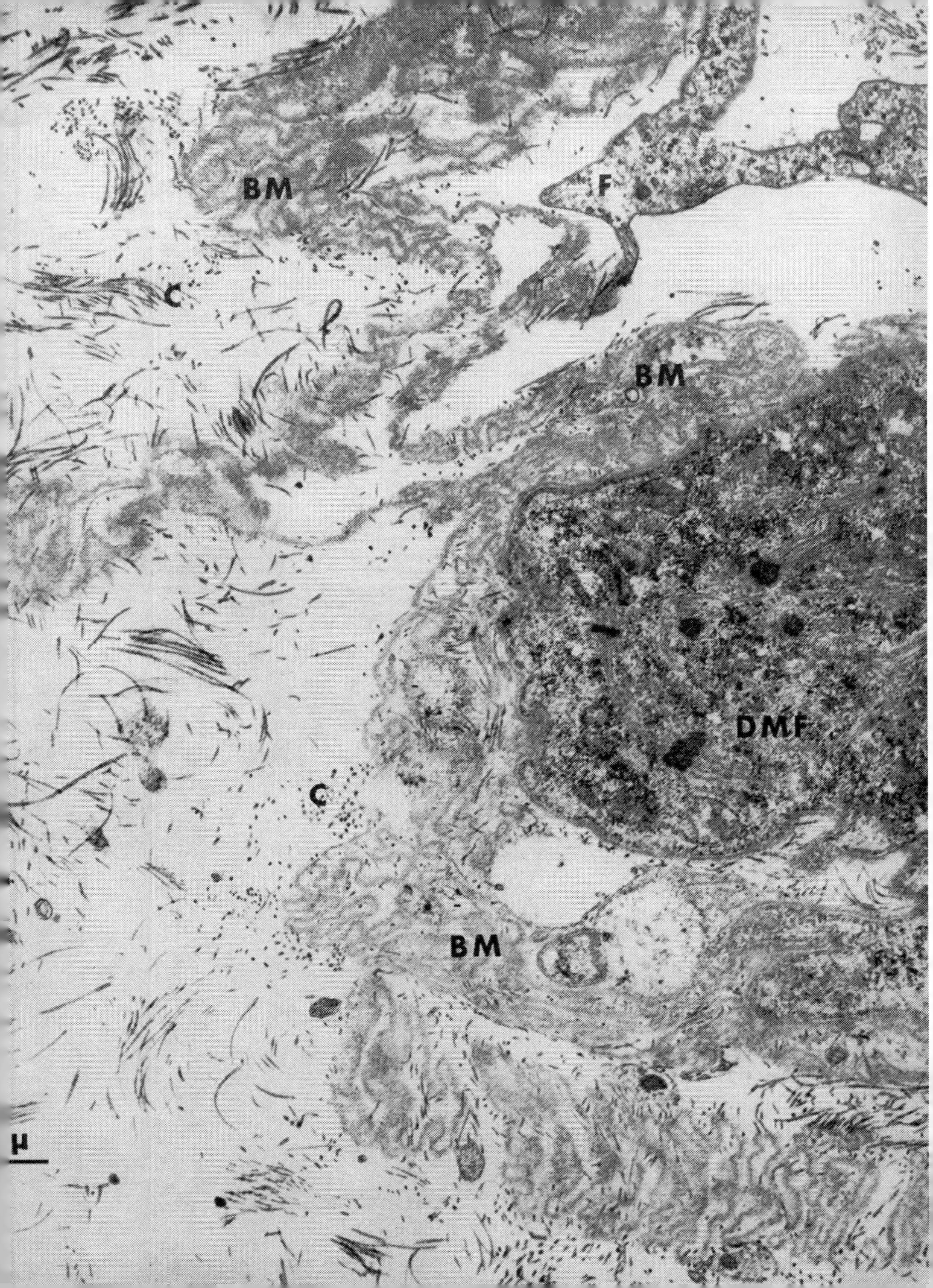
BM
F
C
ℓ
BM
DMF
C
BM
μ

PLATE 51. SATELLITE CELLS IN MUSCLE FIBRES

UPPER. In the lower half of the illustration is a satellite cell which is cut through its nucleus. The cell lies inside the basement membrane of the muscle fibre: no basement membrane separates the muscle fibre and the satellite: in both, the plasma membranes are distinct. The chromatin of the satellite cell nucleus is distributed in masses around its periphery. The nucleus is large and occupies almost the width of the cell. Above this muscle fibre with the satellite lie collagen and processes of fibroblasts and part of a muscle fibre. In addition, amongst the collagen is a prominent blood capillary which has been cut through the nucleus of one of its endothelial cells. Electron dense desmosomes lie at the junctions of the endothelial cells. The basement membrane around the capillary is thick. In a cleft in the basement membrane is a cytoplasmic process of a pericyte. The I- and A-bands and the Z-lines of the muscle fibre are distinct.

MAGNIFICATION 14,000 ×.

From a patient with vitamin E deficiency.

LOWER. A satellite cell lies within the basement membrane of the muscle fibre. The nucleus of the satellite cell is indented and the cytoplasm contains vesicles, polysomes and ribosomes and occasional mitochondria. The outer nuclear membranes of the satellite cell and the muscle fibre are distinct. The nucleus of the muscle fibre is less electron dense than that of the satellite. Slight changes are evident in the filaments of the I-band and there is some distortion of the Z-lines of the myofibrils. Vesicles are numerous under the plasma membrane of the muscle fibre and there are also considerable collections of glycogen at the surface of the fibre and between the myofibrils. A few strands of collagen and a large amount of amorphous material lie outside the muscle fibre.

MAGNIFICATION 15,000 ×.

From a patient with dermatomyositis.

BC Blood capillary
BM Basement membrane
C Collagen
F Fibroblast
G Glycogen
I I-band
N Nucleus
NM Nuclear membrane
PM Plasma membrane
S Satellite cell

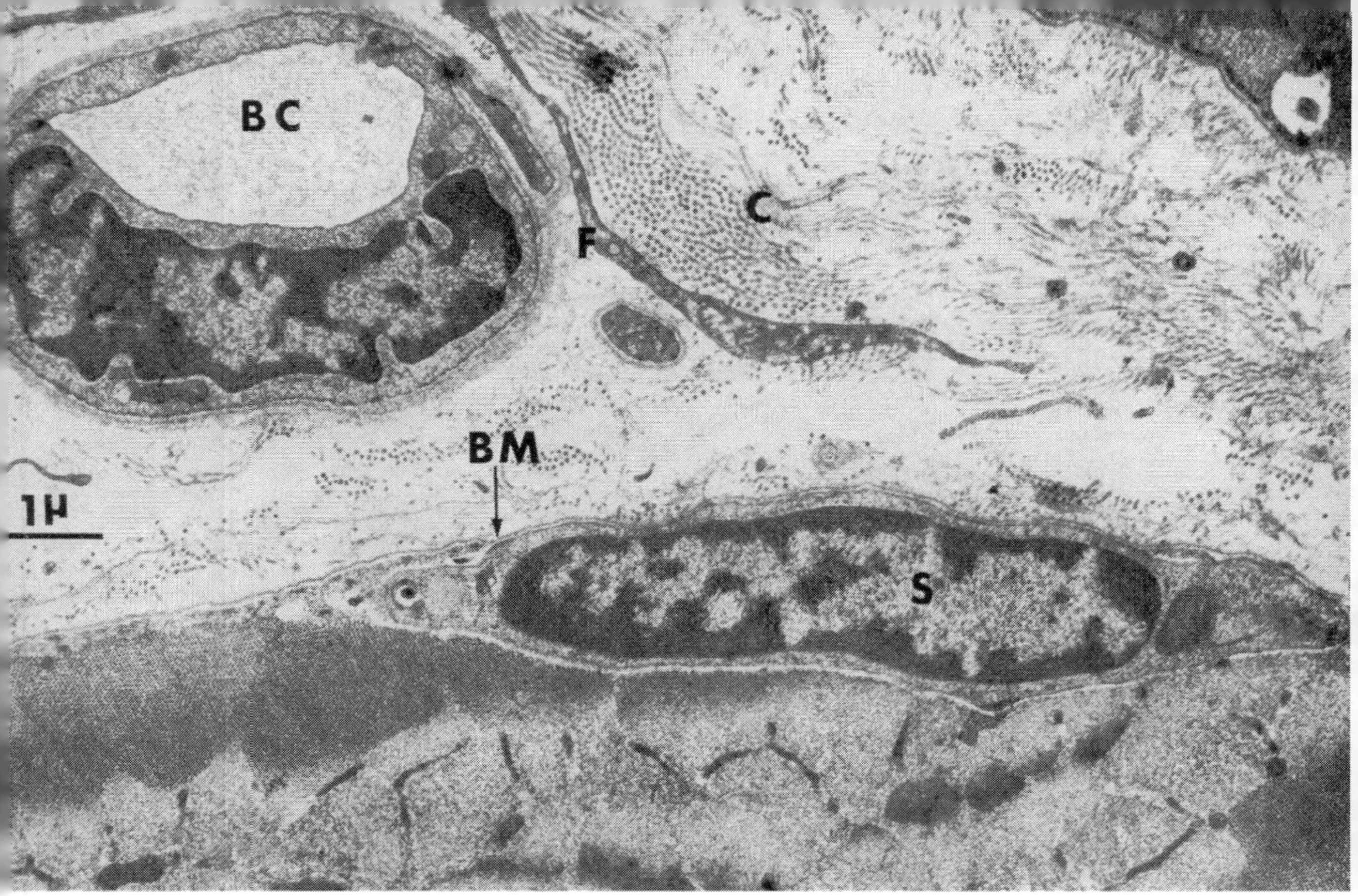
BC
C
F
BM
1μ
S

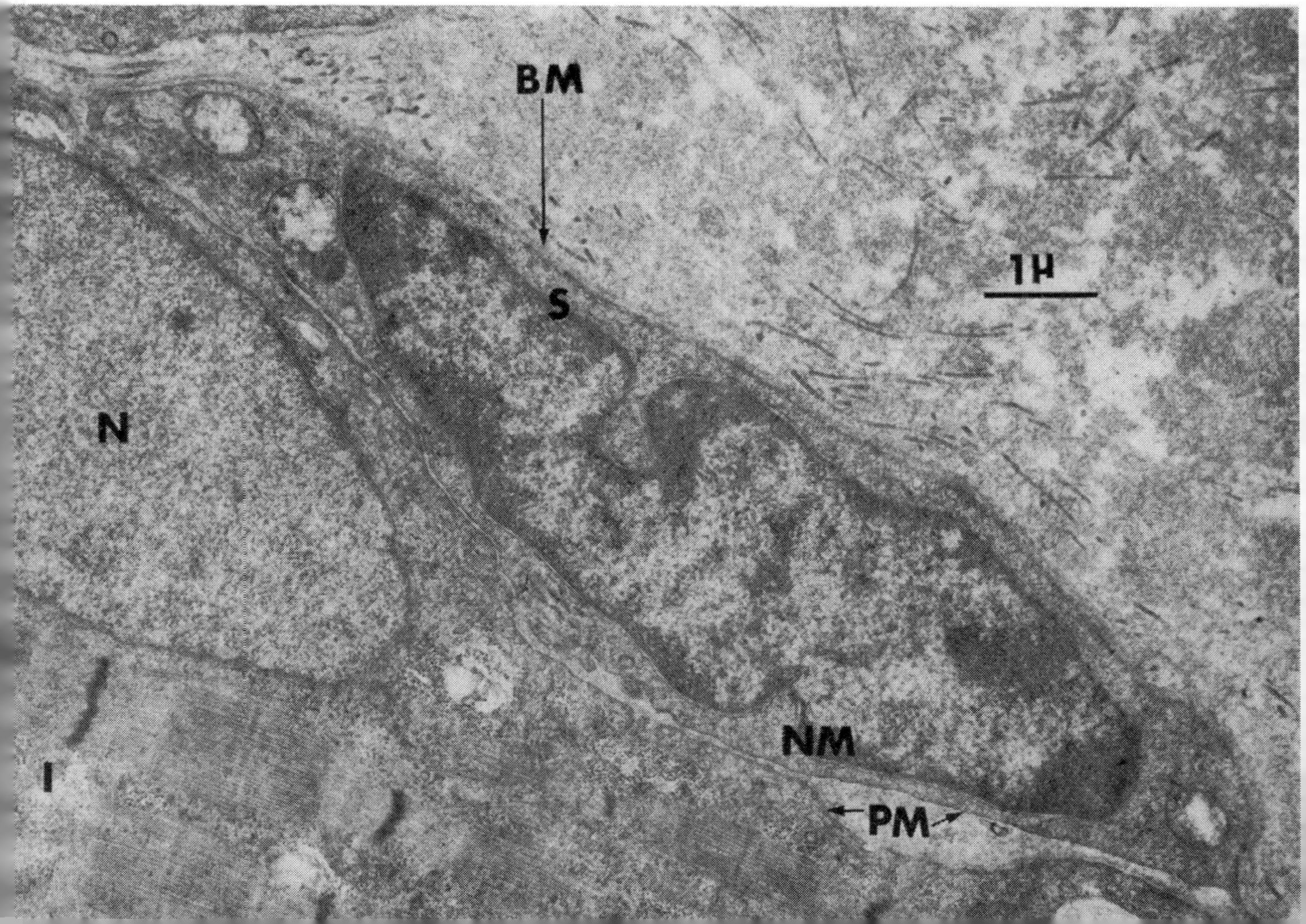
BM
1μ
S
N
I
NM
PM

PLATE 52. REGENERATION OF MUSCLE

UPPER. In inflammatory diseases of muscles there occur as illustrated, fibres in which the myofibrils are well defined even if they may show some structural changes such as irregular expansion of the Z-line. In these fibres the sarcoplasm is unusually rich in polysomes and ribosomes and vesicles occur especially near the plasma membranes. Some randomly disposed myofilaments occur in the sarcoplasm as well as distended sacs of the sarcoplasmic reticulum.

MAGNIFICATION 24,000 ×.

LOWER. Other muscle fibres present myofibrils with fine granules attached to some of the myofilaments. Scattered throughout the sarcoplasm are polysomes, ribosomes, vesicles and numerous thick and thin myofilaments.

It is difficult to be certain if these fibres are in a stage of degeneration or regeneration.

MAGNIFICATION 26,500 ×.

Both are from a patient with dermatomyositis.

C	Collagen	Po	Polysomes
G	Glycogen	PM	Plasma membrane
Mi	Mitochondria	R	Ribosomes
Mf	Myofibrils	V	Vesicles
My	Myofilaments	Z	Z-line

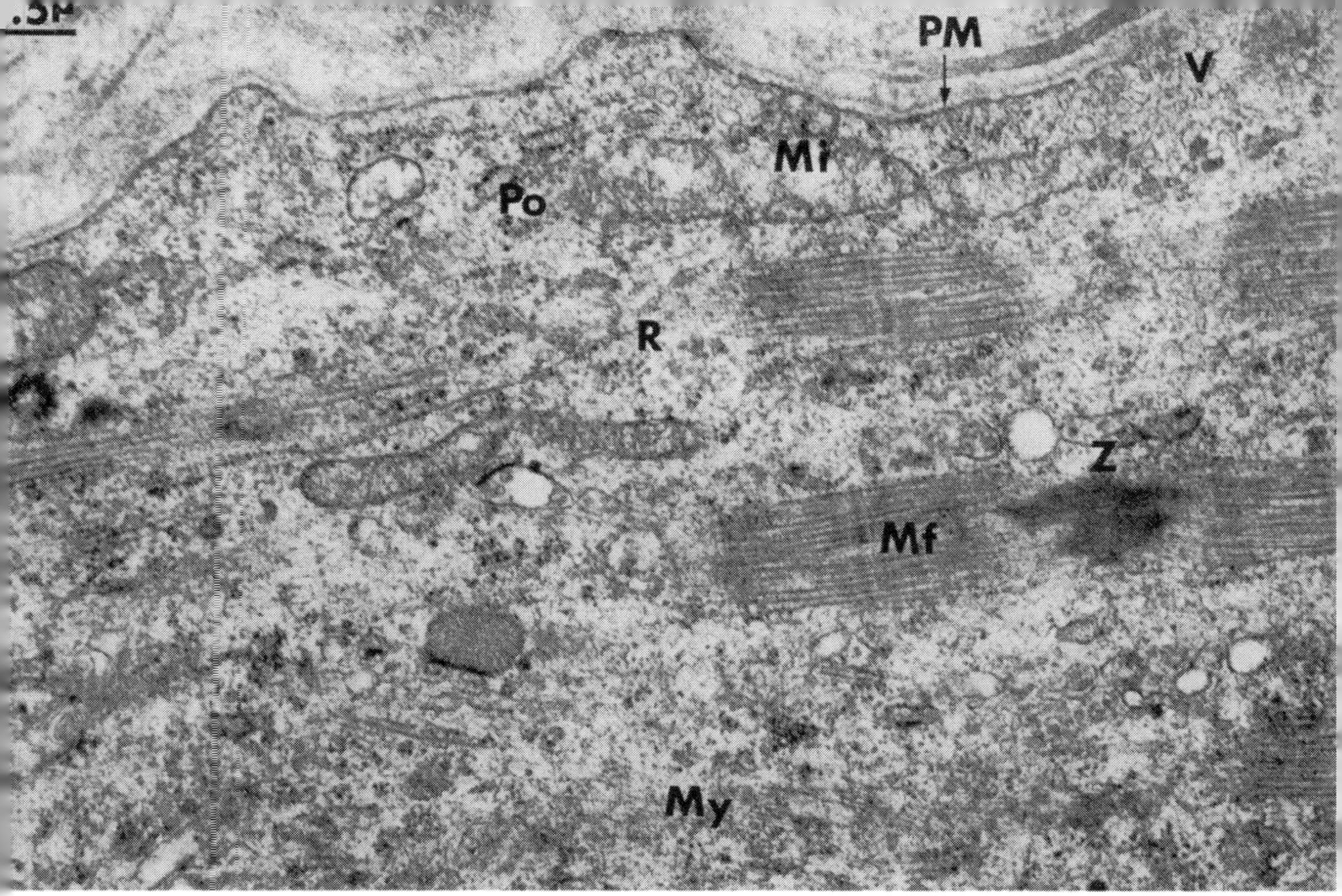
.5μ
PM
V
Mi
Po
R
Z
Mf
My

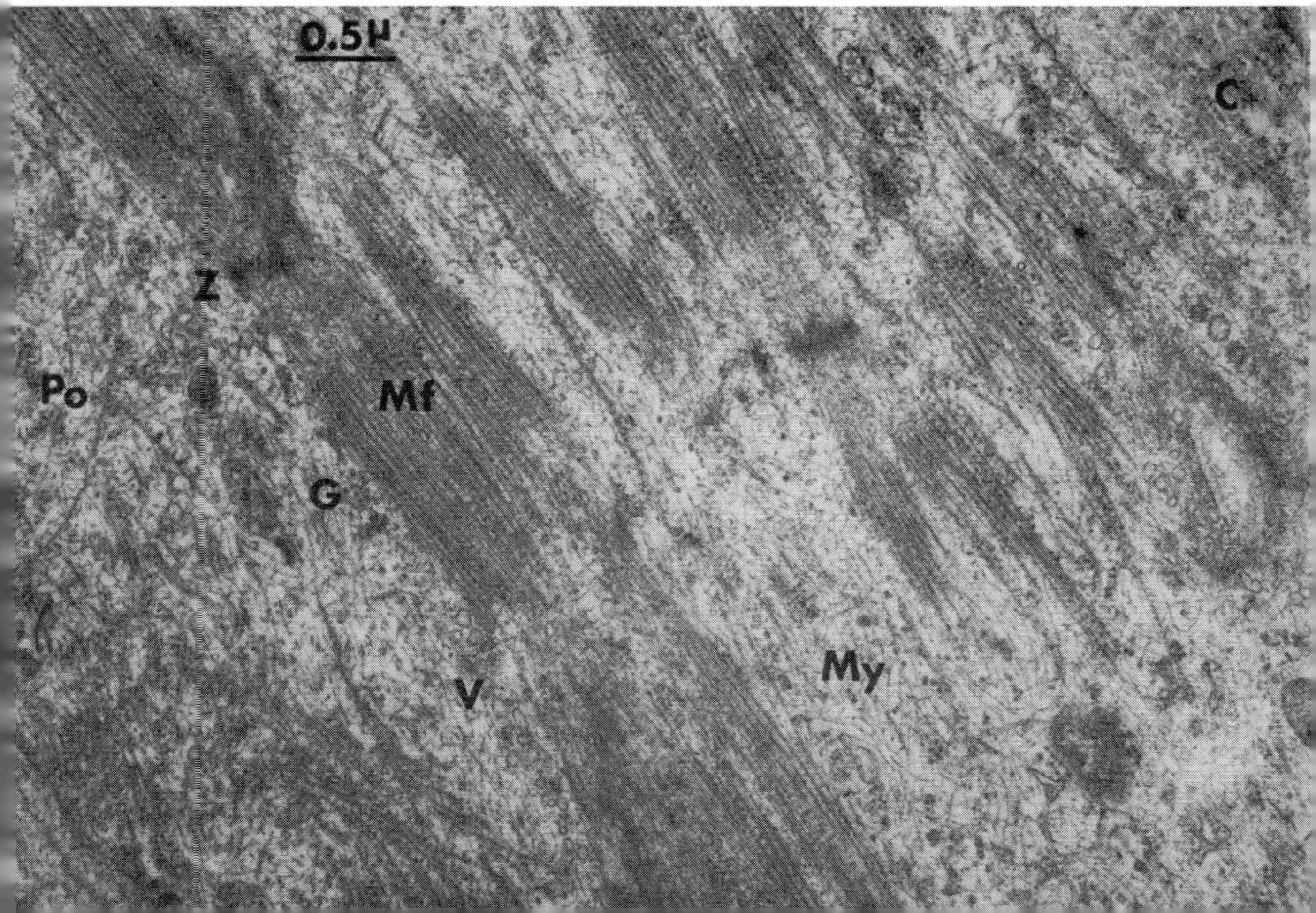
0.5μ
C
Z
Po
Mf
G
V
My

PLATE 53. REGENERATION OF MUSCLE

UPPER. The muscle fibre shows between the myofibrils an increased amount of sarcoplasm containing glycogen granules, polysomes and flattened tubules of the Golgi apparatus. It is difficult to be certain what these alterations in the sarcoplasm imply, whether it be degeneration or regeneration.

MAGNIFICATION 28,000 ×.

LOWER. Similar activity of the satellite cell cytoplasm may occur where the abundance of ribosomes and polysomes is evident as well as the presence of flattened tubules of the Golgi apparatus and the vesicles associated with it. Mitochondria are also relatively numerous. This activity of the satellite cell suggests that it may be differentiating into a more mature form. In the muscle fibre is a vacuole containing granular material.

MAGNIFICATION 36,000 ×.

From two different patients with polymyositis.

G	Glycogen	Po	Polysomes
Go	Golgi apparatus	R	Ribosomes
LB	Lipid body	S	Satellite cell
Mi	Mitochondria	Tr	Triad
MF	Muscle fibre	Va	Vacuole
N	Nucleus		

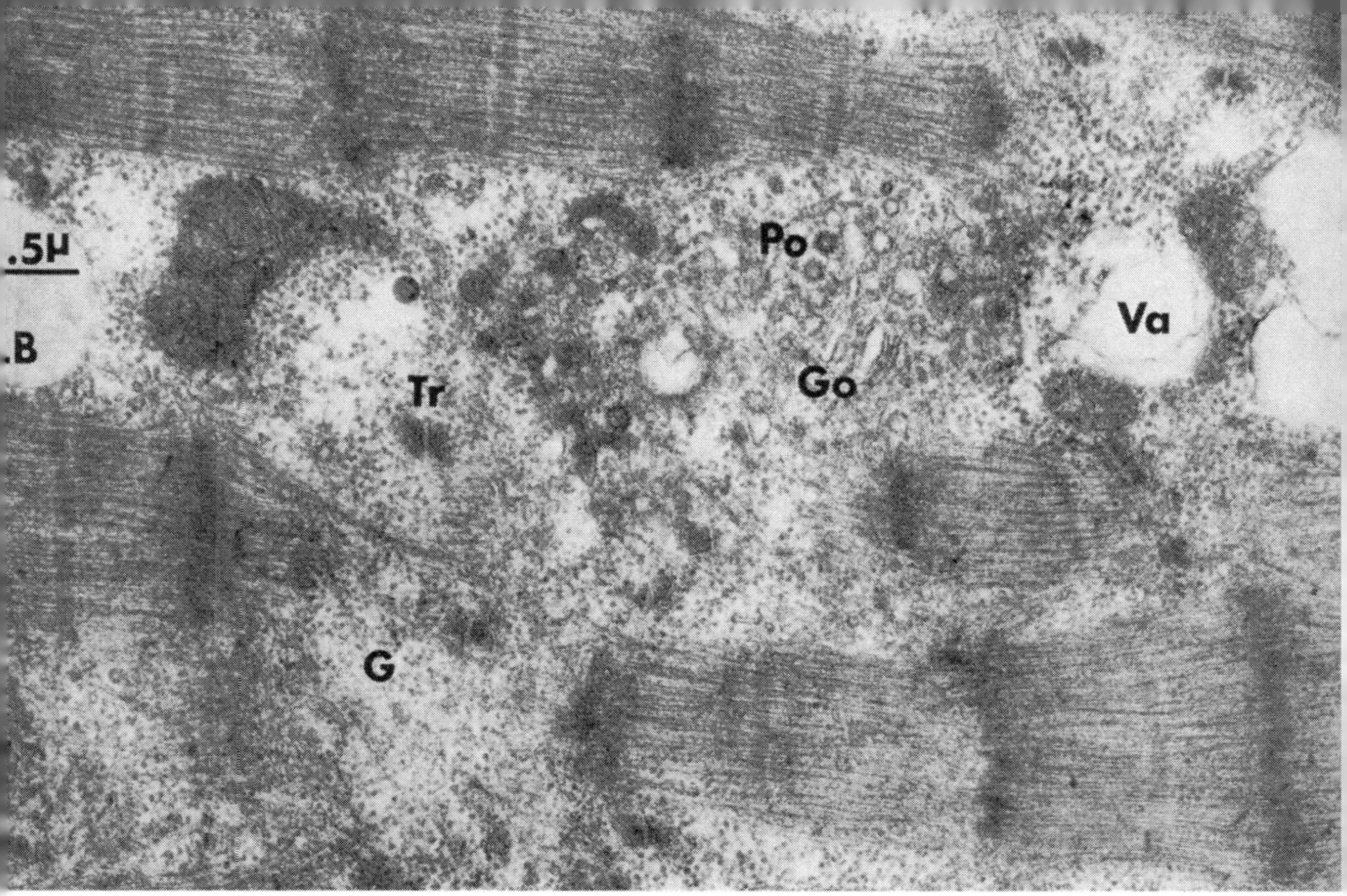

.5μ
.B
Po
Va
Tr
Go
G

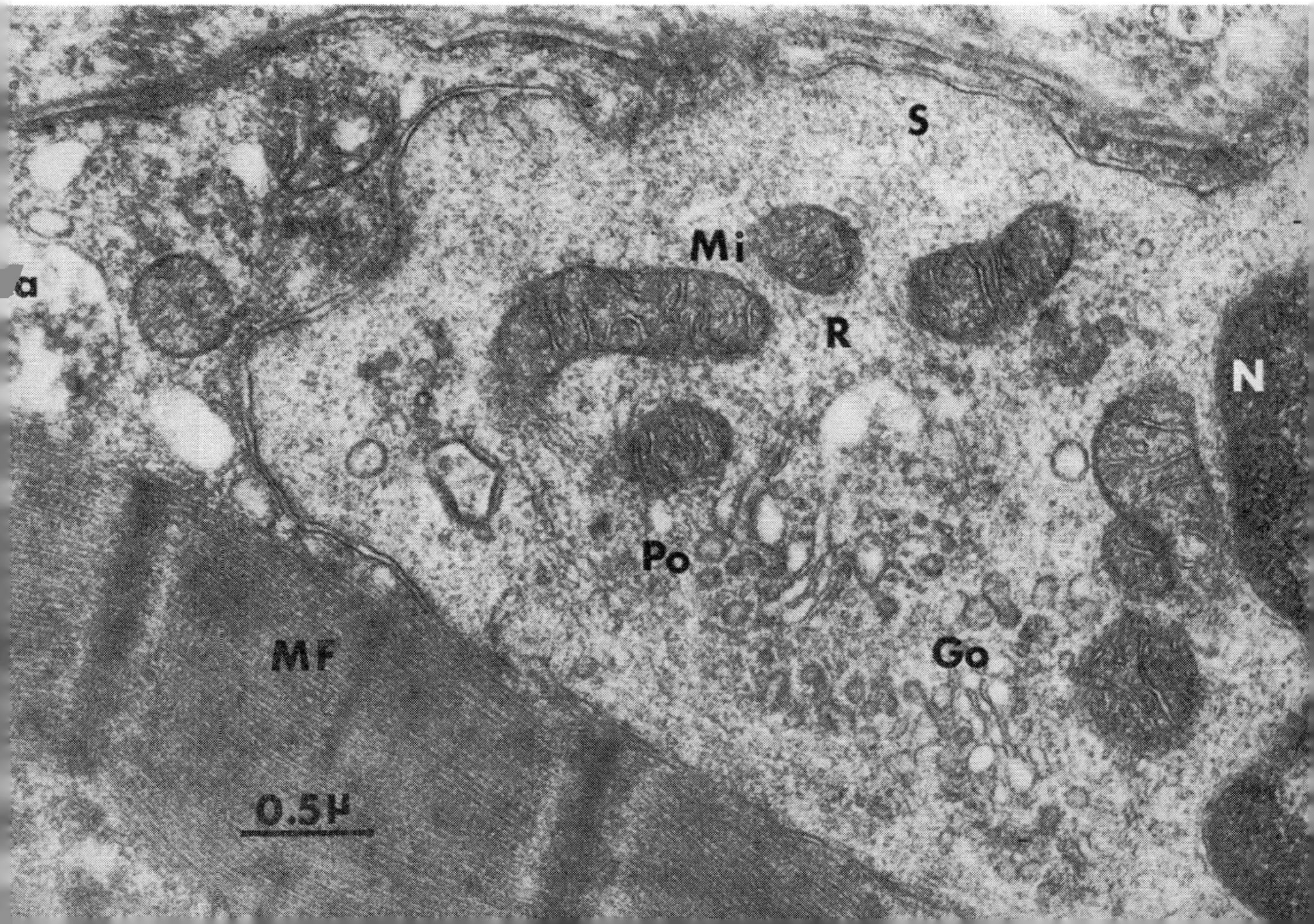

S
Mi
a
R
N
Tr
Po
Go
MF
0.5μ

PLATE 54. REGENERATION OF MUSCLE

UPPER. Collagen and fine filaments lie between a phagocyte at the top of the illustration and a muscle fibre. Within the basement membrane of the fibre lies a satellite cell containing numerous fine filaments. No basement membrane intervenes between the apposed plasma membranes of the satellite and the muscle fibre.

MAGNIFICATION 16,000 ×.

From a patient with rheumatoid arthritis and polymyositis.

LOWER. Within a common basement membrane lie two cells, each of them containing well-differentiated myofibrils, ribosomes and polysomes. In addition the upper cell, a differentiating satellite cell, contains rough endoplasmic reticulum as do developing foetal muscle fibres. The arrowed adjacent plasma membranes have no basement membrane between them.

MAGNIFICATION 17,000 ×.

Muscle from a patient with dermatomyositis.

C	Collagen	Ph	Phagocyte
Fi	Filaments	Po	Polysome
Mf	Myofibril	RER	Rough endoplasmic reticulum
MF	Muscle fibre	S	Satellite cell

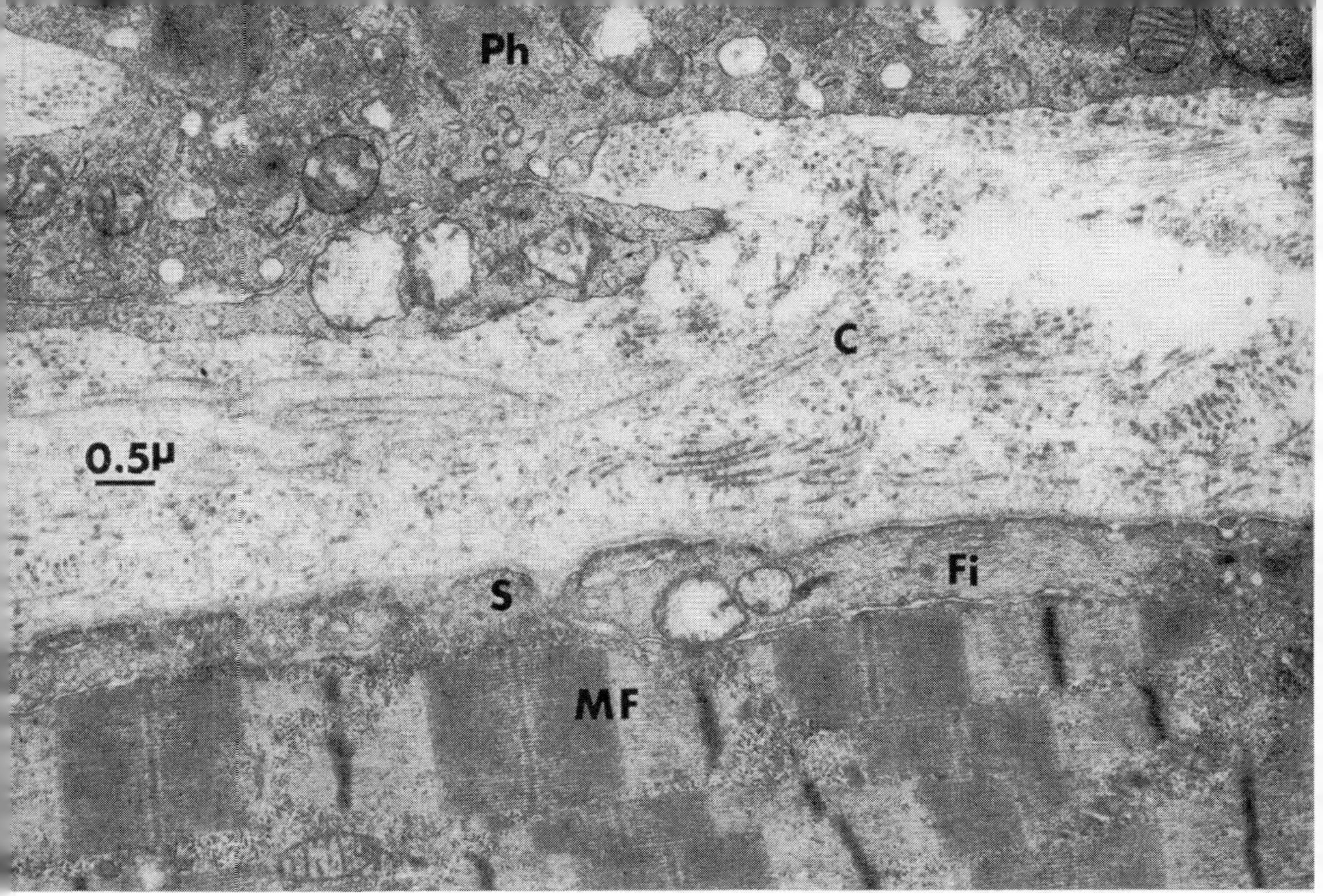
Ph
C
0.5μ
S
Fi
MF

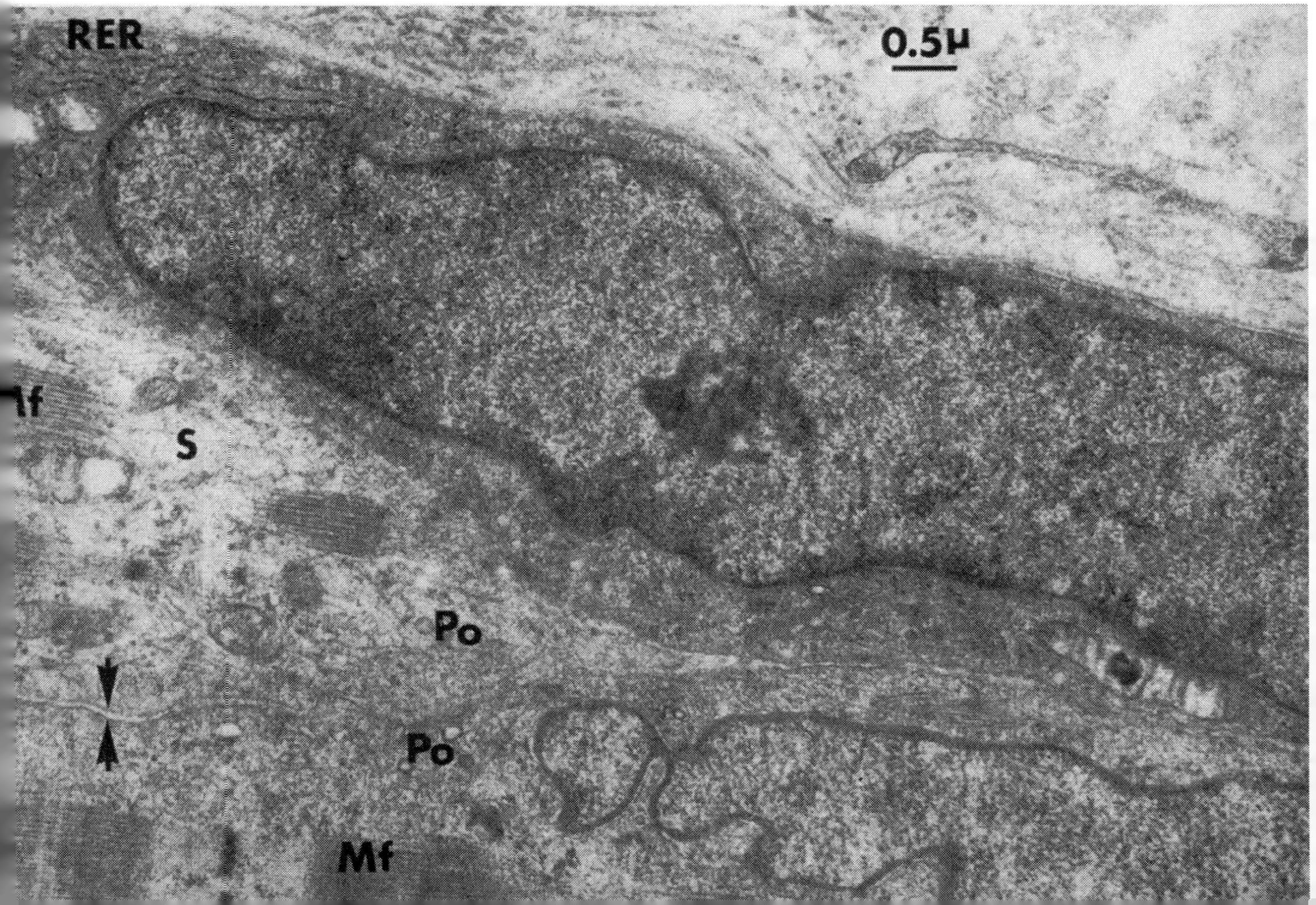
RER
0.5μ
S
Po
Po
Mf

PLATE 55. REGENERATION OF MUSCLE

UPPER. Satellite cells occur frequently in inflammatory diseases of muscle and more than one satellite may accompany one muscle fibre as illustrated here. Basement membrane does not occur between the satellite cells, nor between the satellites and the muscle fibre; the two satellites and the muscle fibre have a common basement membrane. The cytoplasm of the satellites contains mitochondria, rough endoplasmic reticulum and numerous granules. A phagocyte is located amongst the collagen between the two adjacent muscle fibres.

MAGNIFICATION 17,000 ×.

LOWER. Within a common basement membrane lie two muscle fibres and a satellite cell. The muscle fibres have well-differentiated myofibrils. One of the muscle fibres is of small diameter with sarcoplasm rich in polysomes and containing some lipid material, a readily identifiable triad and some mitochondria. The nucleus of the satellite almost fills the transverse section of the cell. Its cytoplasm contains a prominent Golgi apparatus, some mitochondria and some rough endoplasmic reticulum. The occurrence of the satellite and the small muscle fibre within the same basement membrane as the more mature muscle fibre imply regeneration of muscle. Collagen, granular material and a leucocyte lie outside the muscle fibre.

MAGNIFICATION 10,000 ×.

Both are from a patient with dermatomyositis.

BM Basement membrane
C Collagen
Go Golgi apparatus
Le Leucocyte
MF Muscle fibre
Ph Phagocyte
PM Plasma membrane
RER Rough endoplasmic reticulum
S Satellite cell

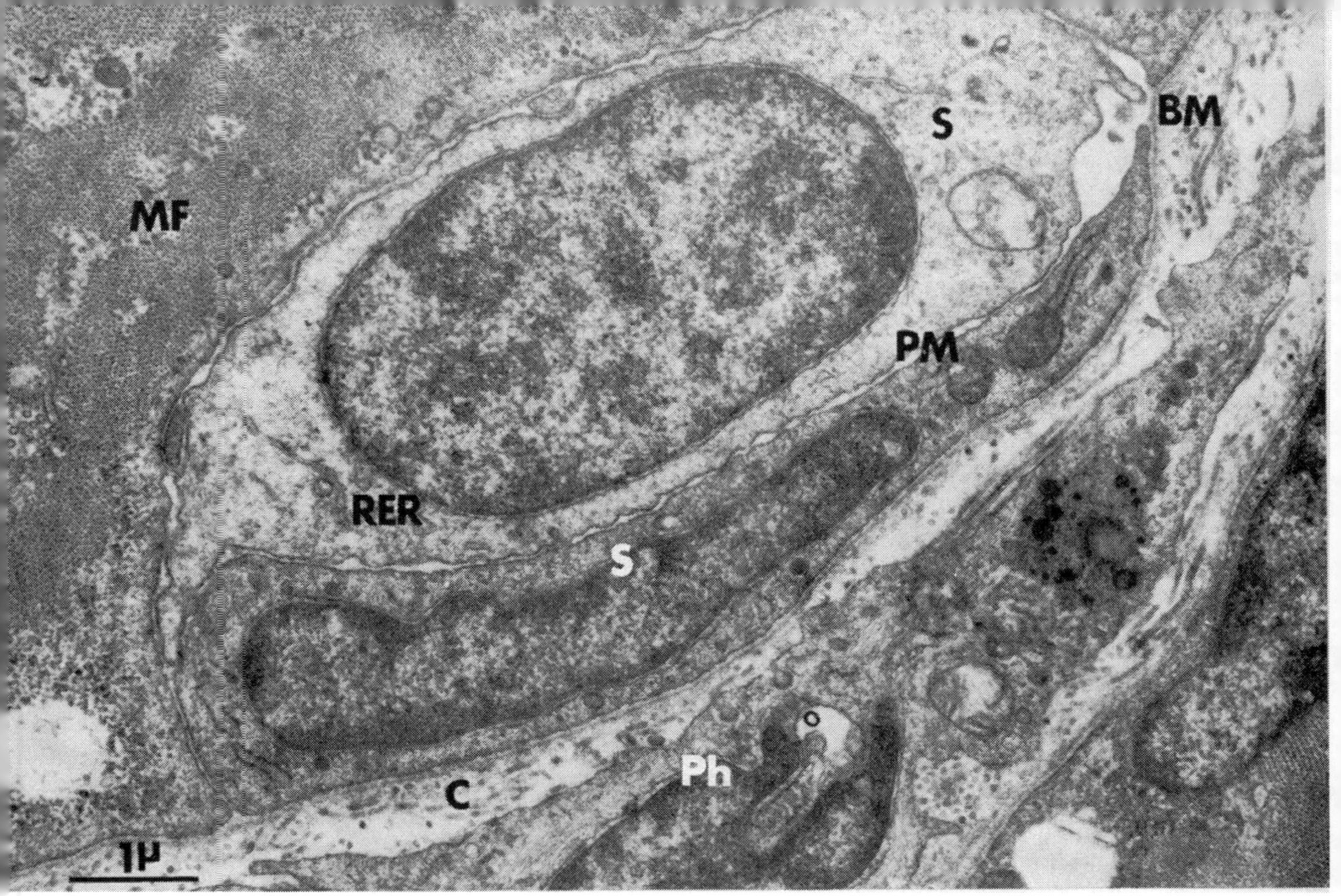
MF
S
BM
PM
RER
S
Ph
C
1μ

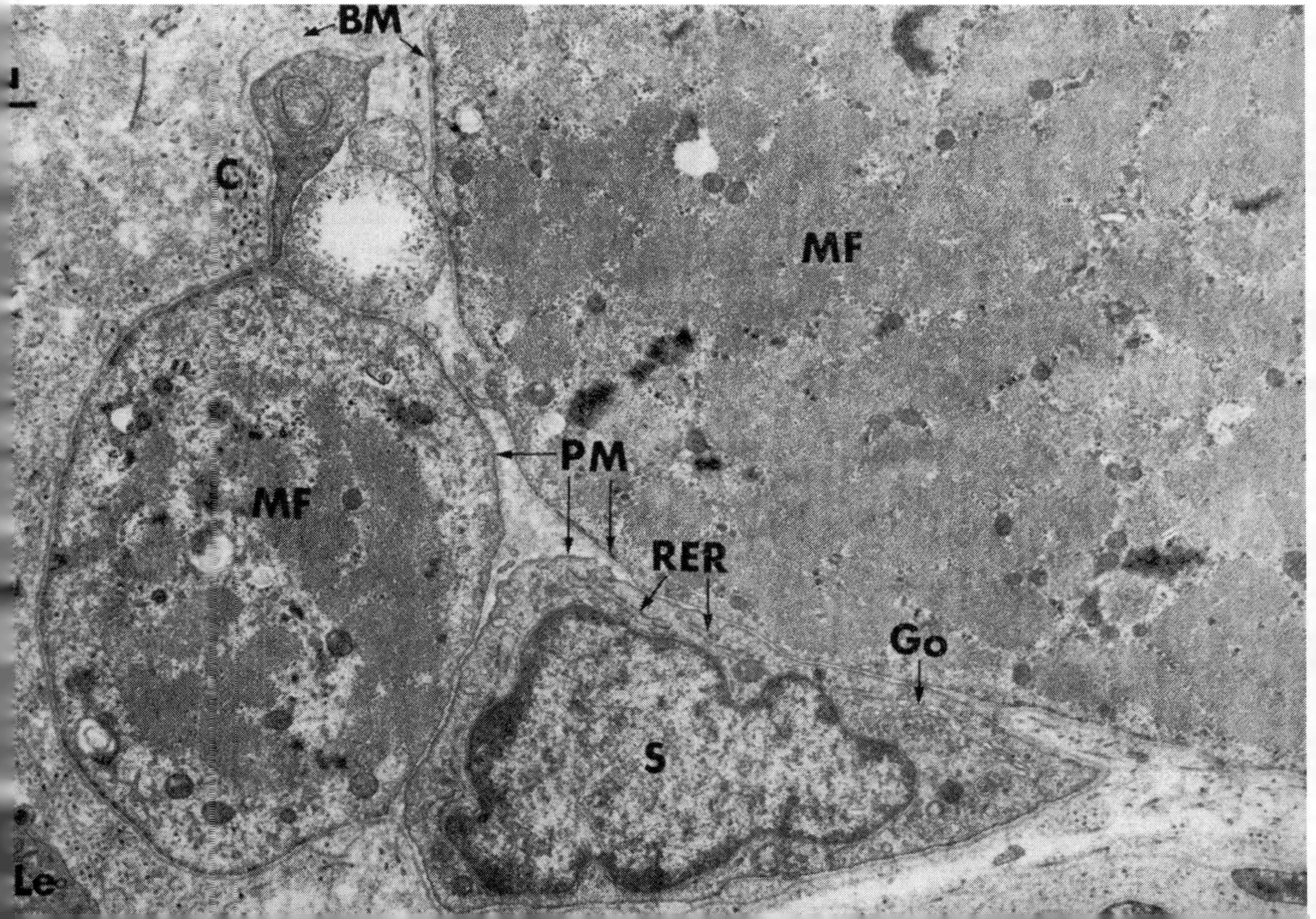
BM
C
MF
PM
MF
RER
Go
S
Le

CHAPTER 3

Changes in Blood Capillaries and Interstitial Tissue of Muscle

BLOOD CAPILLARIES

The blood vessels which supply the muscles may be affected in any of the diseases which involve the vascular system. The most striking changes in the *blood capillaries* are met in polymyositis and allied conditions in which they increase markedly in number and undergo structural changes. All the elements which take part in their formation, namely the endothelial cells, basement membrane and pericytes, may exhibit changes.

The endothelial cells undergo hypertrophy and hyperplasia and in such circumstances exhibit a great increase in number of pinocytotic vesicles at their margins and throughout their cytoplasm (Plates 56 and 58). Tiny depressions on the free edge of the endothelial cells and projections of their cytoplasm which may rejoin the endothelial cell cytoplasm (Plate 58) may be more numerous than in the normal capillaries (p. 6). Besides numerous pinocytotic vesicles, large vacuoles (Plate 76), some of them autophagic vacuoles containing material of various shapes and electron density, may occur in the endothelial cells.

The nucleus of the endothelial cell becomes much larger in size and may be irregular in shape, having several indentations on its surface. The chromatin is most dense around the periphery of the nucleus, the outer membrane of which may be very apparent. Near the nucleus lie numerous tubules of the Golgi apparatus, some of them distended, and, in addition, centrioles may be found in their neighbourhood as illustrated in cross section in Plate 56 and in longitudinal section in Plate 57. The centrioles may be more readily observed in conditions where proliferation of the endothelial cells takes place as they play an important role in cell division.

The number of mitochondria in the endothelial cells is not usually marked. Some of those present may show alterations of their cristae and the formation of membranous bodies as illustrated in the muscle of a patient with muscular dystrophy of the Duchenne type (Plate 58). In this same illustration is a lipid body with a laminated pattern. Osmophilic bodies which may be lipid in nature may be very prominent in the endothelial cell cytoplasm, especially in inflammatory conditions as illustrated in the muscle of a patient with polymyositis (Plate 59 lower part).

The capillary is lined with a single layer of endothelial cells. Adjacent endothelial cells lie in close apposition without any intervening spaces. Areas of the plasma membrane of adjacent cells show thickening of the plasma membrane and increased electron density (Plate 58): these are the desmosomes. Besides the increase in size of individual cells, the number of cells constituting the single endothelial cell layer of capillary endothelium may be greatly increased, especially in inflammatory diseases (Plate 59).

The basement membrane which is closely applied to the outer surface of the endothelial cells may be increased in thickness (Plate 57) and may exhibit reduplication (Plate 59), which is very common in inflammatory conditions. Numerous pericytes appear in the clefts in the basement membrane (Plates 57, 75 and 76).

The ultrastructure of the vascular changes in polymyositis was reported by Shafiq, Milhorat and Gorycki (1967a) and by several others.

The changes in the basement membrane of the intramuscular blood capillaries are prominent in diabetes mellitus as has been reported by Zacks, Pegues and Elliott (1962), Bencosme *et al.* (1966), Siperstein, Unger and Madison (1968), Naccarato *et al.* (1970) and Vracko (1970a). Kniffen and Quick (1970) reported on the intramuscular blood capillaries in patients with amyotrophic lateral sclerosis and diabetes: in both groups there occurs similar thickening of the basement membrane, but this was not so in some other neuromuscular diseases studied by these authors.

LEUCOCYTIC INFILTRATION AND PHAGOCYTOSIS OF THE MUSCLE FIBRES

Leucocytic infiltration and phagocytosis of the muscle fibres is seen predominantly in inflammatory conditions which affect the muscle where leucocytes may lie in collections around the blood capillaries. Various types of leucocytes may occur in these collections as demonstrated in Plates 60, 61, 62, 75 and 77. Leucocytes may be seen occasionally in muscular dystrophy (Plate 73) and also in denervation atrophy of the muscle. The cytoplasm of some leucocytes is rich in lysosomes and vacuoles, containing bodies of various form and electron density: these are the phagocytes. In some of them pseudopodia may be very evident as illustrated in Plates 63 and 84.

Most workers describe the leucocytes as being devoid of basement membrane: they have, however, a distinct plasma membrane.

Different types of leucocytes may be identified at various stages in the inflammatory process. In the early stages polymorphonuclear leucocytes are common and are easily identified by their lobed nucleus. The predominant feature of their cytoplasm is the abundance of dense granules of varying size and shape which are thought to be lysosomes: the Golgi apparatus may be very apparent, many mitochondria may occur and numerous pseudopodia may extend from the cell body as illustrated in the uppermost part of Plate 60. Eosinophil polymorphs sometimes occur in the muscle, particularly in collagen diseases. They are identified in electron micrographs by the presence of elliptical or round membrane bound granules of larger dimensions (0·3 to 1·2 μ) than those of the neutrophil polymorphs as illustrated in the lower left of Plate 60 and upper part of Plate 62. In human eosinophils as in other mammals, crystalline inclusions were demonstrated inside the granules by Miller, de Harven and Pallade (1966). Basophil polymorphs are rarely found in muscle biopsies. They have membrane bound granules of various size, some large up to 0·8 μ in diameter and may contain crystalline inclusions (Watanabe, Donahue and Hoggatt, 1967). Lymphocytes are identified by their relatively large rounded nucleus compared with their small amount of cytoplasm which may contain mitochondria and small electron dense bodies. The nucleus often contains a nucleolus as illustrated in Plate 60 (upper part). Plasma cells are commonly found in subacute or chronic inflammatory muscle disorders. The plasma cells (Plate 61) have a typical rounded, eccentric nucleus with the chromatin disposed in dense masses around its periphery. The cytoplasm is relatively large in amount and contains many concentric or parallel layers of rough endoplasmic reticulum, amongst which may occur large mitochondria, rough coated vesicles and the Golgi apparatus. In some of the plasma cells large vacuoles may occur which contain rounded or irregular shaped electron dense material as illustrated in the lower part of Plate 61. Mast cells whose cytoplasm is filled with typical large, round, membrane bound bodies as illustrated in the lower part of Plate 60 may be found in subacute and chronic inflammatory processes of muscle. Many of the mononucleated cells as those unlabelled in the lower part of Plate 60 are difficult to classify. The leucocytes multiply by mitotic division as illustrated in the lower part of Plate 62.

Leucocytes with phagocytic properties may lie in close proximity to muscle fibres which show early evidence of degenerative change. Where the phagocytes and the muscle fibres lie in close contact, the basement membrane of the muscle fibre may disappear but persists over the rest of the muscle fibre as illustrated in the upper part of Plate 63. However, it is much more common to find phagocytes already within degenerating muscle fibres and the plasma membrane of these fibres has already disappeared, but their basement membrane persists as is illustrated in the lower part of Plate 63 and in Plate 73.

Phagocytosis of the muscle fibre is common in inflammatory diseases of muscle, but may occur also in other conditions such as muscular dystrophy as is illustrated in Plate 73.

FIBROBLASTS AND COLLAGEN

Increased activity of the *fibroblasts* between the muscle fibres and in the neighbourhood of the vessels and nerves within muscles is most apparent in inflammatory conditions. The fibroblasts increase in size and their cytoplasm contains more rough endoplasmic reticulum and mitochondria than normal. The number of fibroblasts also increases. Associated with the increase in activity of the fibroblasts is the deposition of an increased amount of *collagen*. In addition to the strands of collagen there appears, particularly in inflammatory conditions, a considerable amount of amorphous material which may be a precursor of collagen (Plates 40 and 51 lower part). In muscular dystrophy and denervation of muscle (Plates 34 and 69) the increased activity of the fibroblasts and the deposition of large amounts of collagen is generally much less striking. Only in the Duchenne type of muscular dystrophy is there a marked degree of fibroblast proliferation with accompanying increase in collagen production as illustrated in Plate 70 lower part.

AMYLOID FIBRILS

In primary amyloid neuropathy, a familial disease which was described first by Andrade (1952), there occur amongst the strands of collagen between the muscle fibres, collections of *amyloid fibrils* as illustrated in Plate 64. The amyloid fibrils found between muscle fibres in amyloid neuropathy are similar to those found in other tissues and are about 100 Å thick, but their thickness may vary from 50 to 250 Å (Hirschl, 1969). We did not find any amyloid fibrils within the muscle fibres, but they are found in the nerves.

PLATE 56. CENTRIOLE IN THE ENDOTHELIAL CELL OF AN INTRAMUSCULAR BLOOD CAPILLARY

UPPER. A blood capillary between two muscle fibres presents hyperplastic endothelial cells which contain numerous vesicles. Numerous tubules of the Golgi apparatus lie near the nucleus and in addition a well-defined centriole seen in cross section with nine sets of tubules around its periphery. Pericyte cytoplasm lies in the clefts of the basement membrane around the capillary. A fibroblast close by the capillary contains numerous polysomes. A muscle fibre with an aggregation of mitochondria near its surface lies at the bottom of the illustration.

MAGNIFICATION 16,000 ×.

LOWER. Part of the nucleus, the centriole, the Golgi apparatus and vesicles are seen at higher magnification.

MAGNIFICATION 63,000 ×.

From a patient with Behçet's disease with neuropathy.

BC	Blood capillary	Mi	Mitochondria
BM	Basement membrane	Pe	Pericyte
Ce	Centriole	Po	Polysomes
E	Endothelial cell	N	Nucleus
F	Fibroblast	V	Vesicles
Go	Golgi apparatus		

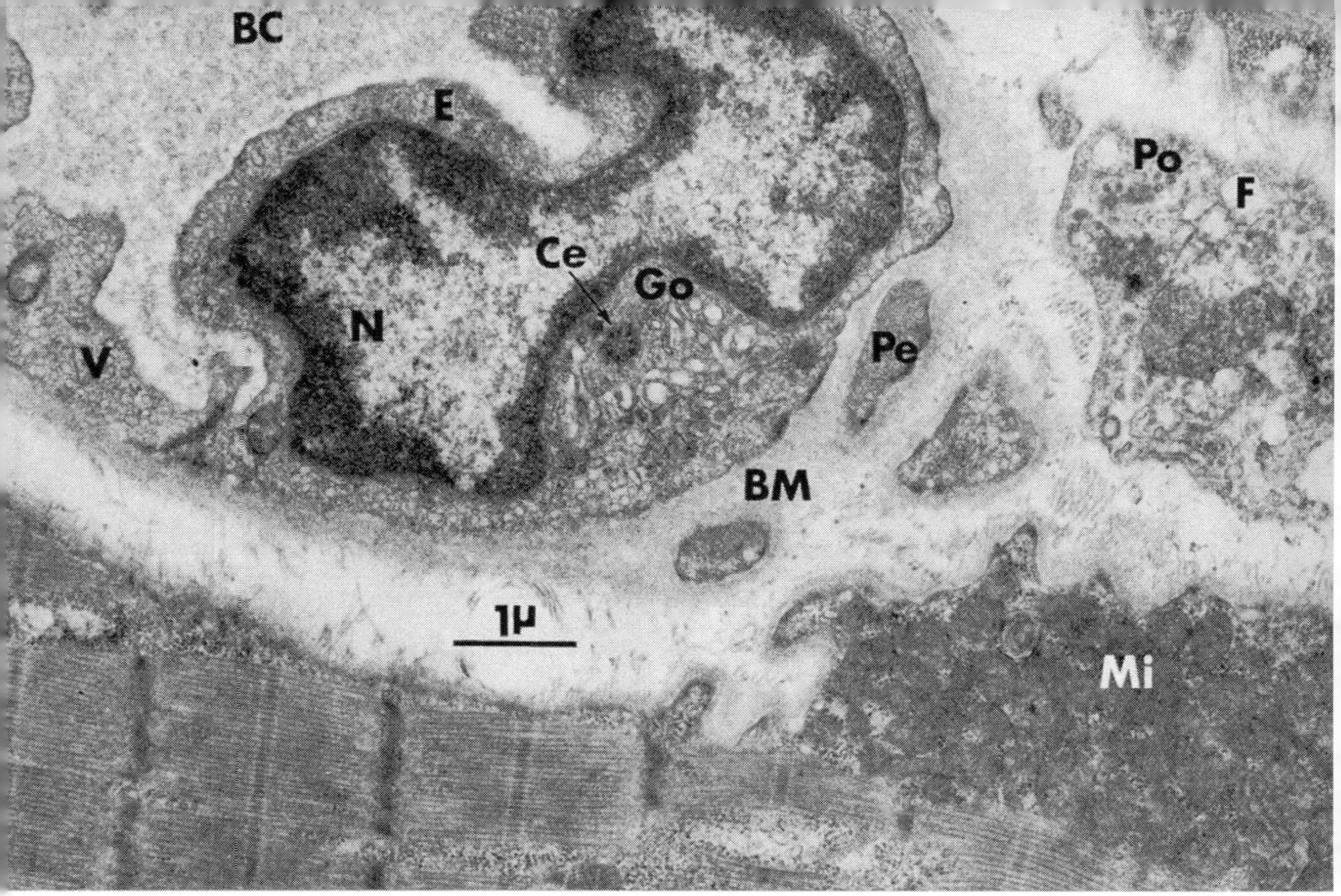
BC
E
Po
F
Ce
Go
N
V
Pe
BM
1μ
Mi

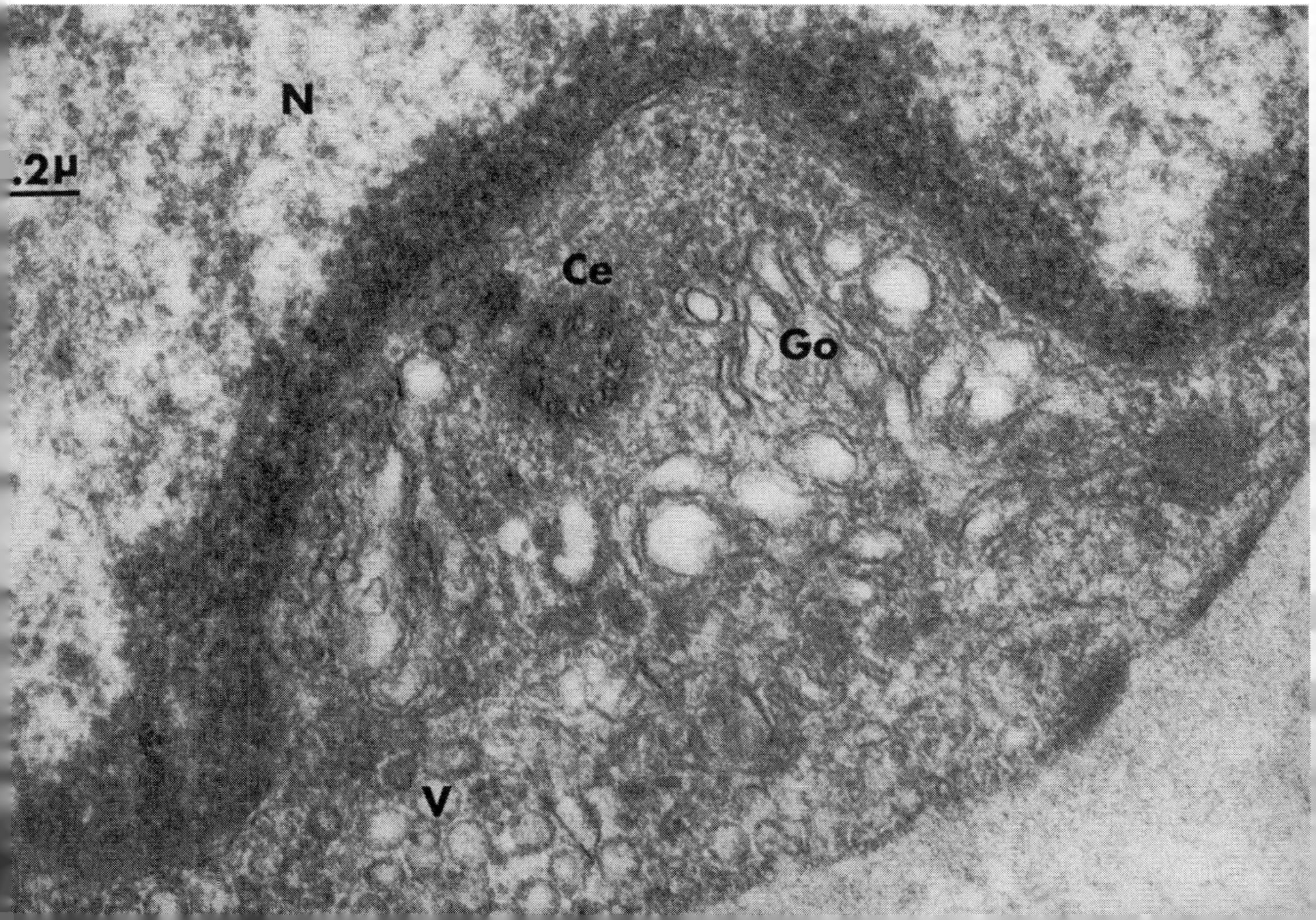
N
.2μ
Ce
Go
V

PLATE 57. CENTRIOLES IN THE ENDOTHELIAL CELL OF AN INTRAMUSCULAR BLOOD CAPILLARY

UPPER. A blood capillary between muscle fibres is covered by a much thicker layer of basement membrane than normal and in places is reduplicated. The endothelial cells are hypertrophied and contain many vesicles. One exhibits a prominent Golgi apparatus and two centrioles cut longitudinally. The clefts in the basement membrane contain pericyte cytoplasm: a red blood corpuscle is present in the capillary lumen. Collagen and basement membrane folds surround the muscle fibre above the blood capillary.

MAGNIFICATION 12,000 ×.

LOWER. The nucleus, Golgi apparatus and the centriole are seen at higher magnification.

MAGNIFICATION 42,000 ×.

From a patient with polyneuropathy of unknown aetiology.

BM	Basement membrane	MF	Muscle fibre
C	Collagen	N	Nucleus
Ce	Centriole	Pe	Pericyte
Go	Golgi apparatus	RBC	Red blood corpuscle

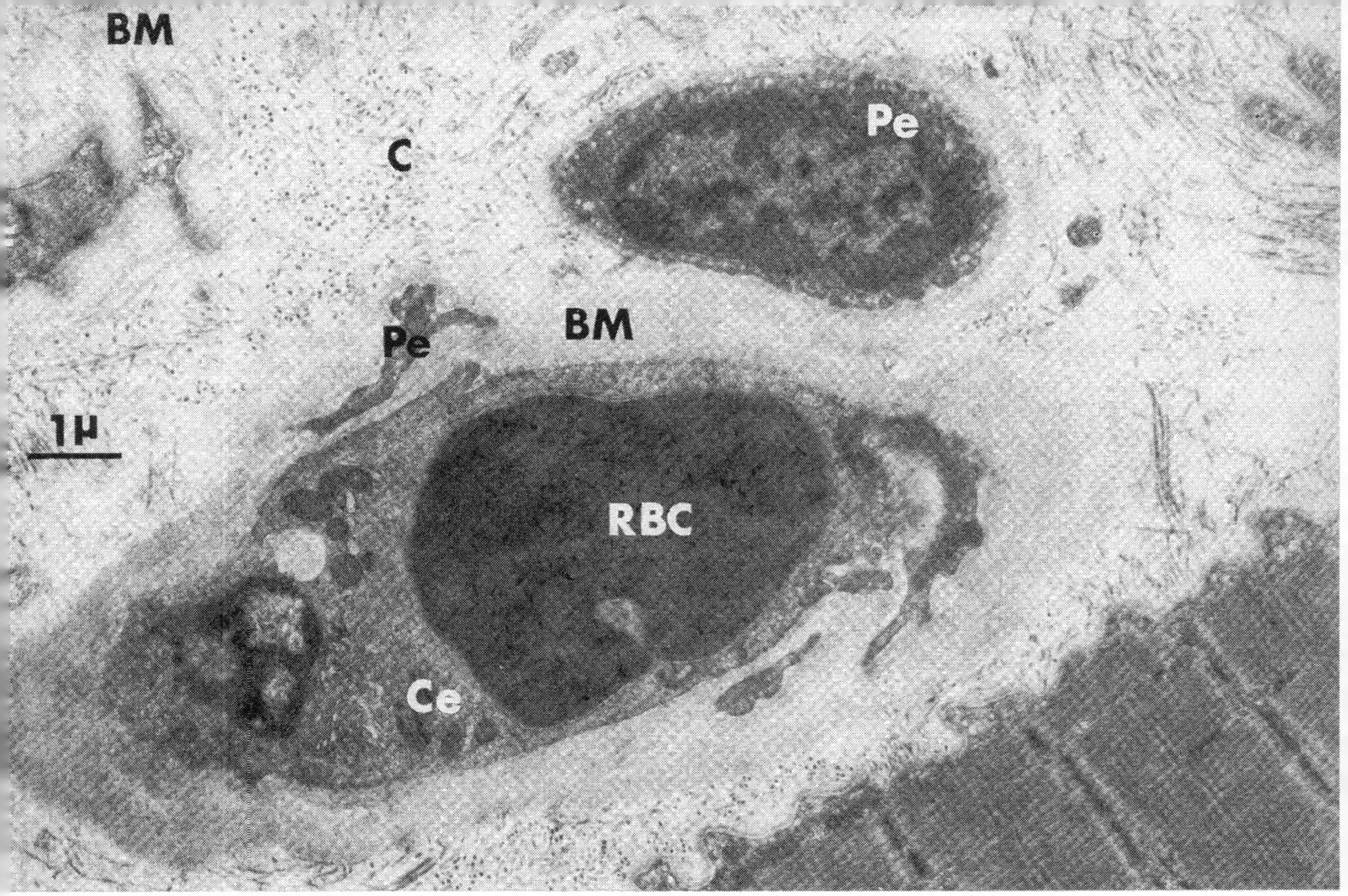
BM
C
Pe
Pe
BM
1μ
RBC
Ce

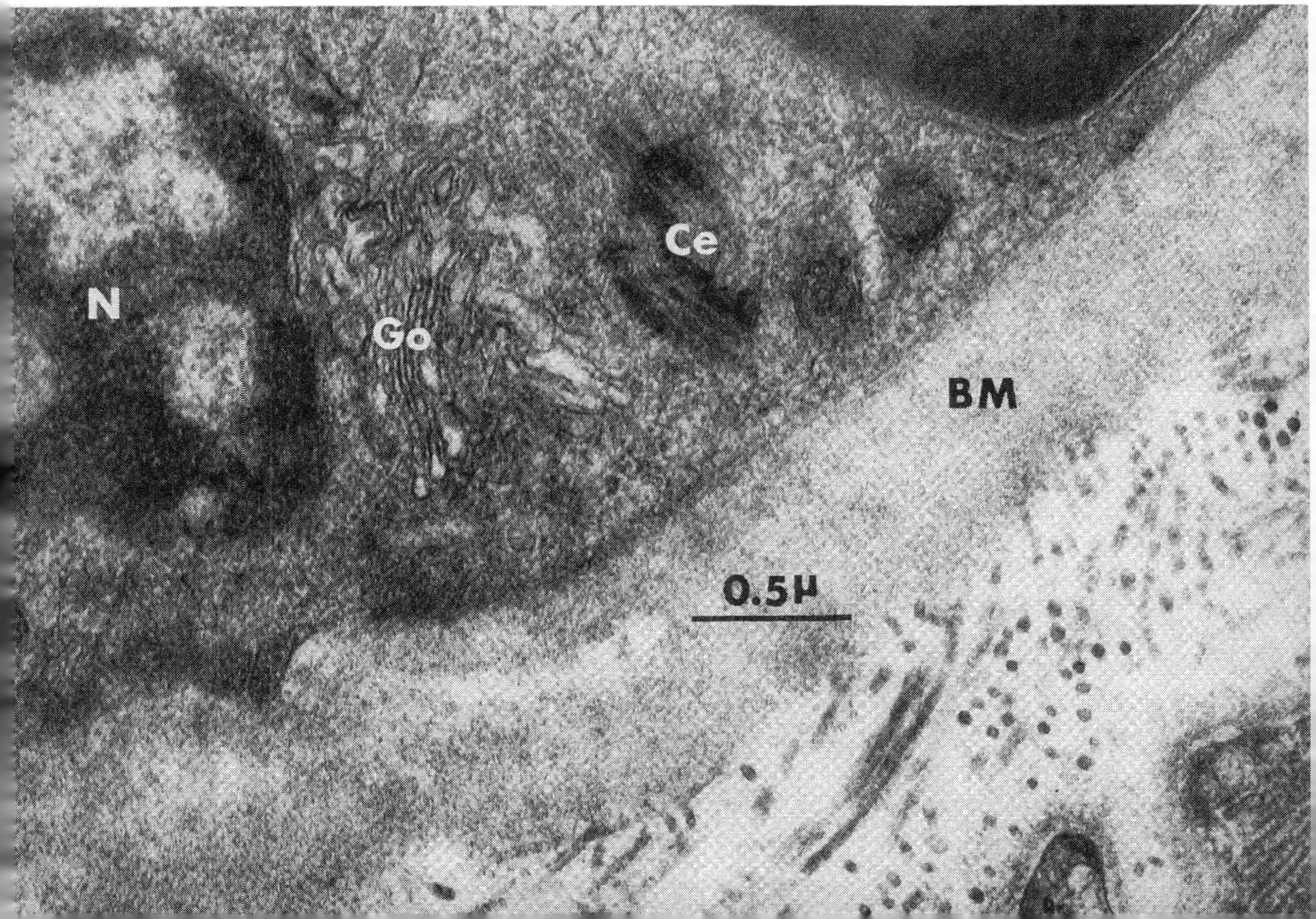
N
Go
Ce
BM
0.5μ

PLATE 58. LAMINATED LIPID INCLUSION IN THICKENED CAPILLARY ENDOTHELIUM

A blood capillary close by a muscle fibre is lined by two endothelial cells: one is cut through its nucleus. The plasma membranes at the junction of the two endothelial cells show thickening and increased electron density. These electron dense areas are called desmosomes. Membranous and myelin bodies, a laminated lipid inclusion and numerous vesicles occur in the endothelial cell cytoplasm, extensions of which project into the capillary lumen. Basement membrane lies in contact with the outer surface of the endothelial cell. A cleft in the basement membrane contains cytoplasm of a pericyte. The muscle fibre below the capillary shows normal myofibrils, prominent T-systems of the triads, a considerable amount of glycogen, and indentations of the plasma membrane (arrowed) which has vesicles immediately below it. The mitochondria near the surface of the muscle fibre exhibit zones of increased electron density in their matrix.

MAGNIFICATION 20,000 ×.

The *inset*, top left, shows a higher magnification of the laminated lipid inclusion.

MAGNIFICATION 50,000 ×.

From a patient with muscular dystrophy (Duchenne type).

BM	Basement membrane	L	Lumen
D	Desmosome	Mit	Mitochondria
Ex	Extension of the endothelial cytoplasm	MB	Myelin body
F	Fibroblast	P	Pericyte
G	Glycogen	T	T-system
I	Inclusion	Ve	Vesicles

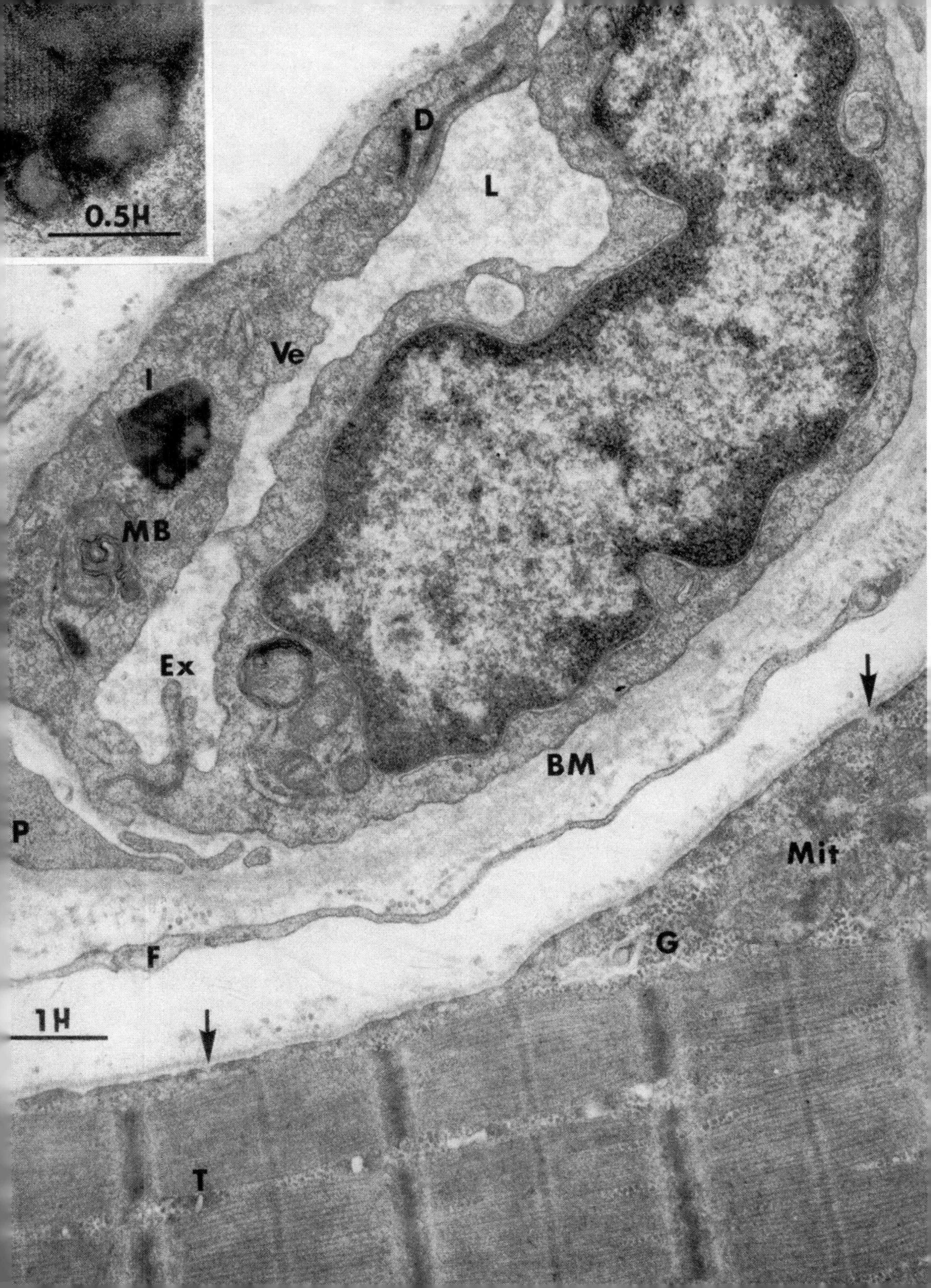
0.5μ
D
L
Ve
I
MB
Ex
BM
P
Mit
G
F
1μ
T

PLATE 59. HYPERTROPHY AND HYPERPLASIA OF THE ENDOTHELIAL CELLS OF THE BLOOD CAPILLARIES

UPPER. An intramuscular capillary shows hypertrophy and hyperplasia of the endothelial cells lining it. The cytoplasm of the cells contains some osmophilic bodies, mitochondria and a large amount of granular material. In three of the adjacent cells the nuclei are prominent. The lumen of the capillary is reduced.

MAGNIFICATION 10,500 ×.

From a patient with periarteritis nodosa.

LOWER. The endothelial cell cytoplasm of a blood capillary containing red blood corpuscles is rich in osmophilic bodies and granular material. Numerous loose folds of basement membrane surround the capillary. Between some of the spaces in the basement membrane are processes of pericytes. Collagen and fibroblast processes lie between the capillary and the degenerating muscle fibre at the bottom of the illustration.

MAGNIFICATION 5,000 ×.

From a patient with polymyositis.

BM	Basement membrane	L	Lumen
C	Collagen	P	Pericyte process
E	Endothelial cell	RBC	Red blood corpuscle
MF	Muscle fibre		

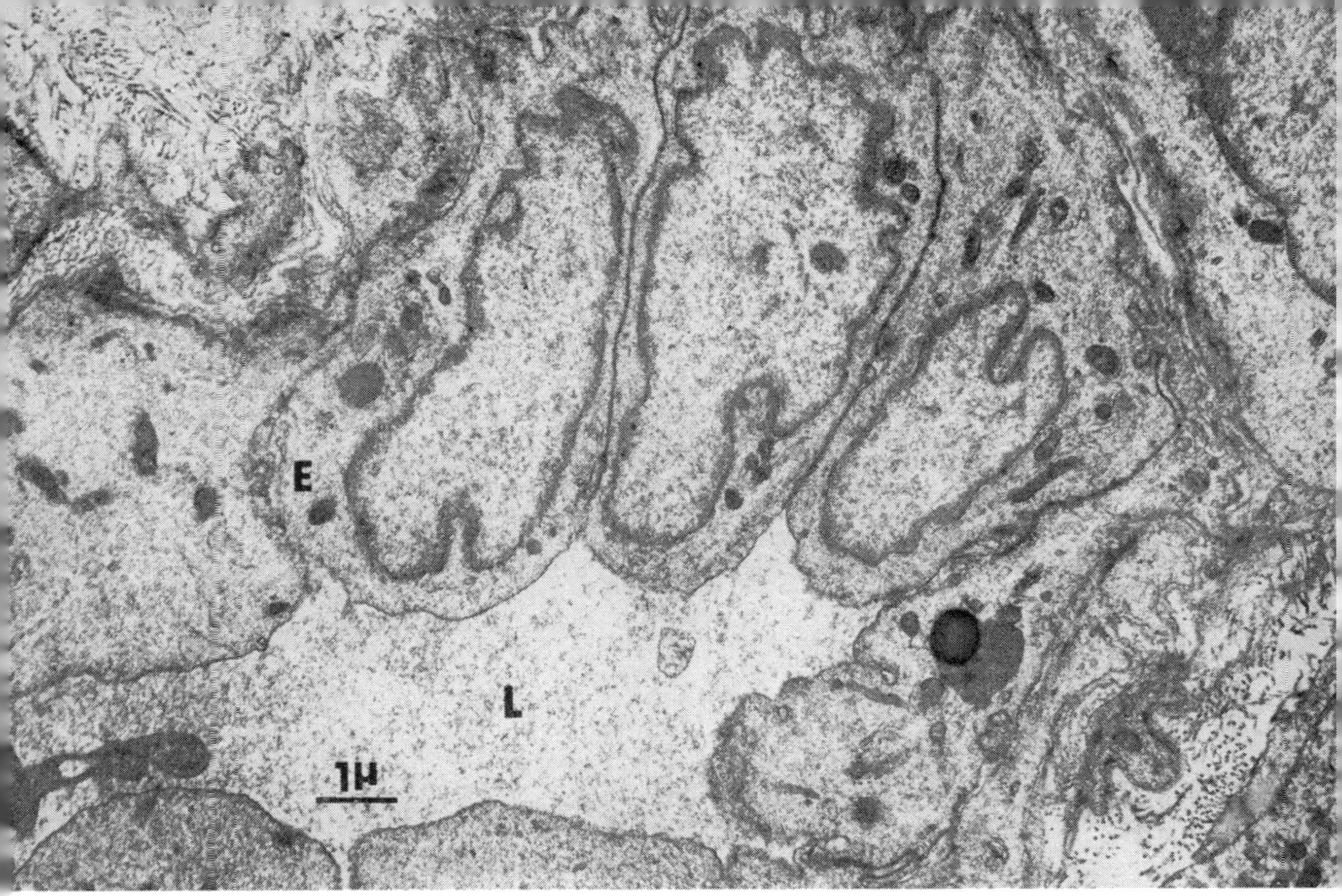
E
L
1μ

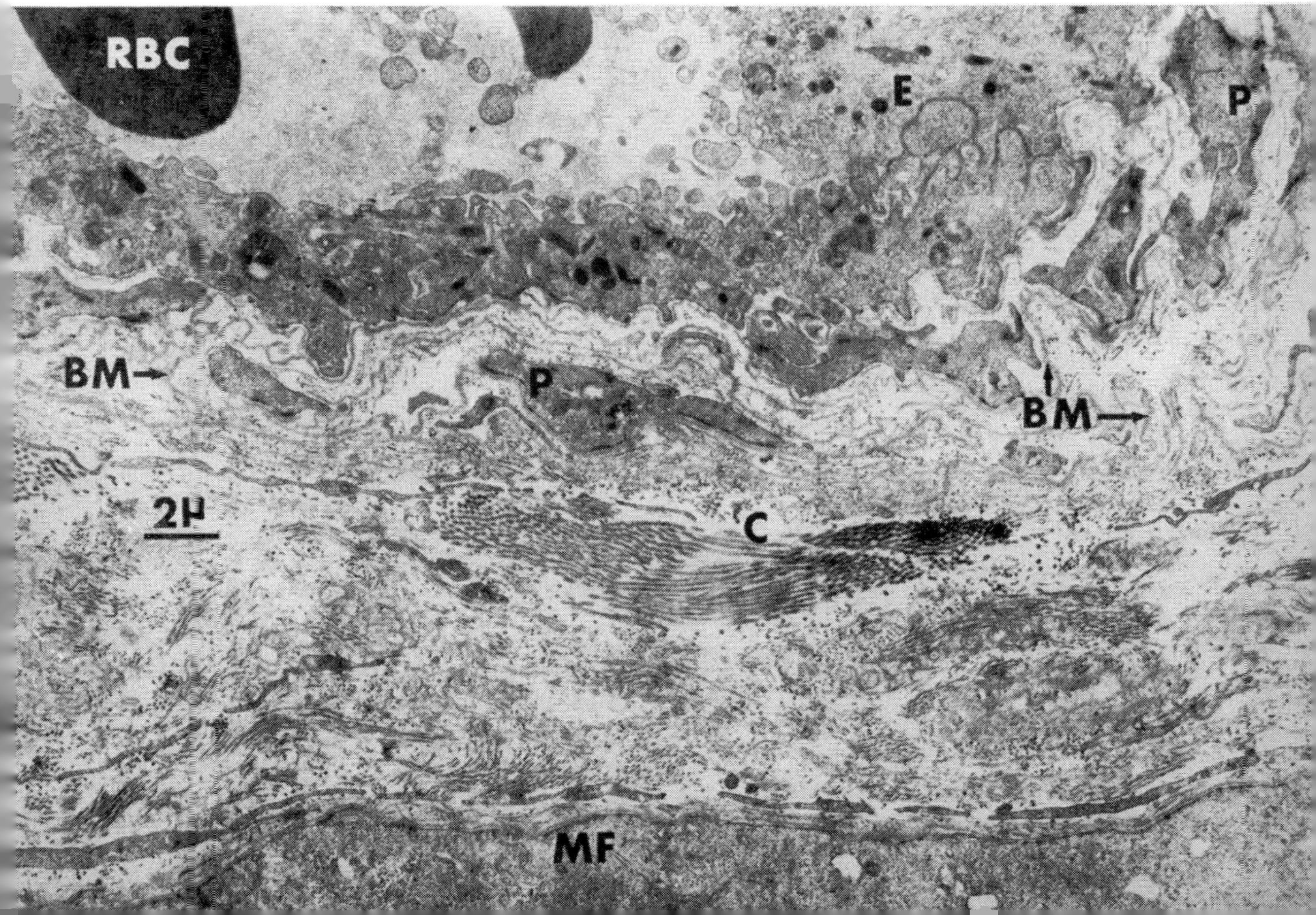
RBC
E
P
BM→
P
BM→
2μ
C
MF

PLATE 60. LEUCOCYTES IN POLYMYOSITIS

UPPER. Leucocytes occur amongst the collagen between the muscle fibres. The cell containing numerous osmophilic bodies of varying size is a neutrophil polymorph. To the left of the illustration is a lymphocyte with a round nucleus and scanty cytoplasm in which there are some varying sized osmophilic bodies. Processes of fibroblasts with prominent rough endoplasmic reticulum and mitochondria are also present.

MAGNIFICATION 5,000 ×.

LOWER. Different types of leucocytes are present in the exudate between the muscle fibres. To the left is a polymorph with numerous osmophilic bodies in its cytoplasm: it is probably an eosinophil. A plasma cell with the typical eccentric nucleus and large amount of rough endoplasmic reticulum lies adjacent to a mast cell containing numerous large, round, membrane bound bodies. Mononucleated cells which cannot be classified accurately are also present in the exudate.

MAGNIFICATION 5,000 ×.

Lym Lymphocyte
MC Mast cell
MF Muscle fibre
Poly Polymorph
PC Plasma cell

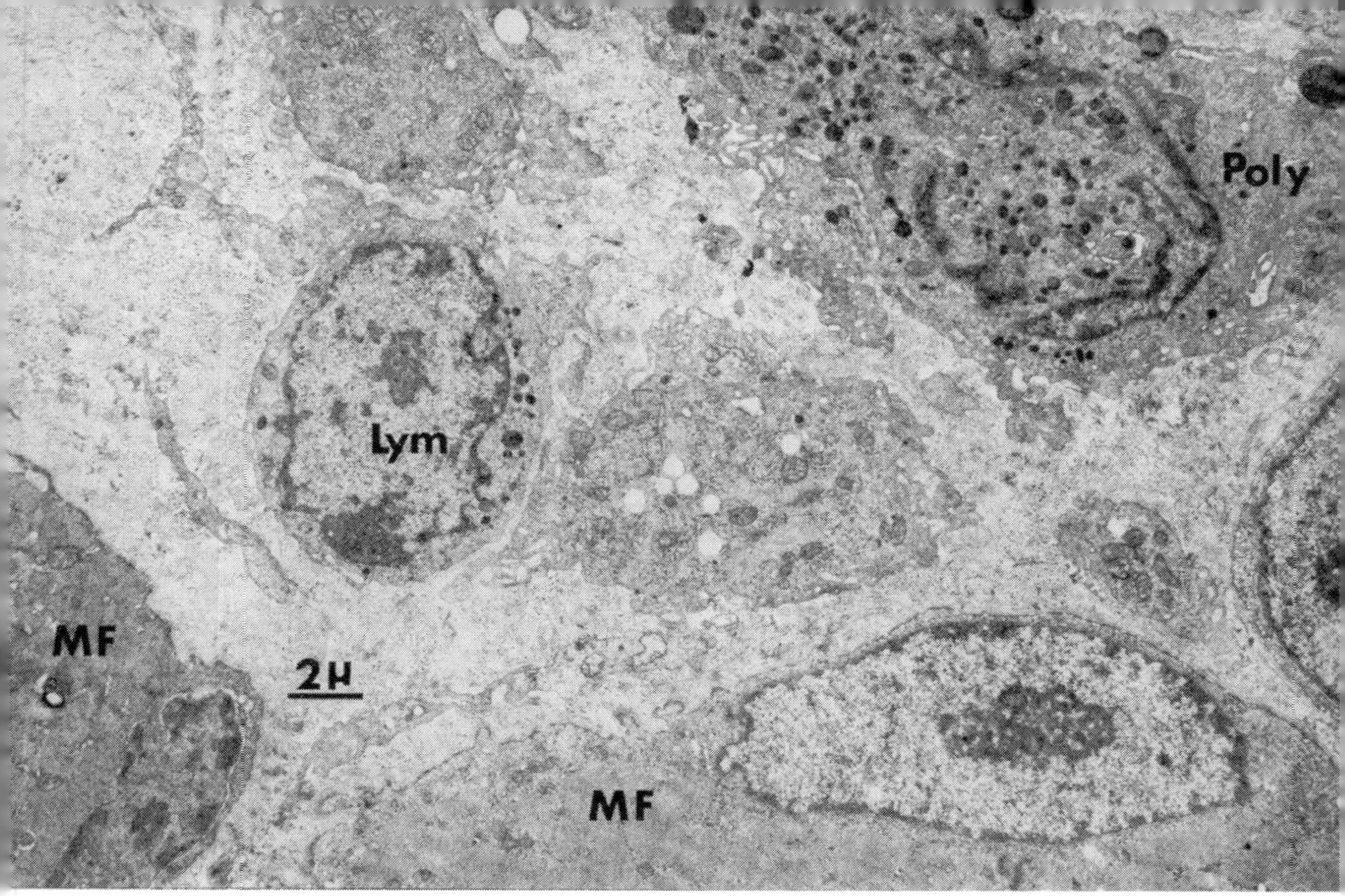
Poly
Lym
MF
2μ
MF

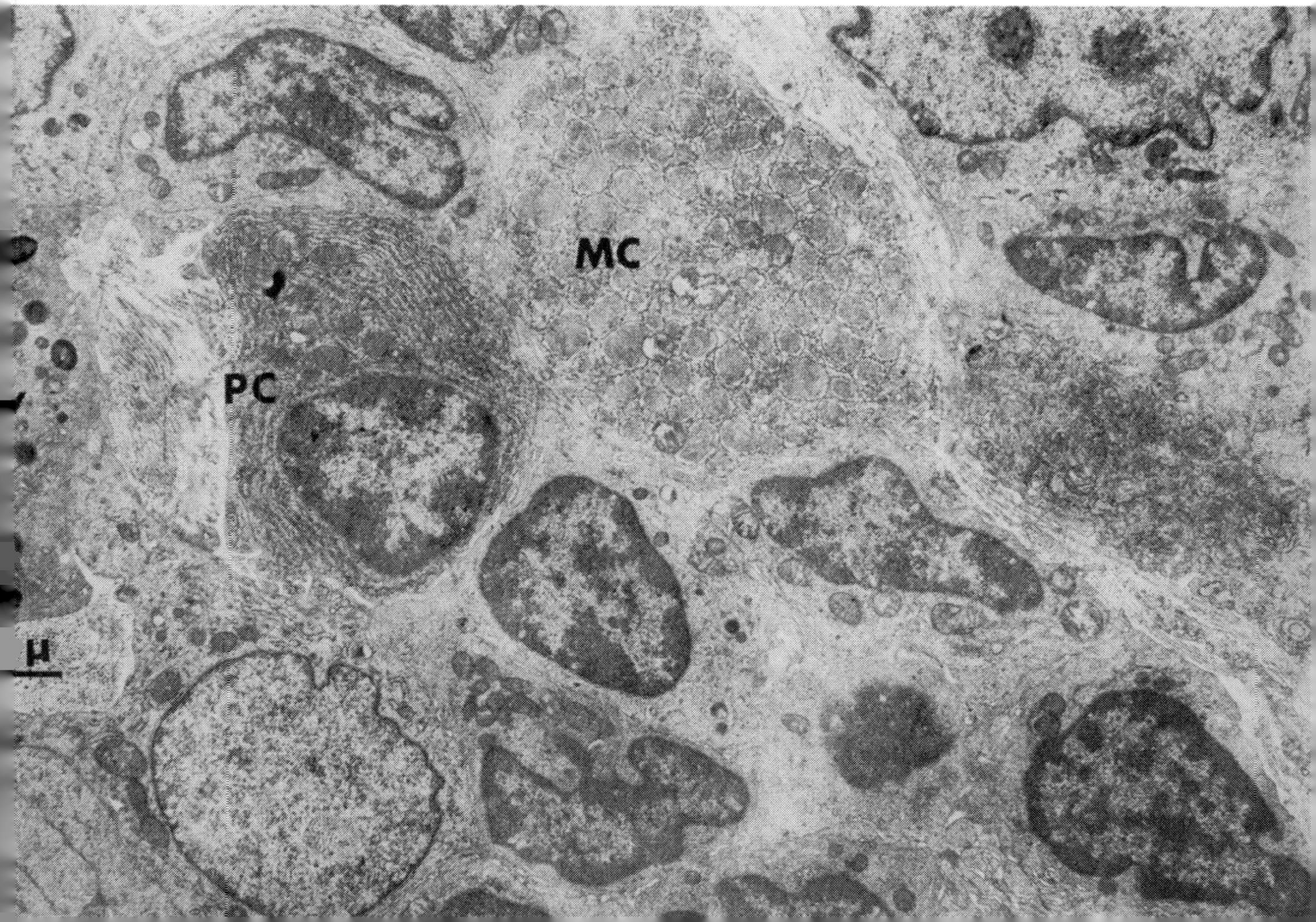
MC
PC
μ

PLATE 61. PLASMA CELLS IN POLYMYOSITIS

UPPER. Plasma cells are commonly found in subacute and chronic inflammatory conditions of muscle. Their ultrastructural features are characterised by the eccentric nucleus and the distribution of a large amount of rough endoplasmic reticulum throughout their cytoplasm. Some of the tubules of the endoplasmic reticulum are distended with electron opaque material. Numerous vesicles and ribosomes are present in the cytoplasm as well as some electron dense bodies and mitochondria some of which are swollen.

MAGNIFICATION 15,000 ×.

LOWER. In this plasma cell the eccentric nucleus has masses of chromatin around the periphery. The cytoplasm contains a large amount of rough endoplasmic reticulum whose tubules are in places arranged concentrically. Vacuoles containing various shaped bodies of differing electron density are also present in the cytoplasm. Around the plasma cell lie collagen and a large amount of granular material. The muscle fibre on the right is undergoing degeneration. Its plasma membrane is thickened. Vacuoles, membranous bodies and glycogen granules are present at the edge of the fibre.

MAGNIFICATION 12,000 ×.

ER Endoplasmic reticulum
MF Muscle fibre
Va Vacuole

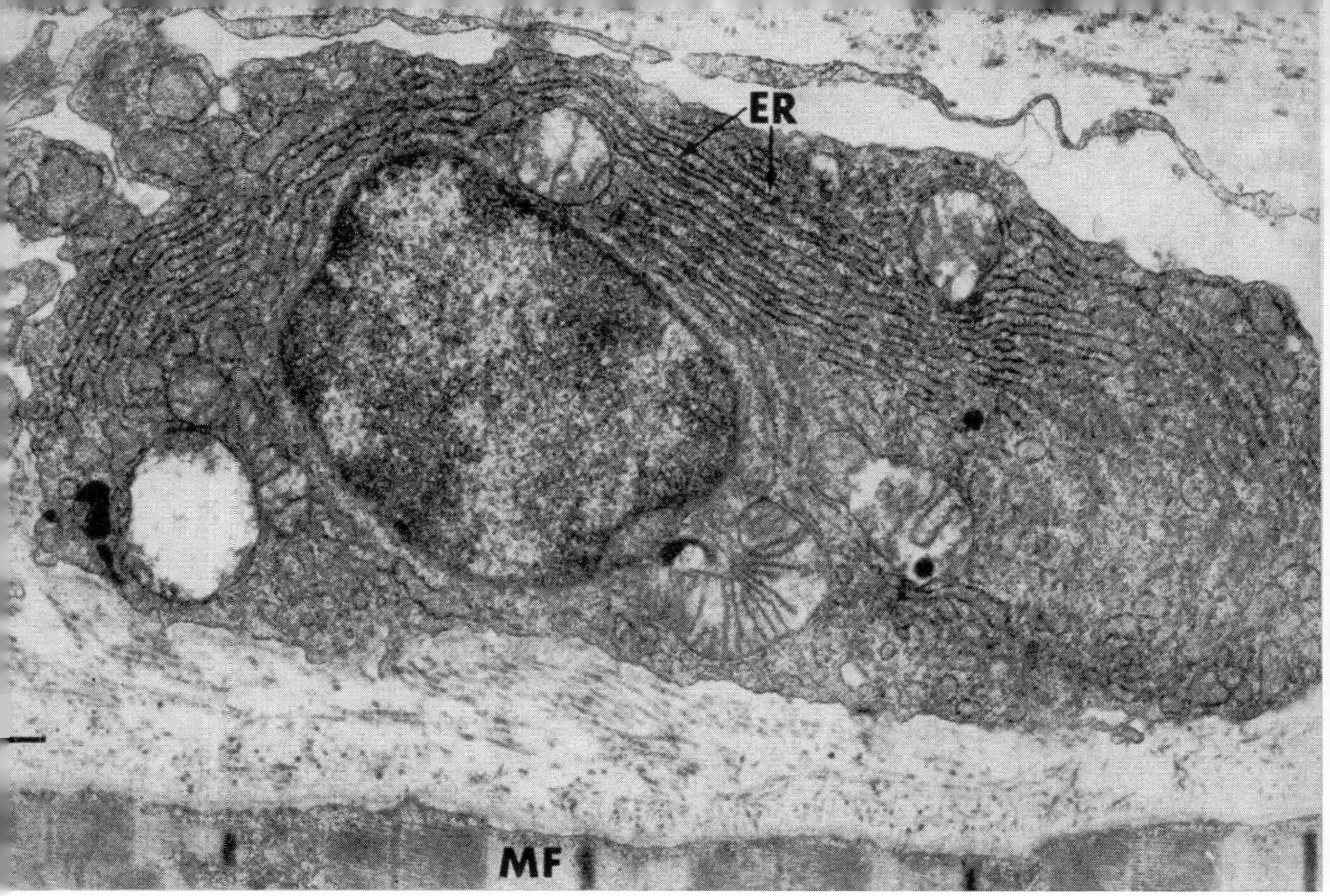
ER
MF

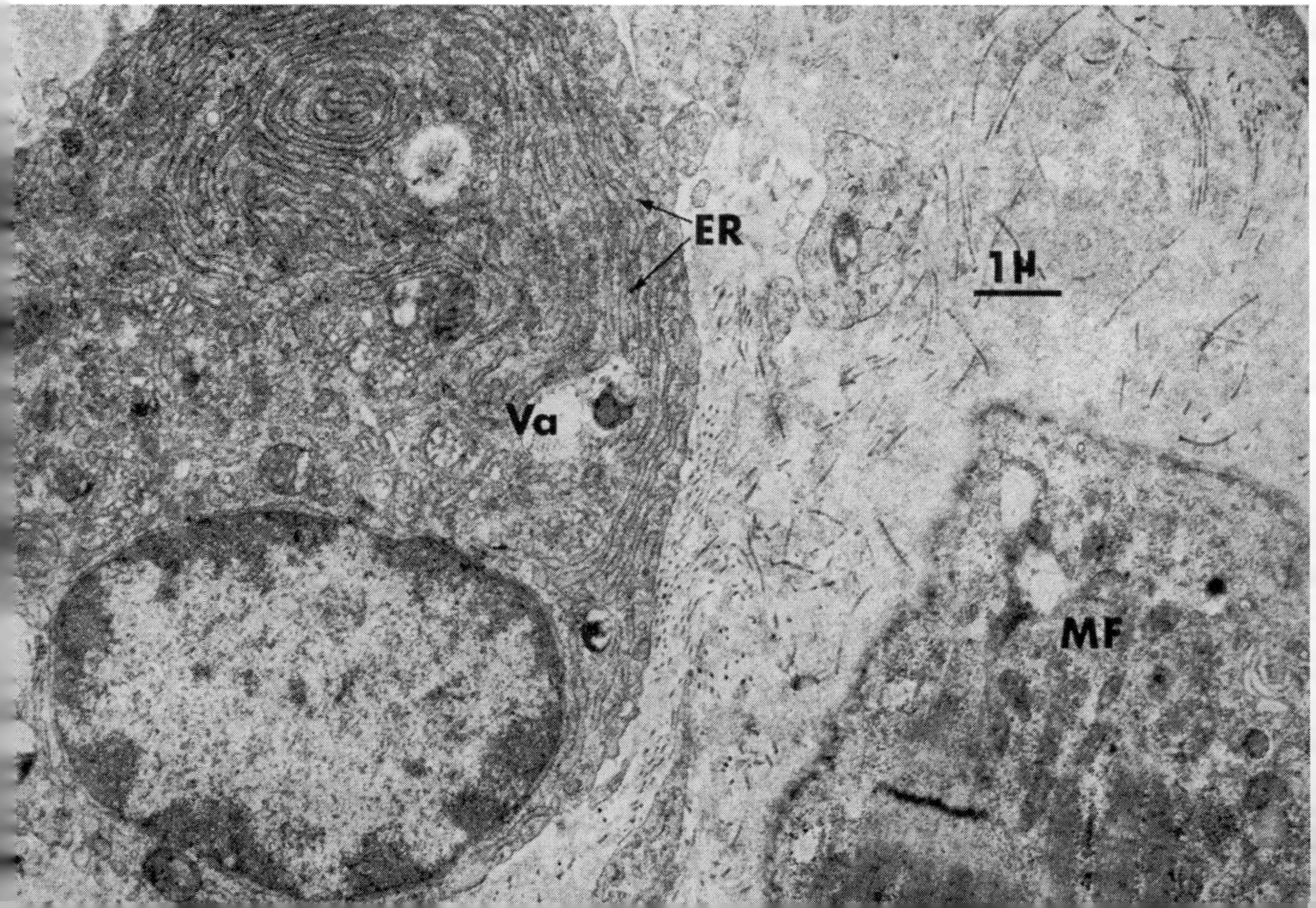
ER
1μ
Va
MF

PLATE 62. LEUCOCYTES IN POLYMYOSITIS
A LEUCOCYTE IN MITOSIS

UPPER. A group of leucocytes with clearly defined plasma membranes are separated from two muscle fibres by collagen and the elongated cytoplasmic expansions of fibroblasts. Another leucocyte lies in the collagen between the two muscle fibres. The cytoplasm of the leucocytes contains many fine granules and small vesicles and some leucocytes contain prominent electron dense lipid bodies. The plasma membranes of the muscle fibres show electron dense beading (arrowed) and numerous subjacent pinocytotic vesicles. Many mitochondria lie between the plasma membrane and the myofibrils of the fibre on the right.

MAGNIFICATION 7,000 ×.

LOWER. Close to a muscle fibre is a leucocyte in mitosis: several of its chromosomes are evident. The cytoplasm contains in addition, numerous mitochondria, rough endoplasmic reticulum, ribosomes and polysomes. Another leucocyte lies to the right of the cell in mitosis.

MAGNIFICATION 12,000 ×.

C Collagen
Ch Chromosomes
ER Endoplasmic reticulum
F Fibroblast
Le Leucocyte
Mit Mitochondria
MF Muscle fibre

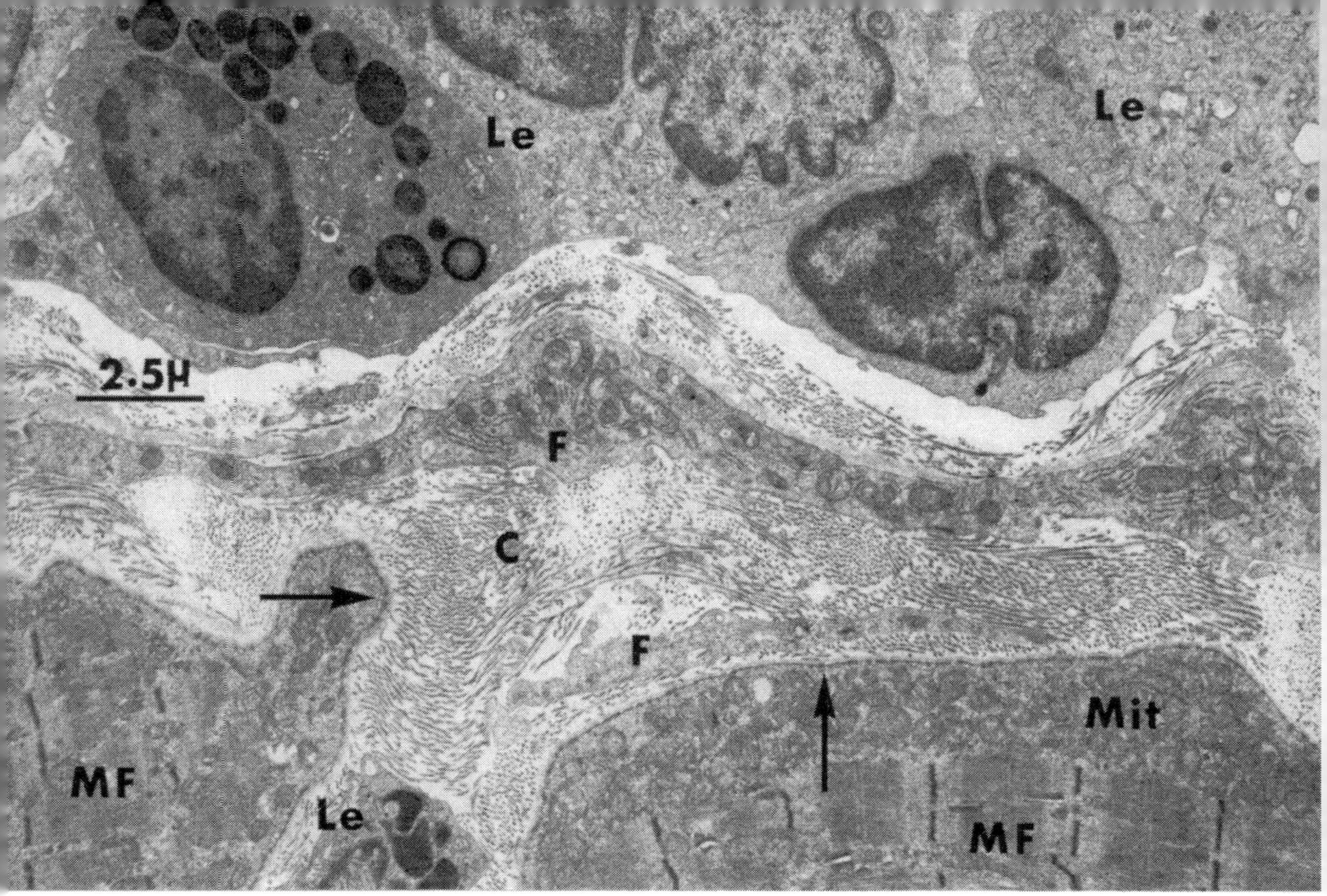
Le
Le
2.5μ
F
C
F
Mit
MF
Le
MF

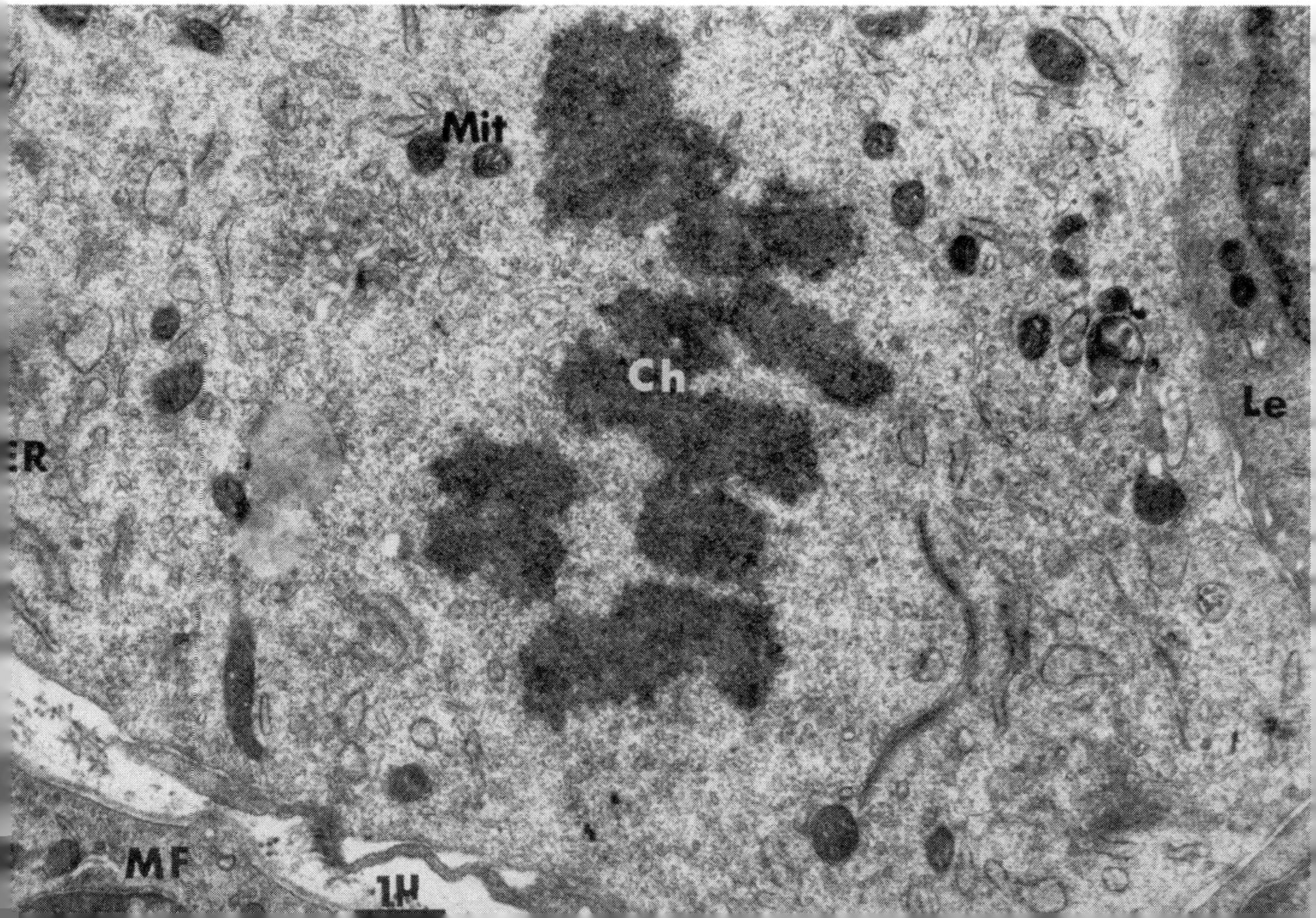
Mit
Ch
Le
ER
MF
1μ

PLATE 63. PHAGOCYTOSIS OF MUSCLE FIBRES IN POLYMYOSITIS

UPPER. Phagocytes are in close apposition to a muscle fibre showing early evidence of degenerative change, namely migration of the subsarcolemmal nucleus to the centre of the fibre and disintegration of the myofibrils near its surface. Where the phagocyte and the muscle fibre are in close contact the basement membrane of the muscle fibre has disappeared but persists over the rest of the muscle fibre. Other leucocytes and strands of collagen overlie the muscle fibre.

MAGNIFICATION 7,000 ×.

LOWER. It is much more common to find phagocytes already within the degenerating muscle fibre whose plasma membrane has disappeared but whose basement membrane persists. The phagocytes below the basement membrane are within the muscle fibre, while outside it are strands of collagen and another phagocyte. The phagocytes have numerous pseudopodia.

MAGNIFICATION 10,000 ×.

BM	Basement membrane	N	Nucleus
C	Collagen	Ph	Phagocyte
DMF	Degenerating muscle fibre	Ps	Pseudopodia

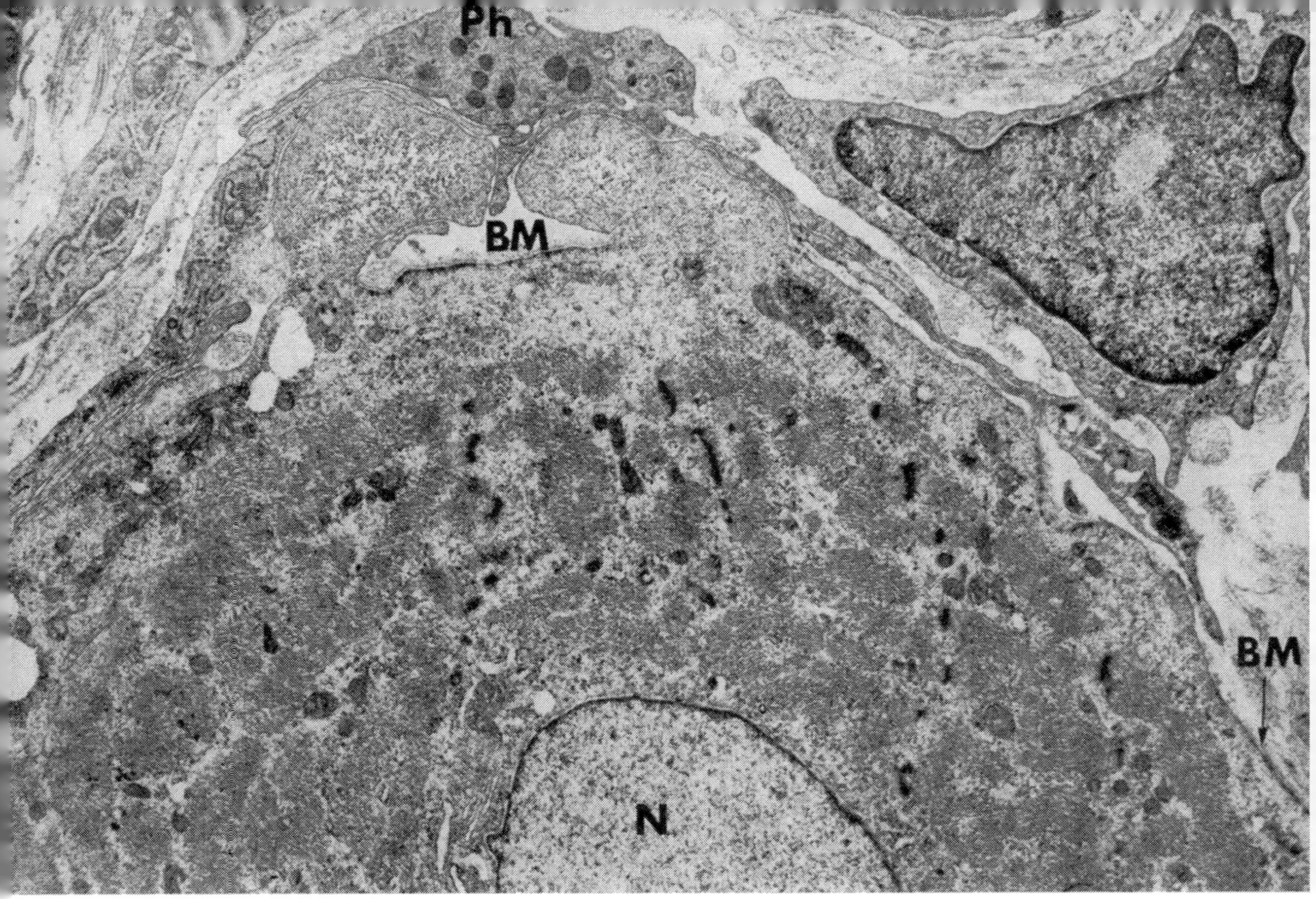
Ph
BM
BM
N

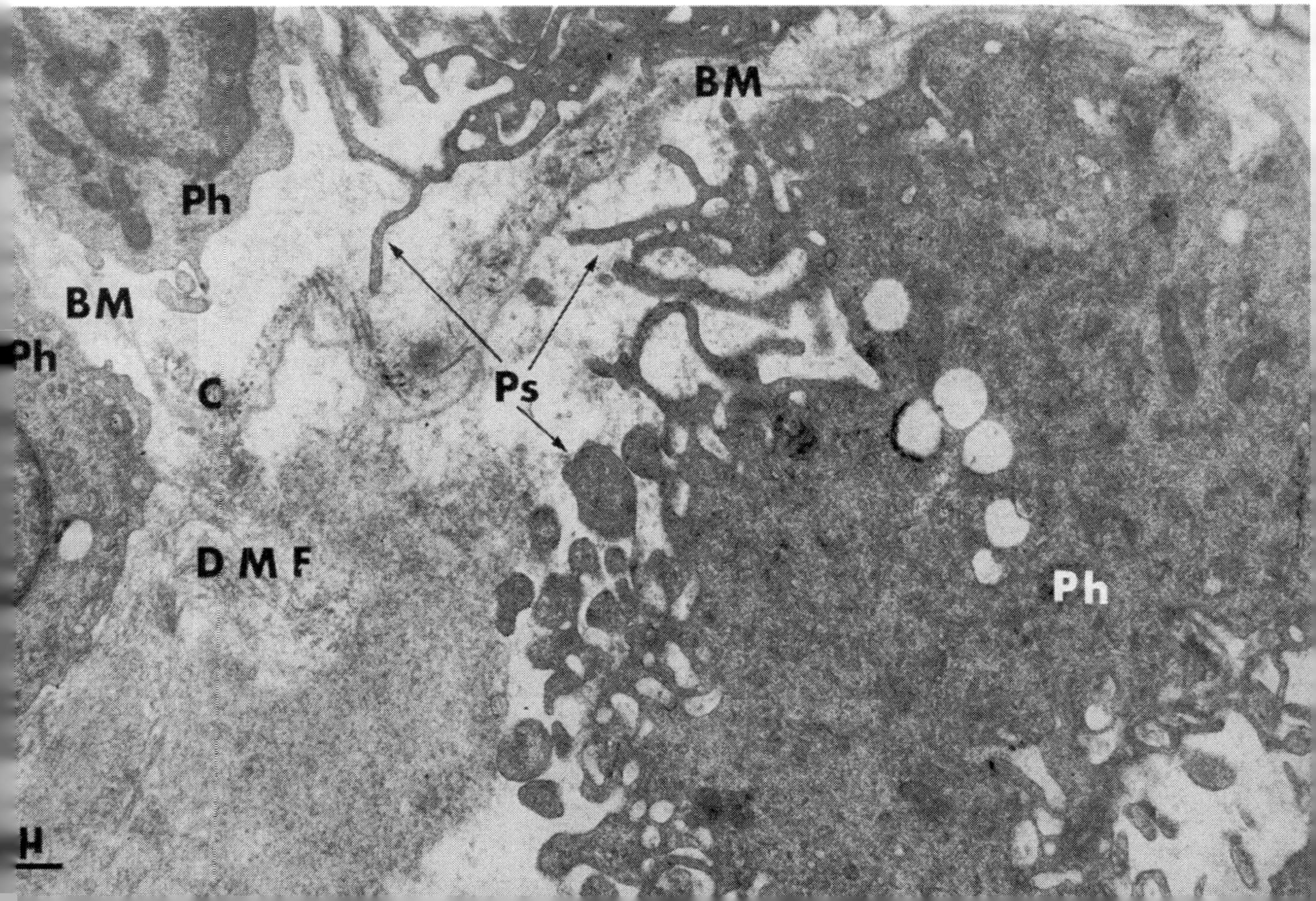
BM
Ph
BM
Ph
C
Ps
D M F
Ph

PLATE 64. AMYLOID FIBRILS

Two adjacent muscle fibres which are in an advanced stage of degeneration are covered with a fairly thick layer of basement membrane. They contain vesicles and numerous electron dense granules: the fibre on the right presents several lipid bodies with zones of different electron density. Between the muscle fibres lie bundles of collagen and between these bundles of collagen are collections of very slender filaments about 100 Å in diameter which are amyloid fibrils.

MAGNIFICATION 15,000 ×.

From a patient with primary amyloid neuropathy.

Am Amyloid
BM Basement membrane
C Collagen
LB Lipid body
MF Muscle fibre

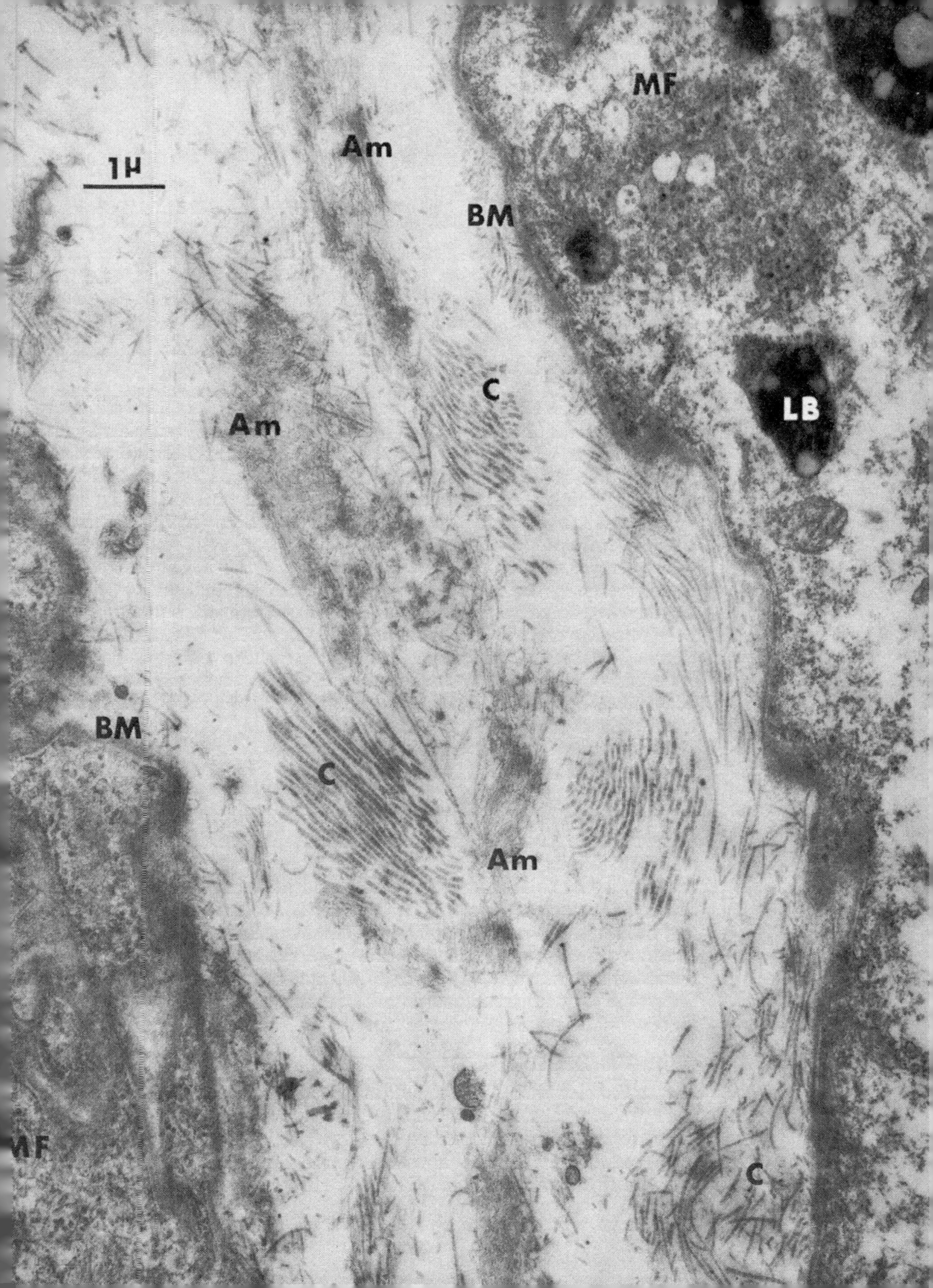

MF
Am
1μ
BM
C
LB
Am
BM
C
Am
MF
C

CHAPTER 4

Changes in Nerves, Motor End Plates and Muscle Spindles

CHANGES IN NERVES

In human muscle biopsies, nerves are not commonly found in the small amount of tissue taken for electron microscopy unless the biopsy has been taken from the motor points as determined by electrical stimulation. In pathological conditions of the muscle in man, the ultrastructure of intramuscular nerves has not been extensively studied, but has been studied in experimental animals by various workers including Thomas (1964), Thomas and Slatford (1964), Ichikawa and Okajima (1969) and Prineas (1969 b and c).

The changes which occur affect the axon, myelin sheath, Schwann cell, perineurial cells and the collagen surrounding the nerve fibres. In the axons undergoing degenerative changes, the synaptic vesicles form clumps and structures having a honeycomb appearance. The mitochondria show swelling with breaking of the cristae. The myelin disintegrates. Lamellar material and electron dense bodies occur in the Schwann cell cytoplasm. Eventually the axons and sometimes the Schwann cells disappear, leaving empty basement membrane tubes. The collagen around the nerve fibre increases in amount.

Many workers including Reger (1959), Birks, Katz and Miledi (1960), Bauer, Blumberg and Zacks (1962), Iwayama (1968), Song (1968), Prineas (1969 b and c), Gutmann, Tuček and Hanzlíková (1969), Babel, Bischoff and Spoendlin (1970), Song and Anderson (1970), and Miledi and Slater (1970), have studied the ultrastructure of the terminal axons and the neuromuscular junction in various experimental animals. In the terminal axons also the synaptic vesicles may form clumps or they may diminish in numbers and the mitochondria undergo degenerative changes. The axons may eventually disappear and then the Schwann cell cytoplasm may lie in contact with the synaptic clefts of the muscle fibre. At a later stage the Schwann cell may no longer be found in association with the synaptic cleft. Eventually the synaptic clefts begin to disrupt and with time they disappear. Changes in the subsynaptic sarcoplasmic structures also take place and extend to the rest of the sarcoplasmic components.

CHANGES IN MOTOR END PLATES

Many authors have studied the ultrastructure of the neuromuscular junction in man under pathological conditions and their reports were reviewed by Zacks (1964). More recent studies have been reported by Woolf (1966), Iwayama and Ohta (1969) and Edwards (1970) in myasthenia gravis, by Fardeau and Godet-Guillain (1970) in myasthenia gravis and chloroquine myopathy, by Allen, Johnson and

Woolf (1969) in dystrophia myotonica, by Agostini and Noetzel (1970) in tetanus, by De Recondo (1970a) in peroneal muscular atrophy and by Stoebner *et al.* (1970) in chronic myastheniform polymyositis. It is difficult to make a correct assessment of what the changes may signify since there is considerable variation in the ultrastructure of the motor end plate in normal muscle. Differences in the structural features occur from section to section in the same motor end plate as well as in different motor end plates of the same biopsy specimen. Regarding the changes which may occur, mention should be made of the area occupied by the motor end plate. In atrophied fibres, both in denervation (Plate 65 lower part) and in muscular dystrophy (Plate 27 lower part), the area of the motor end plate may be small and the synaptic clefts few in number with little evidence of ramification, but sometimes in muscular dystrophy the synaptic area may be large and extends over more than 40 μ as illustrated in Plate 66 upper part. In addition, as in this case, the secondary synaptic clefts are numerous and show many branches. It should be stated, however, that it is well known that in advanced cases of muscular dystrophy where most of the muscle fibres have degenerated, intramuscular nerves containing myelinated nerve fibres may still be identified. In the case of polymyositis illustrated in Plate 67 the area of the motor end plate is also large: the synaptic clefts are numerous but few mitochondria are seen in the subsynaptic region. However, it is difficult to assess the significance of this finding.

In myasthenia gravis, which is a disorder of neuromuscular transmission, changes might be expected in the motor end plates. Several ultrastructural alterations have been described, but Edwards (1970) reports that the only constant findings are changes in the secondary synaptic clefts which are widened and sometimes severely reduced in number. Few reports are available on the ultrastructure of the muscle fibre in myasthenia gravis. They include that of Mitin *et al.* (1969).

CHANGES IN MUSCLE SPINDLES

The changes in the muscle spindles in pathological conditions in man have been studied by various workers. Batten (1897) reported that 'the muscle spindle under various pathological conditions' was unaffected and this has been the view of many subsequent workers. However, Grünbaum (1897) noted in a case of pseudohypertrophic paralysis 'a diminution in size of an intrafusal fibre with deposit of hyaline material around'. In more recent years several authors have reported various abnormalities in the muscle spindle studied by light microscopy. These include Daniel and Strich (1964), who demonstrated changes in the various elements of the spindle in dystrophia myotonica, and Lapresle and Milhaud (1964), Patel, Lalitha and Dastur (1968) and Cazzato and Walton (1968) reported alterations in the muscle spindle in a very varied group of muscular disorders.

The ultrastructure of muscle spindles in pathological conditions has not been adequately studied. The report of Gruner (1961) on two cases of muscular dystrophy and one of amyotrophic lateral sclerosis is well known. Gruner, however, was of the opinion that many more cases must be studied to distinguish the normal from the pathological muscle spindle.

PLATE 65. MOTOR END PLATES IN DENERVATED MUSCLE

UPPER. A terminal axon lies in the primary synaptic cleft. To the right of the axon is Schwann cell cytoplasm and outside it multiple layers of basement membrane with occasional strands of collagen between them. The axon contains many mitochondria and neurofilaments as well as numerous coated vesicles. The plasma and basement membranes in relation to the axon in the upper and central parts of the primary synaptic cleft are clearly defined but in the lower part are obscure. Some of the secondary synaptic clefts are distended. Many mitochondria lie between the secondary synaptic clefts and the myofibrils.

MAGNIFICATION 18,500 ×.

From a patient with polyneuropathy.

LOWER. This shows a very degenerate motor end plate in an atrophied muscle fibre. The secondary synaptic clefts, although few in number, can be readily identified but no axon or Schwann cell was found in relation to them. The sarcoplasm around the secondary synaptic clefts is abundant and contains many vesicles and granules and a few mitochondria. Some broken-down myofilaments lie in relation to it.

MAGNIFICATION 17,000 ×.

From a patient with primary amyloid neuropathy.

Ax	Axon	Nf	Neurofilaments
BM	Basement membrane	PSC	Primary synaptic cleft
Mf	Myofibril	SCC	Schwann cell cytoplasm
Mi	Mitochondria	SSC	Secondary synaptic cleft
My	Myofilaments		

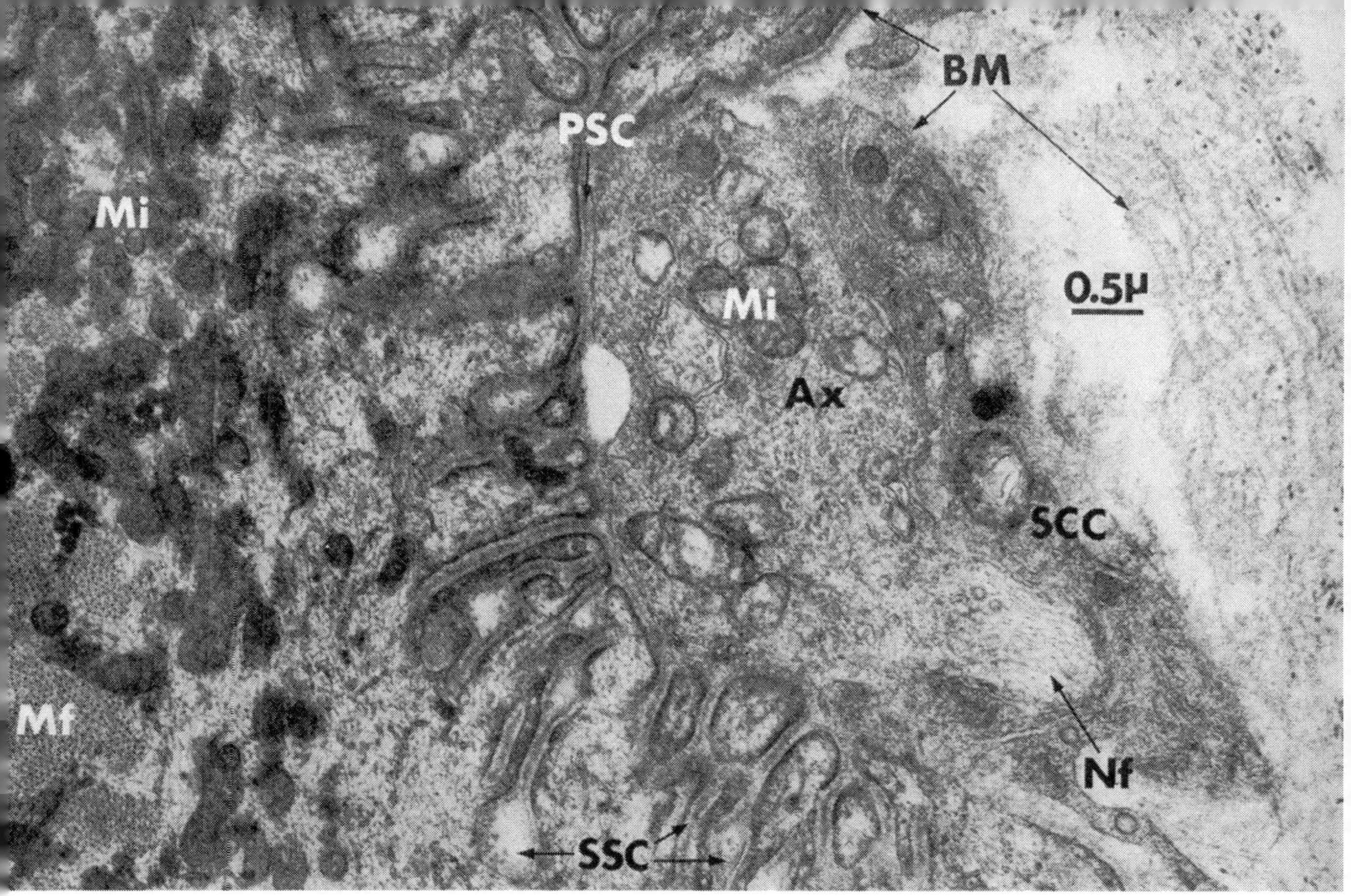
BM
PSC
Mi
0.5μ
Mi
Ax
SCC
Mf
Nf
SSC

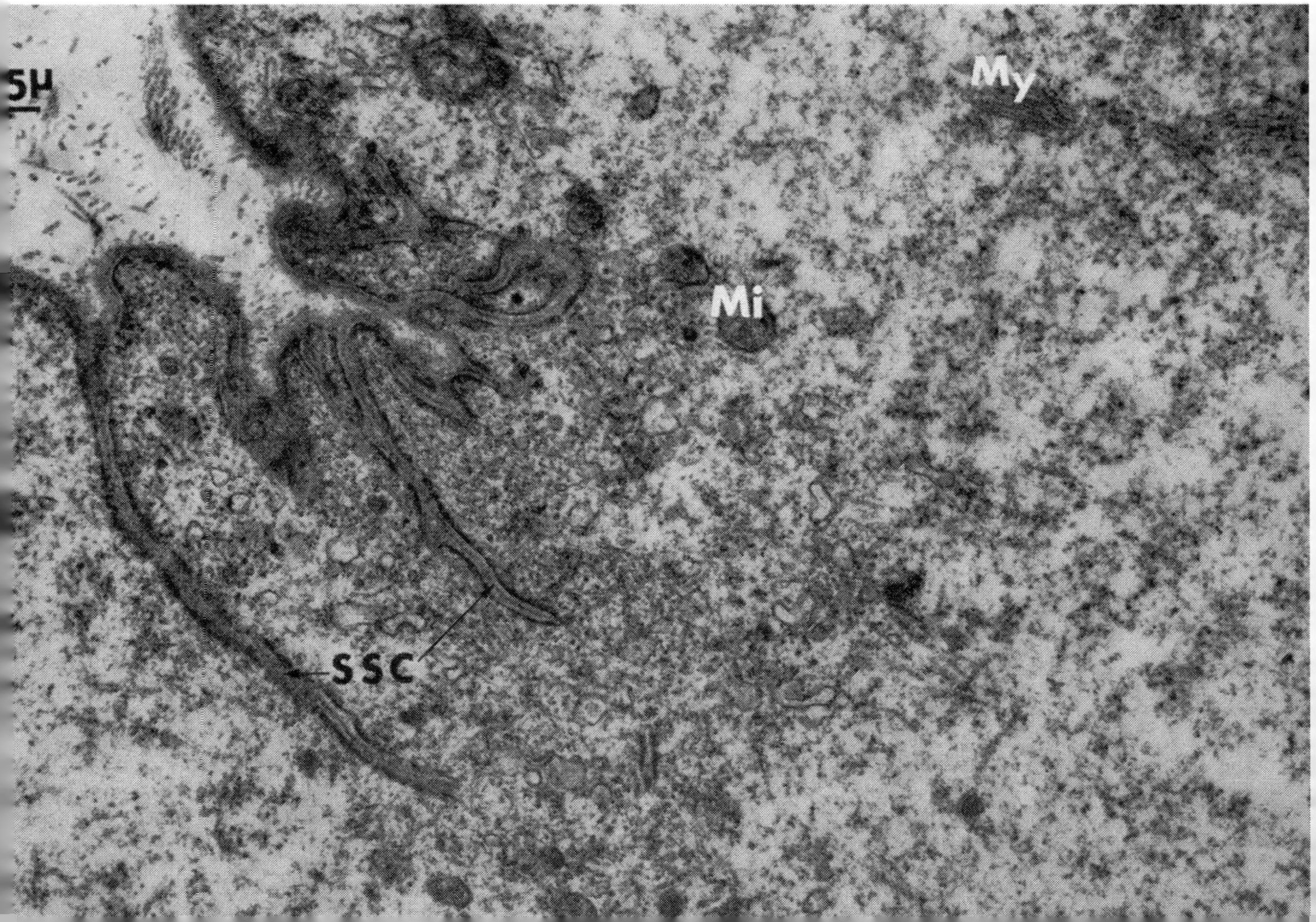
5μ
My
Mi
SSC

PLATE 66. MOTOR END PLATE IN MUSCULAR DYSTROPHY

UPPER. Between two muscle fibres lie thin elongated portions of perineurial cells and collagen related to them. On the lower muscle fibre is a motor end plate which extends over more than 20 sarcomeres. The axon cut at several levels, lies in the primary synaptic cleft. The secondary synaptic clefts are very numerous and mitochondria occur near those on the left of the illustration, where they lie near a satellite cell with a prominent nucleus. Few alterations are seen in the two muscle fibres.

MAGNIFICATION 5,500 ×.

LOWER. The right part of the motor end plate above is seen in more detail. Mitochondria, vesicles and tubules can be seen in the terminal axon which is covered by Schwann cell cytoplasm and empty folds of basement membrane. The plasma membrane of the muscle fibre bounding the secondary synaptic clefts shows increased electron density. Many granules, some vesicles and microtubules lie in the sarcoplasm around the secondary synaptic clefts. Myofibrils and triads are seen in the lower part of the illustration.

MAGNIFICATION 16,500 ×.

Ax	Axon	S	Satellite cell
BM	Basement membrane	SCC	Schwann cell cytoplasm
Mf	Myofibril	SSC	Secondary synaptic clefts
Mi	Mitochondria	Tu	Tubules
PN	Perineurial cell	V	Vesicles
PSC	Primary synaptic cleft		

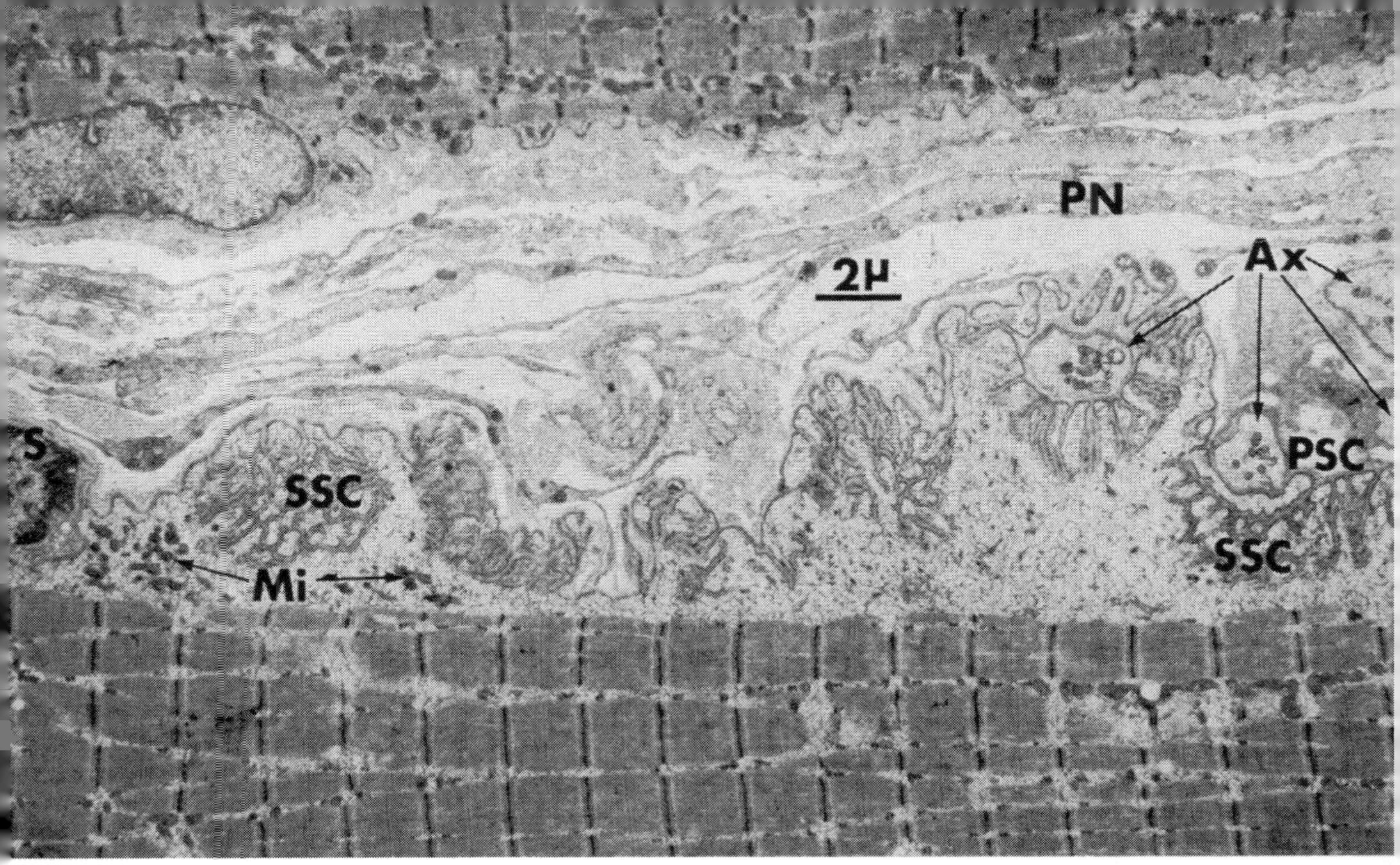
PN
2μ
Ax
PSC
SSC
SSC
Mi
S

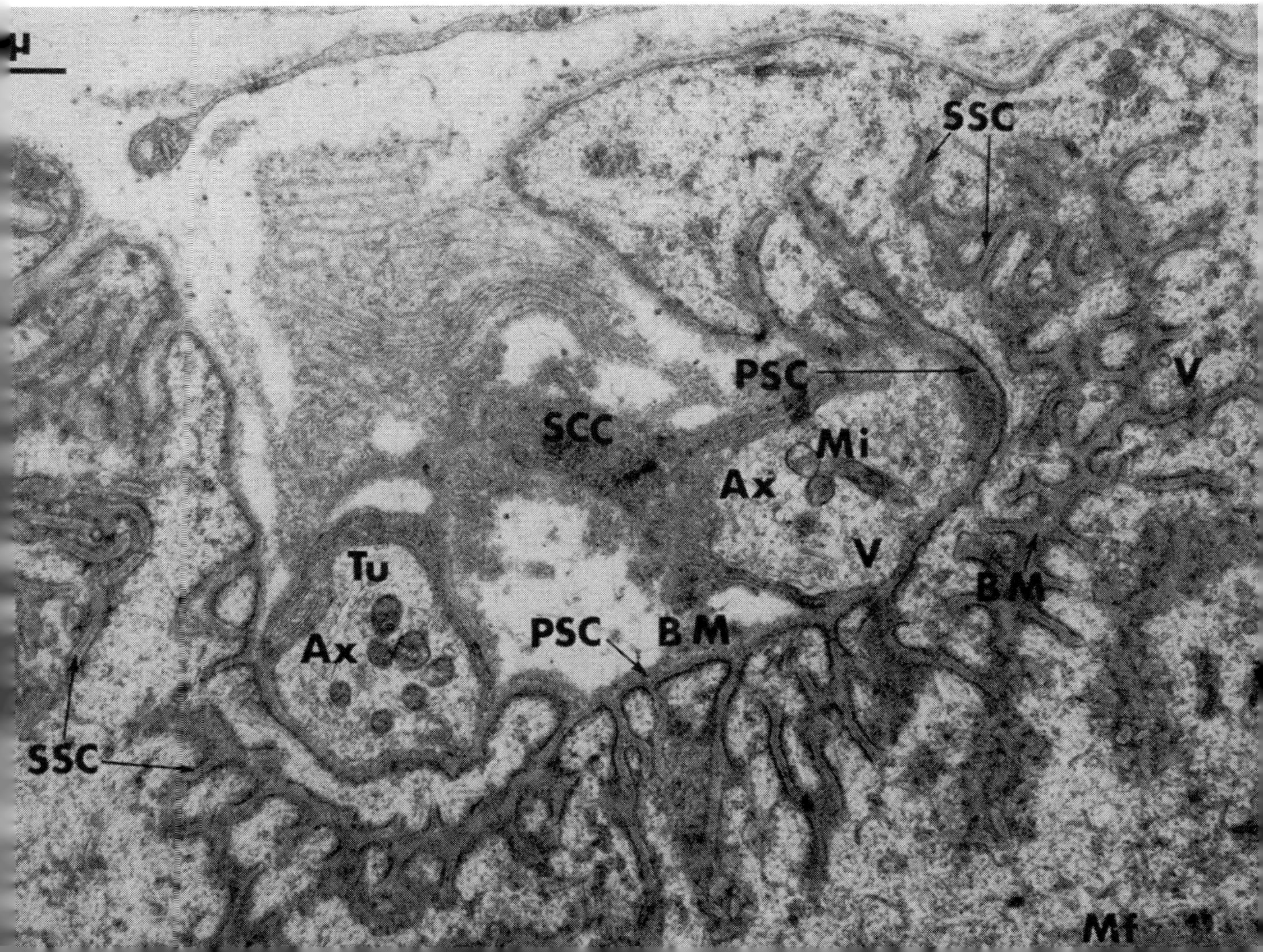
μ
SSC
PSC
V
SCC
Mi
Ax
V
Tu
Ax
PSC
B M
B M
SSC
Mf

PLATE 67. MOTOR END PLATES IN POLYMYOSITIS

UPPER. To the right is a myelinated nerve surrounded by perineurial cells and close by is a motor end plate, the axon of which is covered on its outer aspect by Schwann cell cytoplasm and in turn by layers of basement membrane. The axon contains many synaptic vesicles and lies in the primary synaptic cleft being separated from the muscle by basement membrane. Numerous secondary clefts containing basement membrane extend from the primary synaptic cleft and indent the surface of the muscle fibre. To the left of the motor end plate lies a nucleus of the muscle fibre. Some vesicles, fine filaments and numerous granules, some of which are glycogen, lie around the secondary clefts. Mitochondria are not present in this section of the motor end plate: this is most probably a chance finding without pathological significance.

MAGNIFICATION 10,000 ×.

LOWER. A terminal axon lying in the primary synaptic cleft on the surface of the muscle fibre is partly surrounded by Schwann cell cytoplasm. The axon contains neurofilaments and mitochondria and where it lies next to the muscle fibre presents numerous synaptic vesicles. Basement membrane lines the primary synaptic cleft and dips into the secondary clefts indenting the surface of the muscle fibre. In the sarcoplasm around the synaptic clefts are numerous granules, microtubules, vesicles and a few mitochondria.

MAGNIFICATION 34,000 ×.

Both are from a patient with polymyositis associated with carcinoma of the breast.

Ax	Axon	PM	Plasma membrane
BM	Basement membrane	PN	Perineurial cells
Mi	Mitochondria	PSC	Primary synaptic cleft
MF	Muscle fibre	SCC	Schwann cell cytoplasm
MN	Myelinated nerve	SSC	Secondary synaptic cleft
N	Nucleus	V	Vesicles
Nf	Neurofilaments		

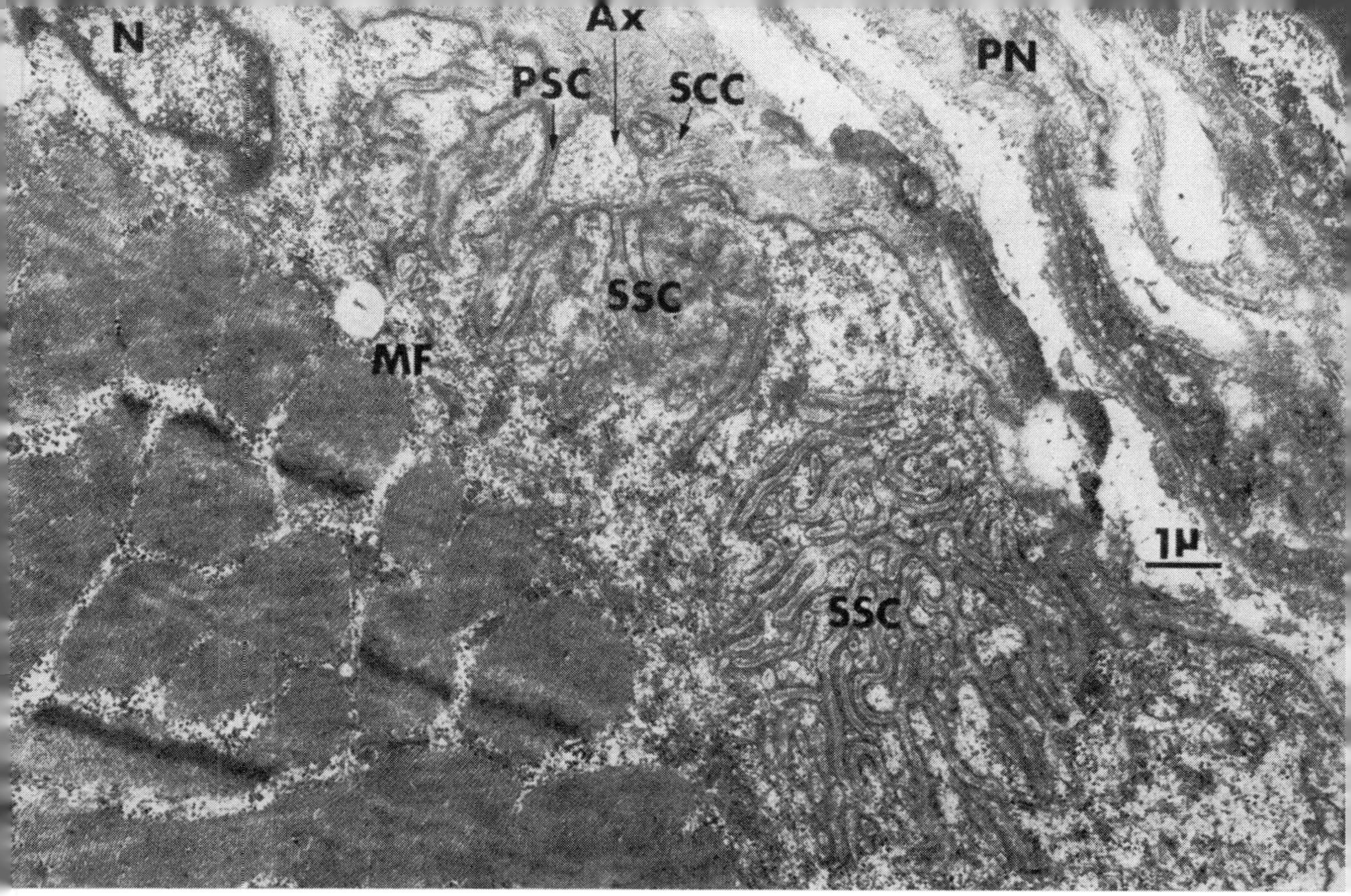
N
Ax
PN
PSC
SCC
SSC
MF
1μ
SSC

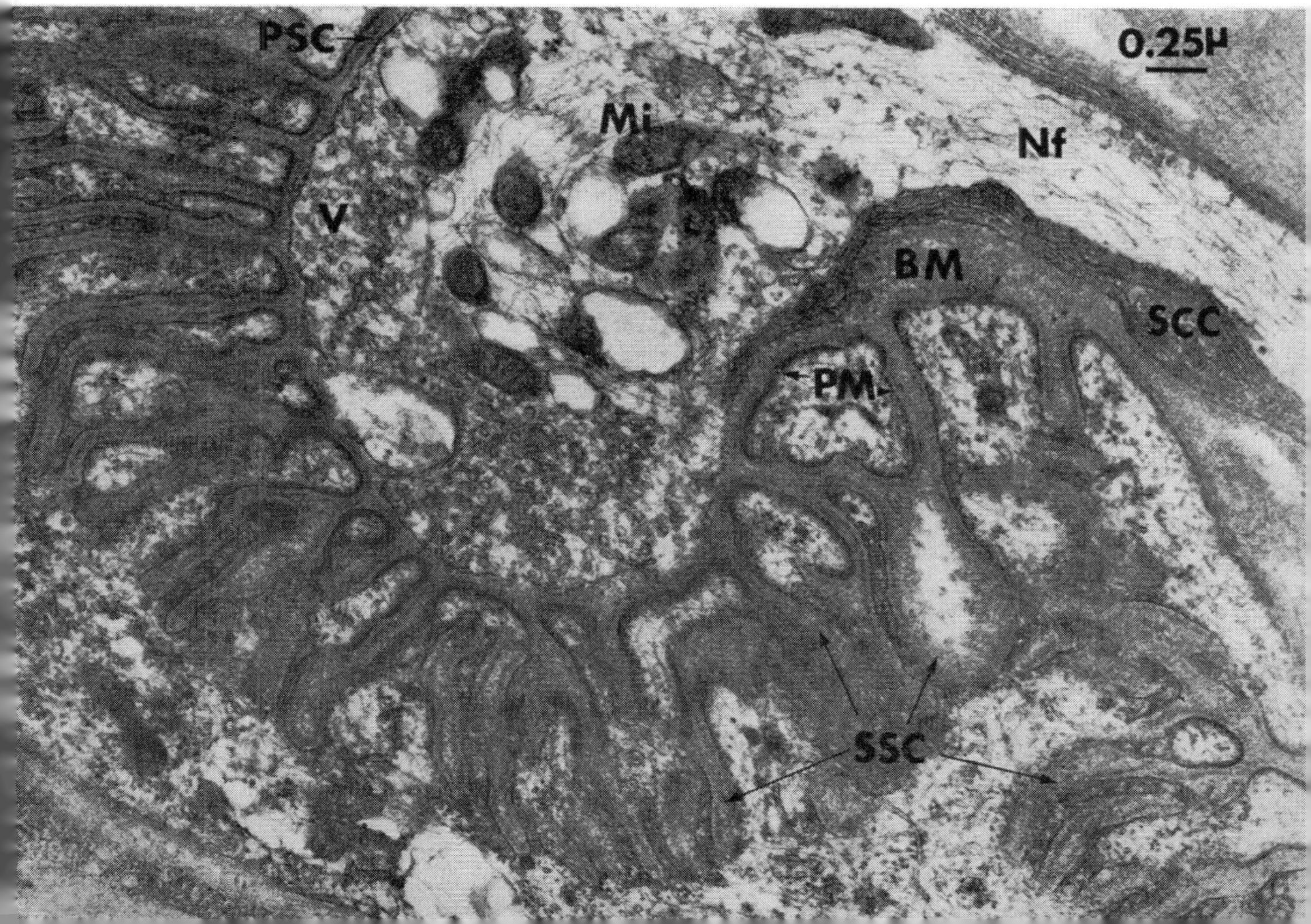
PSC
0.25μ
Mi
Nf
V
BM
SCC
PM
SSC

CHAPTER 5

Changes in Various Muscle Diseases

Muscle when affected by disease presents many ultrastructural changes which are common to many disorders, but certain patterns of change take place which may help to distinguish different diseases. As would be expected, the changes exhibited by the muscle may vary according to the stage of the disease process affecting it. An effort has been made to outline some of the patterns which tend to occur in particular diseases.

DENERVATION ATROPHY OF MUSCLE

In denervated muscle, groups of small muscle fibres may be found (Plates 22 lower part, 34 and 68) and may contain many nuclei of varying size, shape and electron density, lying peripherally or centrally in the muscle fibre (Plate 69). Around these nuclei occur collections of glycogen granules, some lipid bodies and disorganised myofibrils. In affected fibres some myofilaments have disappeared and those remaining are often randomly distributed and do not present the normal sarcomere pattern (Plate 69). The Z-lines are frequently thickened and distorted and in some fibres 'target' zones are found (Plate 24 upper part). Collections of triads may occur in the fibre as well as large vacuoles (Plate 36). In addition the sarcoplasmic reticulum may be distended with electron dense material (Plate 37). Membranous and myelin bodies may be found in affected fibres (Plate 68 lower part) as well as collections of concentric tubules (Plate 45), concentric laminated bodies (Plate 44), honeycomb structures (Plate 38) and cytoplasmic bodies (Plate 27 upper part). As in any other disease affecting muscle the mitochondria may be altered. Satellite cells occur but are not usually frequent. Loose folds of basement membrane project from some atrophying muscle fibres and sometimes only empty basement membrane tubes remain, the muscle fibre having completely degenerated. The collagen around the muscle fibre in advanced stages of degeneration may be increased but not in the early stages. Phagocytes are occasionally found between muscle fibres. The changes in the nerve and motor end plates are described in Chapter 4.

Various authors have reported the ultrastructural changes in denervated muscles in man and these include Wechsler and Hager (1962), Thiébaut *et al.* (1963), Pearce (1964), Roth *et al.* (1964 and 1965), Fardeau (1965), Sluga-Gasser (1965), De Recondo, Fardeau and Lapresle (1966), Afifi *et al.* (1966), Fisher, Cohn and Danowski (1966), Shafiq, Milhorat and Gorycki (1967b), Hausmanova-Petrusewicz *et al.* (1968), Sato and Tsubaki (1968), Hudgson and Pearce (1969), Hughes and Brownell (1969) and De Recondo (1970b).

In experimental animals the ultrastructure of denervated muscle has been extensively studied by many authors; some of these are Birks, Katz and Miledi (1959), Wechsler and Hager (1960 and 1961a), Pellegrino and Franzini (1963), Lee (1963), Lee and Altschull (1963), Muscatello, Margreth and Aloisi (1965), Wechsler (1966), Schrodt and Walter (1966), Song (1968), Miledi and Slater (1969) Ichikawa and Okajima (1969).

MUSCULAR DYSTROPHIES

The structural changes which take place in the various types of muscular dystrophy cannot be regarded as specific for them since similar changes may occur in other muscle disorders. At the onset of muscular dystrophy the changes in the muscle may differ markedly from those present in its later stages. Biopsies from muscles which are only slightly affected may show few pathological changes: those commonly seen are degeneration of the myofilaments of one or more sarcomeres of a myofibril. The I-band is affected early in the disease but the Z-line may persist (Plates 19 and 70 upper parts). The sarcoplasm between the myofibrils appears to be increased and aggregates of mitochondria tend to occur and the amount of lipid droplets may be increased. In very occasional cases the mitochondria may exhibit crystalline inclusions (Plate 32). The amount of glycogen granules in the muscle fibre is increased, especially in the more advanced stages of the disease (Plate 33). In some cases the Z-lines become tortuous and thickened and occasionally double Z-lines may be found (Plate 71). The T-systems and the sarcoplasmic reticulum may be very apparent. Membranous and myelin bodies may occur, the membranous bodies being sometimes within mitochondria which may be distended and contain some glycogen granules (Plate 30). Eventually the mitochondria may rupture and disintegrate. Sarcoplasmic masses (Plate 21) and ring fibres (Plates 17 and 18) may be found. The muscle fibres become shrunken and contain aggregates of nuclei situated either peripherally or centrally (Plate 74). Cytoplasmic and filamentous bodies (Plates 27 and 28 lower parts respectively) may be found in the degenerating muscle fibre. Another feature of the atrophied fibres are empty basement membrane folds projecting from their surface (Plates 50 and 72). In late stages of the disease loss of myofilaments and other organelles is severe and autophagic vacuoles may be present in the fibre. Phagocytes may be seen occasionally within degenerating muscle fibres and also between the muscle fibres (Plate 73). In degenerate muscle fibres containing clusters of nuclei there may also be found occasional groups of electron dense round particles of doubtful origin and significance (Plate 74 and page 56). Satellite cells are found, but less frequently than in inflammatory conditions of muscle, and the satellites may occur in fibres showing obvious ultrastructural degenerative changes (Plate 19 lower part) as well as in fibres which appear to be normal. In many cases of muscular dystrophy there is relatively little increase of fibroblasts and collagen around the degenerating muscle fibres, but a feature of the Duchenne type of muscular dystrophy is the great increase of fibroblasts and collagen which is seen around the muscle fibres as illustrated in the lower part of Plate 70.

The nerves may show little change in muscular dystrophy. The changes in the motor end plate are described on page 161 and are illustrated in Plate 66.

The ultrastructural changes in muscular dystrophy have been extensively studied by van Breemen (1960b), Mölbert (1960), Pearce (1963 and 1966), Laguens (1963), Lapresle, Fardeau and Milhaud (1964 and 1966), Wechsler (1966), Fisher, Cohn and Danowski (1966), Hudgson, Pearce and Walton (1967), Hudgson (1968), Sato and Tsubaki (1968), Santa (1969), Hudgson and Pearce (1969), Milhorat and Goldstone (1969), Papadimitriou, Mastaglia and Kakulas (1969), Mastaglia, Papadimitriou and Kakulas (1969b), Fardeau (1970), Monticone, Gabella and Bergamini (1970) and various other authors.

The ultrastructure of the muscle in carriers of muscular dystrophy has been reported by several authors. Amongst the recent studies are those of Roy and Dubowitz (1970) and Beckmann, Kloke and Freund-Mölbert (1970).

The muscular changes in various animals which are affected by muscular dystrophy were reported by many authors including Ross, Pappas and Harman (1958 and 1960), Rigdon (1966), Wechsler (1966), Wechsler and Pabelick (1966), Caulfield (1966), Banker (1967 and 1968) and Johnson and Pearse (1968).

The ultrastructural changes in dystrophia myotonica have been studied by many authors, who report changes which are very similar to those occurring in other muscular dystrophies at a similar stage of evolution. The occurrence of central nuclei (Plate 29), sarcoplasmic masses and ring fibres in dystrophia myotonica has been stressed by various authors. In addition honeycomb structures have been reported by Schroeder and Adams (1968), Schotland (1970) and Mussini, Di Mauro and Angelini (1970). A less common finding is the presence of autophagic vacuoles within the muscle fibre and the extruded contents of these vacuoles in the basement membrane of the fibre as illustrated in Plates 39 and 40.

The ultrastructure of the muscle in dystrophia myotonica has been reported by Wechsler and Hager (1961b), Mahoudeau *et al.* (1961), Thiébaut *et al.* (1963), Aleu and Afifi (1964), Milhaud, Fardeau and Lapresle (1964), Fardeau, Lapresle and Milhaud (1965), Schotland, Spiro and Carmel (1966), Klinkerfuss (1967), Samaha *et al.* (1967), Schroeder and Adams (1968), Sato and Tsubaki (1968), Lapresle and Fardeau (1968), Monticone and Gabella (1969), Allen, Johnson and Woolf (1969), Santa (1969), Mussini, Di Mauro and Angelini (1970), Schotland (1970), Fardeau (1970), Schroeder (1970), Monticone, Gabella and Bergamini (1970), Radu *et al.* (1970) and Ionescu, Radu and Nicolescu (1970).

The ultrastructural changes in the muscle fibres of rats with experimental myotonia were reported by Schroeder and Kuhn (1968).

POLYMYOSITIS AND ALLIED CONDITIONS

Polymyositis is an inflammatory condition of muscle which is sometimes associated with inflammation of the skin and is then referred to as dermatomyositis. The changes in polymyositis and allied conditions such as periarteritis nodosa consist of cellular infiltration around the blood vessels and between the muscle fibres which may present degenerative changes. The infiltrating cells consist usually of polymorphs, lymphocytes, plasma cells and mast cells: some of the polymorphs may be eosinophils (Plates 60, 61, 62 and 75). Similar infiltration may be found within degenerating muscle fibres (Plate 63 lower part). The affected muscle exhibits many more blood capillaries than normal: they show endothelial cell hypertrophy and hyperplasia (Plate 59). The pericytes in the clefts within the basement membrane around the capillaries increase in number and the basement membrane may be thickened and reduplicated. The endothelial cells and the pericytes show evidence of increased cellular activity, their cytoplasm containing numerous ribosomes, vesicles and various bodies as well as autophagic vacuoles. The fibroblasts and collagen between the muscle fibres may be greatly increased, particularly during the healing stage of the disease. In florid cases the degenerative changes in the muscle may be intense and many muscle fibres may be involved; they may show disorganisation and disintegration of the myofibrils (Plates 35 and 76). The sarcoplasm appears to be increased in amount and contains randomly distributed triads (Plate 35), numerous vesicles, abnormal mitochondria (Plate 31 lower part), membranous and myelin bodies (Plate 41) and autophagic vacuoles. The Z-lines may become distorted and thickened (Plate 23 lower part).

In addition some muscle fibres may contain groups of electron dense rods (Plates 35 and 77). Some of the affected muscle fibres exhibit multiple infoldings of their surface (Plate 20 upper part). The nerves and motor end plates may also be affected in inflammatory disorders of muscles, but so far as we know their ultrastructure under such circumstances has not been extensively studied. Motor end plates in a case of polymyositis are illustrated in Plate 67, but in this case there is little evidence of structural alteration.

In inflammatory conditions of muscle, regeneration of muscle fibres very often accompanies their degeneration (Plates 52, 53, 54 and 55). Satellite cells are found much more frequently than in other muscle diseases. Some of the satellite cells present myofilaments which are forming myofibrils (Plate 54). The satellite cells may also exhibit degenerative changes.

Ultrastructural changes in polymyositis have been illustrated by various authors including Palmeiro, Behrend and Wechsler (1966), Rose, Walton and Pearce (1967), Shafiq, Milhorat and Gorycki (1967a), Mintz, Gonzáles-Angulo and Fraga (1968), Chou (1967 a and b and 1969), Hudgson and Pearce (1969), Stoebner *et al.* (1970), and Mastaglia and Walton (1970).

Palmeiro *et al.* (1966) demonstrated tubular structures which might possibly be altered virus particles in the sarcoplasm of a case of polymyositis.

Chou (1967b and 1968) described myxovirus-like structures in the nucleus and cytoplasm of the muscle fibres in chronic polymyositis, and later Chou and Gutmann (1970) and Mastaglia and Walton (1970) described picornavirus-like particles in the cytoplasm of muscle fibres in subacute polymyositis. Norris *et al.* (1969) described virus-like particles in the muscle biopsies of two patients who had myositis associated with herpes zoster. These findings may suggest that a virus may play a role in the aetiology of polymyositis, but we should add that we have seen structures similar to these reported by Norris *et al.* in a case of muscular dystrophy as illustrated in Plate 74.

In scleroderma the muscle may also be affected and the changes in its ultrastructure were reported by Michalowsky and Kudejko (1966).

Changes similar to these observed in polymyositis were noted in the capillaries, interstitial tissue and the muscle fibres in Behçet's disease by Garcin, Lapresle and Hewitt (1967).

Generalised myositis was induced in rats by the administration of dimethyl paraphenylenediamine by Anderson and Song (1966a) and inflammatory vascular changes and changes in the muscle following the administration of dimethylsulphoxide to rats were reported by Walters, Papadimitriou and Shilkin (1967) and Kakulas (1969).

METABOLIC, ENDOCRINE AND TOXIC MYOPATHIES

Muscle may undergo changes in many metabolic, endocrine and toxic conditions. These include periodic paralysis, glycogen storage diseases, diseases of the thyroid, pituitary and adrenal glands and toxic conditions caused by steroids, chloroquine, vincristine and other therapeutic drugs.

PERIODIC PARALYSIS. The ultrastructure of muscle in cases of periodic paralysis, and particularly of the hypokalaemic type, has been fairly extensively studied. The most obvious ultrastructural change is the presence of large membrane bound vacuoles which may be numerous and are thought to arise from dilatation of the sarcoplasmic reticulum. In addition the myofibrils and the other organelles of the fibre may undergo changes and, as mentioned in Chapter 2, cytoplasmic bodies, honeycomb and tubular structures may appear in the sarcoplasm.

The ultrastructure of the muscle was reported in hypokalaemic periodic paralysis by Gruner and Porte (1959), Shy *et al.* (1961), Pearce (1963), Seitelberger and Stockinger (1965), A. G. Engel (1965 and 1966c), Gruner (1966), Howes *et al.* (1966), Odor, Patel and Pearce (1967), Norris, Panner and Stormont (1968), Mussini, Di Mauro and Margreth (1968), Macdonald, Rewcastle and Humphrey (1969), Brody and Dudley (1969), Biczyskowa, Fidziánska and Jedrzejowska (1969), Schutta and Armitage (1969), Bergman *et al.* (1970) and Dunkle *et al.* (1970); in hyperkalaemic periodic paralysis by Jaffurs *et al.* (1963), van Bogaert *et al.* (1967), Macdonald, Rewcastle and Humphrey (1968); and in hyper and normokalaemic periodic paralysis by Bradley (1969). Paramyotonia congenita, which some authors consider to be the same disease as hyperkalaemic periodic paralysis, was reported by Garcin *et al.* (1966) and Castaigne *et al.* (1970).

Tubular structures which may occur in periodic paralysis (page 54) have been described by Gruner (1966), Odor *et al.* (1967), Macdonald *et al.* (1968 and 1969), Bradley (1969), W. K. Engel, Bishop and Cunningham (1970), Bergman *et al.* (1970), Dunkle *et al.* (1970) and Castaigne *et al.* (1970).

GLYCOGEN STORAGE DISEASES. Glycogen storage diseases are rare conditions in which the metabolism of glycogen is altered due to inherited enzyme deficiencies of which several have been identified. McArdle (1969) considered eight types and in addition refers to phosphohexoisomerase and phosphorylase-b-kinase deficiencies. The skeletal musculature is involved in Types II, III, IV, V, VII and VIII and also in phosphohexoisomerase deficiency. The myocardium is involved in Types II, III and IV.

The ultrastructural features of the muscle in the glycogenoses consist of an excess of free or membrane bound glycogen in the muscle fibres. Degenerative changes, autophagic vacuoles and various abnormal structures may be found in the sarcoplasm.

Glycogen storage disease may be suspected from the clinical features and the histological examination of the muscle, but a definite diagnosis can be made only with recourse to histochemical and biochemical techniques which may reveal the respective enzyme deficiencies. In some cases more than one enzyme has been found to be deficient.

Reports on the ultrastructure of muscle have been made in Types II, III and V.

Type II (Pompe's Type) which is due to acid maltase deficiency occurs not only in young children but also in adults and has been reported by Zellweger *et al.* (1965), Isch *et al.* (1966), Cardiff (1966), Hug *et al.* (1966), Smith, Zellweger and Afifi (1967), Hers and van Hoof (1968), Hudgson *et al.* (1968), Pearce, Adamson and Salter (1968), A. G. Engel and Dale (1968), Garancis (1968), A. G. Engel (1970 a and b) and Bruni and Paluello (1970). The ultrastructure of the myocardium in this condition was reported by Bordiuk *et al.* (1970).

Type III (Cori's or Forbes' Type) is due to amylo-1,6-glucosidase deficiency and occurs in young children and has been reported by Hug *et al.* (1966), Paluello, Bruni and Spiele (1967) and Neustein (1969).

Type V (McArdle's Type) is due to muscle phosphorylase deficiency and is met in children and later in life. It has been reported by Schotland *et al.* (1965), Sluga, Seitelberger and Moser (1967), Schimrigk *et al.* (1967), Salter, Adamson and Pearce (1967), Gruener *et al.* (1968), Pearce, Adamson and Salter (1968), Brownell *et al.* (1969) and Mastaglia, McCollum *et al.* (1970).

THYROID AND PITUITARY GLAND DISORDERS. It is well known that weakness and wasting of muscles may be associated with thyroid disease, especially thyrotoxicosis.

When the thyrotoxic disorder is associated with hypokalaemic periodic paralysis, the muscle changes may be very striking and the ultrastructure of muscle in such conditions has already been mentioned.

The electron microscopy findings in the muscle in hyperthyroid myopathies have been reported in two cases by A. G. Engel (1965 and 1966 b and c). The changes consist of folds of basement membrane protruding from the surface of the muscle fibre, subsarcolemmal deposits of glycogen, collections of vesicles and changes in many of the mitochondria. Some of the T-systems are dilated but the sarcoplasmic reticulum is normal.

Norris and Panner (1966), Bergouignan, Vital and Bataille (1967) and Godet-Guillain and Fardeau (1970) reported the ultrastructural changes in hypothyroid myopathy. They described disorganisation of myofibrils, sarcoplasmic masses, increase of nuclei, rods throughout the sarcoplasm and alterations and inclusions in the mitochondria.

Hypothyroidism may be secondary to deficiency of the pituitary thyrotrophin hormone. Grabow and Chou (1968) reported the ultrastructure of muscle in a patient with peripheral neuropathy due to thyrotrophin deficiency. The changes included variability in the width of the myofibrils, abnormalities of the Z-lines which were sometimes doubled, mitochondrial changes and the presence of vacuoles.

Asbøe-Hansen, Iversen and Wichmann (1952) in a light microscopy study described at the periphery of muscle fibres PAS positive mucopolysaccharide crescentic masses in transverse section and spindle-shaped masses in longitudinal section, in patients with pituitary-thyroid disease. These masses could be identified only after fixation by lead sub-acetate. Iversen, Asbøe-Hansen and Carlsen (1953) illustrated these crescents in electron micrographs of muscle.

Hyperparathyroidism may also be associated with myopathy and the ultrastructure of the muscle of two familial cases was reported by Hudson, Cholod and Haust (1970).

ADRENAL GLAND DISORDERS AND STEROID MYOPATHY. In Cushing's syndrome, aldosteronism and prolonged steroid therapy, symptoms due to the involvement of muscle may occur. We are unaware of any report on the ultrastructure of muscle in Cushing's syndrome or aldosteronism, but reports on myopathy due to steroids have been made by Golding *et al.* (1961), Pearce (1963), A. G. Engel (1965 and 1966b), Afifi, Bergman and Harvey (1968), Mastaglia, McCollum *et al.* (1970) and Jerusalem (1970). The changes affect the myofibrils and the sarcoplasmic reticulum and glycogen accumulates in the muscle fibres. Lipid bodies and myelin bodies occur in the sarcoplasm. The mitochondria undergo various changes: some of them appear to give rise to membranous bodies as illustrated in Plate 78. Prominence of the Golgi apparatus of the muscle fibre and marked thickness of the capillary basement membrane were noted by Afifi *et al.* (1968).

The ultrastructure of two muscle biopsies in patients with myopathy following adrenalectomy for Cushing's syndrome was reported by Prineas *et al.* (1968). The changes consisted of increase of lipid droplets, lipofuscin, glycogen and aggregations of mitochondria.

The ultrastructural changes in the muscle of rabbits treated with steroids were studied by D'Agostino and Chiga (1966 a and b), Ritter (1967), Tice and A. G. Engel (1967), Afifi and Bergman (1969), Freund-Mölbert *et al.* (1970) and Serratice, Toga *et al.* (1970). They reported similar changes as those seen in human steroid myopathy. The ultrastructural changes in the myocardium have been reported by D'Agostino (1964) and D'Agostino and Chiga (1966b).

VINCRISTINE NEUROMYOPATHY. Patients who are treated with vincristine sulphate because of malignant disease may develop neuromyopathy. The muscle of such patients undergoes degeneration and atrophy of the fibres: the intermyofibrillary spaces become widened and filled with glycogen granules, mitochondria and lipid bodies. In some fibres the number of nuclei per field may be increased and they are often vesicular with prominent nucleoli. Near the nucleus lipid bodies may occur

(Plate 79 lower right). Mitochondrial aggregates occur under the plasma membrane and around the nuclei. The mitochondria are frequently distended and their cristae broken: they may contain tubules or membranous and lipid bodies (Plates 31 and 79 upper parts). The membranous bodies may be very striking in some degenerating fibres (Plate 80 upper part). The T-systems are frequently very prominent and their course may be followed over several myofibrils (Plate 79 lower left).

The ultrastructure of vincristine neuromyopathy in man has been reported by Bradley *et al.* (1970).

The muscle in experimental animals exposed to vincristine show somewhat similar but more marked ultrastructural changes than in man. Particularly striking in rats exposed to the drug are the numerous and large spheromembranous bodies (Plate 80 lower part) and also honeycomb structures which may be very numerous in some atrophying fibres. Studies on this subject were carried out in rats by Anderson, Song and Slotwiner (1967) and Morgan-Hughes, Le Quesne and Mair and in guinea pigs by Bradley (1970). Anderson *et al.* described in addition dilated synaptic vesicles in the terminal axon extensions and irregular infolding and evagination of the secondary synaptic clefts of the motor end plate.

CHLOROQUINE MYOPATHY. Prolonged treatment with chloroquine and related drugs may produce myopathy or neuromyopathy.

A very striking feature of muscle biopsies of patients so treated is the presence of numerous vacuoles in the muscle fibres and was first reported in light microscopy by Whisnant *et al.* (1963).

The ultrastructural changes which take place in the muscle consist of atrophy of the muscle fibres, the myofibrils of which become widely spaced with large amounts of glycogen granules (Plate 82) and vesicles between them. The myofibrils eventually undergo degenerative changes and become disarrayed. Aggregates of mitochondria are often prominent, particularly under the plasma membrane (Plate 81 upper part). Very large vacuoles also occur: some appear to be empty while others contain granules of varying size and electron density and myelin bodies which sometimes contain collections of granules. Some of the vacuoles are autophagic vacuoles (Plate 81 lower part). The nucleus of the degenerating fibres may exhibit distensions of the outer nuclear membrane which contain electron dense bodies of varying size (Plate 82 lower part).

Humphrey and Rewcastle (1963), Garcin, Rondot and Fardeau (1964), Rewcastle and Humphrey (1965) and Mair (1965) reported on the ultrastructure of the muscle in patients treated with chloroquine. Rewcastle and Humphrey and Garcin *et al.* demonstrated autophagic vacuoles in the cells of the blood capillaries as well as in the muscle.

Studies on the muscle of animals treated with chloroquine have been reported by several authors and the most recent of these are on rats by Macdonald and A. G. Engel (1970) and on rabbits by Aguayo and Hudgson (1970). Macdonald and A. G. Engel used peroxidase as a marker for the T-systems in their study and deduced that the T-systems may contribute to the membranes limiting the autophagic vacuoles.

OTHER DRUGS AFFECTING MUSCLE. We are unaware of the reports on the ultrastructural changes in muscle in man due to other drugs. However, numerous reports are available on the ultrastructure of muscle following the administration of different drugs to experimental animals. These reports include the effects of plasmocid by Price, Pease and Pearson (1962), D'Agostino (1963) and Anderson and Song (1966b). The effects of emetine were reported by Duane and A. G. Engel (1970), of calvacin by Anderson and Song (1966 a and b), of tri-ortho-cresyl phosphate by Prineas (1969 a and b) and acrylamide by Prineas (1969c), of dimethyl paraphenylenediamine by Anderson and Song (1966a) and of dimethyl sulphoxide by Walters, Papadimitriou and Shilkin (1967) and Kakulas (1969).

ALCOHOLIC MYOPATHY. It is well known that acute or chronic myopathy may occur in alcoholics.

The ultrastructural features of muscle in acute alcoholic myopathy were first reported by Douglas *et al.* (1966) who described distortion of the myofibrils, changes in the mitochondria and discontinuity of the plasma membrane in affected fibres. Klinkerfuss *et al.* (1967) reported the ultrastructural changes of muscle in both acute and chronic alcoholic myopathy in eight biopsies. In acute cases the myofibrils were widely spaced and some of them were undergoing degeneration. In chronic cases they illustrated degeneration of muscle fibres, dense bodies in some mitochondria, an increase of lipid droplets and condensation of the filaments of parts of myofibrils: in these parts, the T-tubules could sometimes be identified but not the other organelles. Morgan-Hughes, Anderson and Mair studied a case of chronic alcoholic myopathy in which the most frequent ultrastructural change in the muscle was replacement of all the elements of one or more adjacent or consecutive sarcomeres by electron dense material: this change is often referred to as streaming of the Z-lines (Plate 23 upper part). Mitochondria were absent from the regions of the muscle fibre affected by this change. Such change in the myofibrils, however, is common to many diseases of muscle. In many muscle fibres the mitochondria contained small, round, electron dense bodies. Collections of tubules were also found near the surface and around the nuclei of the muscle fibres as illustrated in Plate 48 (upper part).

The ultrastructure of the myocardium post mortem was reported in six cases of alcoholic myopathy by Hibbs *et al.* (1965).

VITAMIN E DEFICIENCY. It has long been known that animals develop myopathy when fed on a diet deficient in vitamin E. Vitamin E deficiency in animals and men was reviewed recently in the *Lancet* (1969).

Myopathy due to vitamin E deficiency in animals was reviewed by West (1963) and Blaxter (1969). Reports of the ultrastructure of the muscle in acute vitamin E dystrophy in suckling rats were given by Rumery and Hampton (1959) and of the chronic stages in rats by Howes, Price and Blumberg (1964), in chickens by Cheville (1966) and in rabbits by van Vleet, Hall and Simon (1967 and 1968). In the early stages of vitamin E deficiency the changes may be confined to localised regions of the muscle fibre and consist of alterations of the mitochondria and sarcoplasmic reticulum, accumulations of lipid and glycogen and degeneration of myofibrils.

Membranous and myelin bodies may also be found in the affected muscle fibres and Howes *et al.* illustrated structures with the appearance of autophagic vacuoles in their report. van Vleet *et al.* described also regeneration coexisting with degeneration of muscle.

In a patient with vitamin E deficiency studied by Borgström, Nordén and Ståhl (1971), the muscle was examined by Hendriksson, Nordén and Mair (1971): the nuclei of the muscle fibres had often migrated to the centre (Plate 29 upper part) and many fibres were undergoing degeneration (Plates 83 and 84). Some of them contained prominent collections of tubules (Plate 83 upper part). The myofibrils were sometimes disintegrating or were agglutinated into electron dense masses with large vacuoles between them. Muscle fibres in an advanced stage of degeneration were infiltrated by phagocytes. Empty folds and tubes of basement membrane of muscle fibres frequently occurred and phagocytes were found between the degenerating muscle fibres. In addition many muscle fibres contained satellite cells (Plates 51 upper part and 84 lower part).

CARCINOMATOUS NEUROMYOPATHY. Besides the incidence of dermatomyositis and polymyositis, various clinical manifestations of peripheral neuropathy and myopathy are associated with malignant disease and are generally referred to as carcinomatous neuromyopathies. Studies of the muscle by light microscopy were reported by Henson, Russell and Wilkinson (1954) and other authors and a recent report on this subject is that of Urich and Wilkinson (1970). There are few reports on the ultrastructure of muscle in association with malignant disease and to our knowledge no specific changes have been reported.

CONGENITAL MYOPATHIES

In recent years, some congenital myopathies which are thought to have specific features have been identified as new diseases. These include central core disease, nemaline, myotubular and the so-called mitochondrial myopathies.

CENTRAL CORE DISEASE. Shy and Magee (1956) described, in three generations of the same family, five cases of non-progressive congenital myopathy which later were named central core disease by Greenfield, Corman and Shy (1958). This term was applied because there occurs in almost every fibre 'a central core of more closely set myofibrils which appear more amorphous than the surrounding zone'. Two or three cores were described in some of the fibres and were sometimes more peripheral than central.

Thirteen more cases of this condition have since been reported: four were sporadic (Bethlem and Meyjes, 1960; W. K. Engel *et al.*, 1961; Dubowitz and Platts, 1965; and Mrozek, Strugalska and Fidziánska, 1970) and the others familial (Afifi, Smith and Zellweger, 1965; Gonatas *et al.*, 1965; Bethlem *et al.*, 1966; and Dubowitz and Roy, 1970). The clinical picture was similar in all cases except those of Bethlem *et al.* (1966) and consists of hypotonia, proximal weakness which is most severe in the lower limbs and walking is delayed. The disability remains stationary. The patients reported by Bethlem *et al.* had no hypotonia nor delay of motor development but had mild proximal weakness and muscle cramps after exercise.

Histochemical methods demonstrated that the cores are deficient or devoid of enzyme activity (Dubowitz and Pearse, 1960b; Seitelberger, Wanko and Gavin, 1961; Gonatas *et al.* 1965; Dubowitz and Platts, 1965; Bethlem *et al.*, 1966; W. K. Engel, 1967; and Dubowitz and Roy, 1970). The changes appear to be confined to type I fibres (Dubowitz and Platts, Bethlem *et al.*, W. K. Engel and Dubowitz and Roy). Further, in the cases of W. K. Engel *et al.* (1961) which were studied histochemically by Dubowitz and Pearse (1960b) and by W. K. Engel (1967) and in a case of Dubowitz and Roy almost all the muscle fibres present in the biopsy were type I. In the two cases reported by Gonatas *et al.* all the fibres reacted similarly with the histochemical techniques employed and could not be differentiated into fibre types.

Ultrastructural studies of the muscle in central core disease have been reported by W. K. Engel *et al.* (1961), Seitelberger, Wanko and Gavin (1961), Afifi, Smith and Zellweger (1965), Gonatas *et al.* (1965), Dubowitz and Roy (1970) and Mrozek, Strugalska and Fidziánska (1970). The changes consist of alteration of the sarcomere pattern, the Z-lines being zig-zag or fragmented and the myofibrils more closely packed together. In the altered regions glycogen, mitochondria, sarcoplasmic reticulum and T-systems are reduced in number or are absent. The transition between the cores and the adjacent areas of the muscle fibre is abrupt.

The majority of the cases of central core disease have similar clinical features and all of them present similar morphological change, which favours the view that central core disease may be a definite entity.

Afifi, Smith and Zellweger (1965) reported the ultrastructural features of central core disease and nemaline myopathy in a muscle biopsy of a woman with a non-progressive myopathy whose daughter had a similar congenital myopathy. By light microscopy, central cores were identified in a muscle biopsy from the daughter but nemaline bodies were not found. However electron microscope studies were carried out on the biopsy of the mother only. Because of the incidence of nemaline rods and central cores in the same biopsy Afifi *et al.* suggested that nemaline myopathy and central core disease may be different manifestations of the same disease process. It is interesting in this connection that Shafiq *et al.* (1969) produced central cores and nemaline rods in the same muscle fibre by tenotomy of the soleus muscle in the rat and deduced that these morphological changes were not specific for any particular pathological process.

NEMALINE MYOPATHY. Nemaline myopathy is a congenital condition which is usually non-progressive and may be familial. The disease was so named by Shy *et al.* (1963) because of the presence of rods or thread-like structures (Gk. nema = thread) in many of the muscle fibres. In 1963 the disease was described independently by Conen, Murphy and Donohue, who stated that the ultrastructure of the rods which they called myogranules resembled the recrystallised muscle protein paramyosin. Since 1963 various other cases have been reported. Most cases are congenital and symptoms become manifest early in life, but a few cases have been described in older individuals by W. K. Engel and Resnick (1966), A. G. Engel (1966a) and Hefferman, Rewcastle and Humphrey (1968).

The disease is characterised on pathological grounds by the presence of numerous rods mainly in type I fibres. The ultrastructure of the rods is described on page 48. Apart from the presence of the rods and disruption of the sarcomere pattern of the myofibrils in the immediate neighbourhood of the rods, few other changes have been reported in cases of nemaline myopathy.

Studies on the ultrastructure of the disease have been reported by Shy *et al.* (1963), Conen, Murphy and Donohue (1963), W. K. Engel, Wanko and Fenichel (1964), Price *et al.* (1965), Afifi, Smith and Zellweger (1965), Gonatas, Shy and Godfrey (1966), Gonatas (1966), W. K. Engel and Resnick (1966), A. G. Engel (1966a), Lindsey, Hopkins and Clark (1966), A. G. Engel and Gomez (1967), Shafiq, Dubowitz *et al.* (1967), Hudgson *et al.* (1967), Kolin (1967), Hefferman, Rewcastle and Humphrey (1968) and Fardeau (1969b).

MYOTUBULAR MYOPATHY. Myotubular myopathy was described first by Spiro, Shy and Gonatas (1966) in an adolescent male with insidious progressive generalised muscular weakness, bilateral ptosis, ophthalmoplegia, facial diplegia and other congenital abnormalities. Two muscle biopsies showed large numbers of fibres having nuclei, mitochondria and myelin figures in the centre of the fibres and absence of myofibrils in this central region. The authors regarded these fibres as myotubes and suggested that they indicated arrest in the development of the muscle.

The ultrastructure of myotubular myopathy has been reported by Spiro, Shy and Gonatas (1966), Sher *et al.* (1967), Kinoshita and Cadman (1968), Campbell, Rebeiz and Walton (1969), Badurska *et al.* (1969), Karpati, Carpenter and Nelson (1970), Ortiz de Zarate and Maruffo (1970), and Vital *et al.* (1970).

Sher *et al.* (1967), Bethlem *et al.* (1968 and 1970), and Munsat, Thompson and Coleman (1969) do not think that the muscle fibres with the central nuclei in this condition are really myotubes and refer to the condition as centronuclear myopathy, while Campbell *et al.* and Vital *et al.* prefer the descriptive term peri-centronuclear myopathy.

MITOCHONDRIAL MYOPATHIES. Luft *et al.* (1962) were the first to claim that changes in the mitochondria of muscle were responsible for a clinical syndrome in which there was hypermetabolism which was not due to thyroid hyperactivity. The mitochondria in the muscle were very numerous: some showed structural changes including lamellar inclusions. Luft *et al.* carried out biochemical studies on mitochondria isolated from the muscle of this case and concluded that the hypermetabolism was due to '. . . a defect in the mitochondrial enzyme organisation, resulting in a severely lowered capacity for respiratory control'. Mitochondrial inclusions were reported by Gruner (1963) in two cases: one of slowly progressive distal myopathy of late onset and the other neurogenic muscular atrophy. Two cases of slowly progressive muscular dystrophy with mitochondrial abnormalities were later described by Gonatas and Shy (1966) and Shy, Gonatas and Perez (1966). Both cases were children of 8 years. In one, the mitochondria were very large and contained rectangular or round inclusions. They called the disorder 'megaconial myopathy' because of the unusually large size of the mitochondria. In the other child the mitochondria were small but very numerous and contained round dense inclusions and the disease was termed 'pleoconial myopathy'.

Subsequent to this more than 40 cases of disorders of muscle with mitochondrial inclusions have been described in a variety of clinical conditions by Norris and Panner (1966), De Recondo, Fardeau and Lapresle (1966), Garcin *et al.* (1966), Zintz (1966), Price *et al.* (1967), Shafiq, Milhorat and Gorycki (1967c), Gonatas (1967), Sluga, Seitelberger and Moser (1967), D'Agostino *et al.* (1967 and 1968), Chou (1967a and 1969), van Wijngaarden *et al.* (1967), A. G. Engel and Dale (1968), Sato and Tsubaki (1968), Schutta and Armitage (1969), Fisher and Danowski (1969), Schellens and Ossentjuk (1969), Mastaglia *et al.* (1970), Fardeau (1970), Buscaino, de Giacomo and Mazzarella (1970), Sluga and Moser (1970), Godet-Guillain and Fardeau (1970), Hudgson (1970) and Sluga and Monneron (1970).

We found mitochondrial inclusions in four different clinical conditions: muscular dystrophy of the limb girdle type (Plate 32), muscular dystrophy of the Duchenne type, polymyositis and neuropathy.

Inclusions and various other changes in mitochondria have been reported in many 'normal' and pathological tissues. In muscle these changes occur in a great variety of diseases, and although they may indicate a disturbance in the metabolism of the mitochondria, there is not enough evidence to ascribe the changes to a particular disease.

Spiro, Prineas and Moore (1970) and other authors reported cases of muscular disease in which the mitochondria undergo various changes such as increase in their size and number, etc., and have labelled the condition mitochondrial myopathy. However, Peter, Stempel and Armstrong (1970), following a biochemical and electron microscope study of the mitochondrial fraction isolated from muscle of patients with various muscular disorders, concluded that while the mitochondria may be abnormal little significance could be attributed to this finding.

OTHER CONGENITAL MYOPATHIES. Ultrastructural studies of muscle have been described in cases of various other congenital myopathies and amongst these are the reports of Gubbay, Walton and Pearce (1966), A. G. Engel and Gomez (1966), Zellweger *et al.* (1967 a and b), Hurwitz *et al.* (1969), Afifi (1969), Afifi and Zellweger (1969) and Afifi *et al.* (1969).

The changes in the muscle in these cases, as in many other muscle diseases, are not, however, specific for the conditions and we shall not attempt to enumerate them.

PLATE 68. ABNORMALITIES OF MUSCLE FIBRES IN DENERVATION

UPPER. Here, between two larger muscle fibres, is a very small fibre with collagen on either side of it. The myofibrillary pattern is preserved in all three. In the small fibre, however, the Z-lines are not in evidence, being displaced presumably by the mitochondria and glycogen granules which are apparent between the A-bands of the myofibrils. Some myofilaments cut transversely lie at the upper edge of this fibre. The surfaces of all the fibres are undulating. In the upper and lower fibres a great increase in the glycogen is seen under the plasma membrane and between the myofibrils which show little evidence of structural change.

MAGNIFICATION 13,500 ×.

LOWER. Between two muscle fibres is a third muscle fibre exhibiting an irregular protrusion of the sarcoplasm overlying its myofibrils. The sarcoplasmic protrusion contains a nucleus, collections of lipid, membranous bodies and a large amount of glycogen granules. To the left of the nucleus are parallel membranes running an irregular course and enclosing collections of glycogen, lipid and a membranous body. Another membranous body lies in the fibre (top right).

MAGNIFICATION 21,000 ×.

Both are from a patient with polyneuropathy.

C	Collagen	Mi	Mitochondria
G	Glycogen	MeB	Membranous body
LB	Lipid body	MB	Myelin body
Me	Membranes	N	Nucleus
Mf	Myofibrils	TS	Transverse section

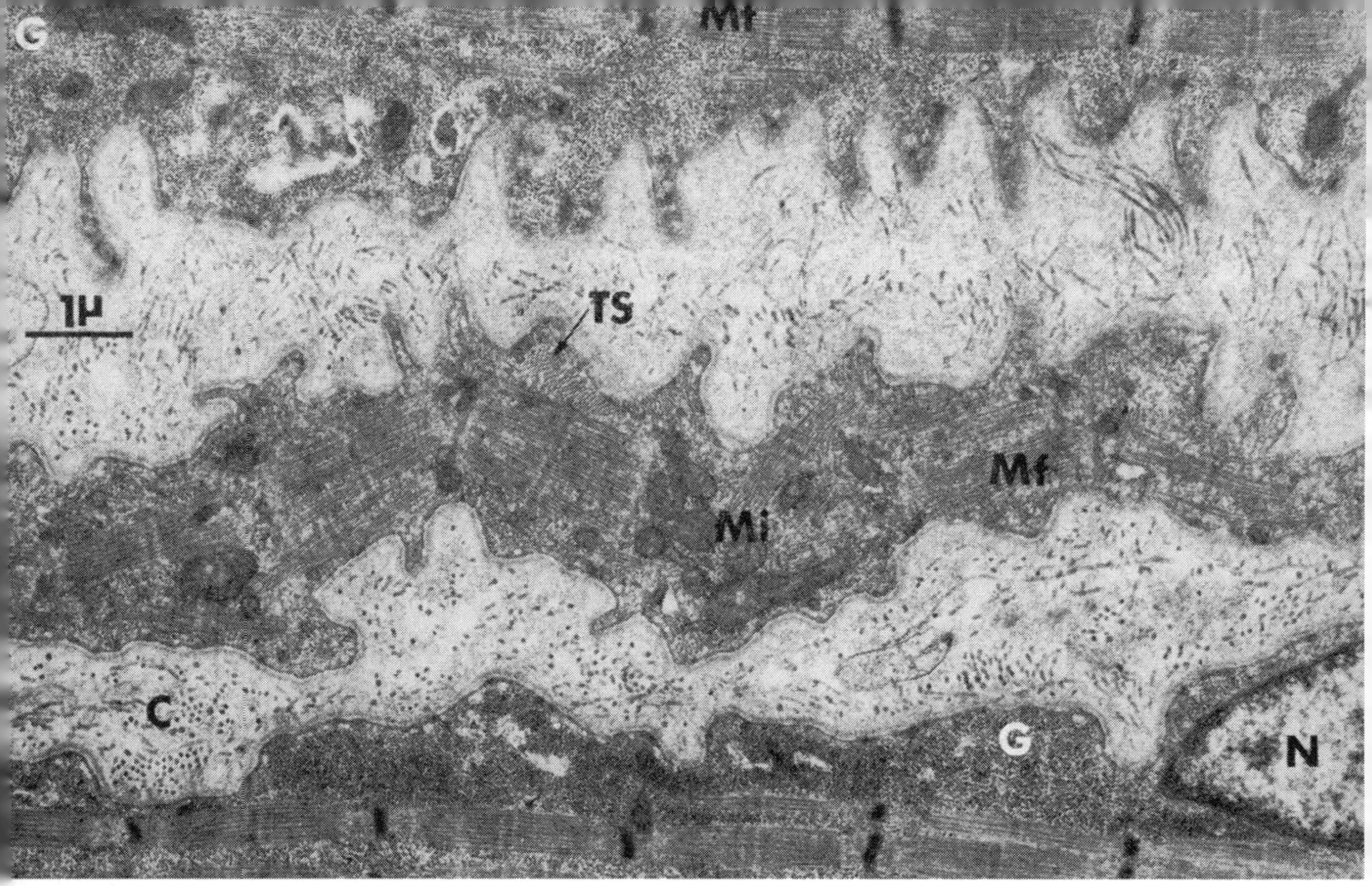
G
1μ
TS
Mf
Mi
C
G
N

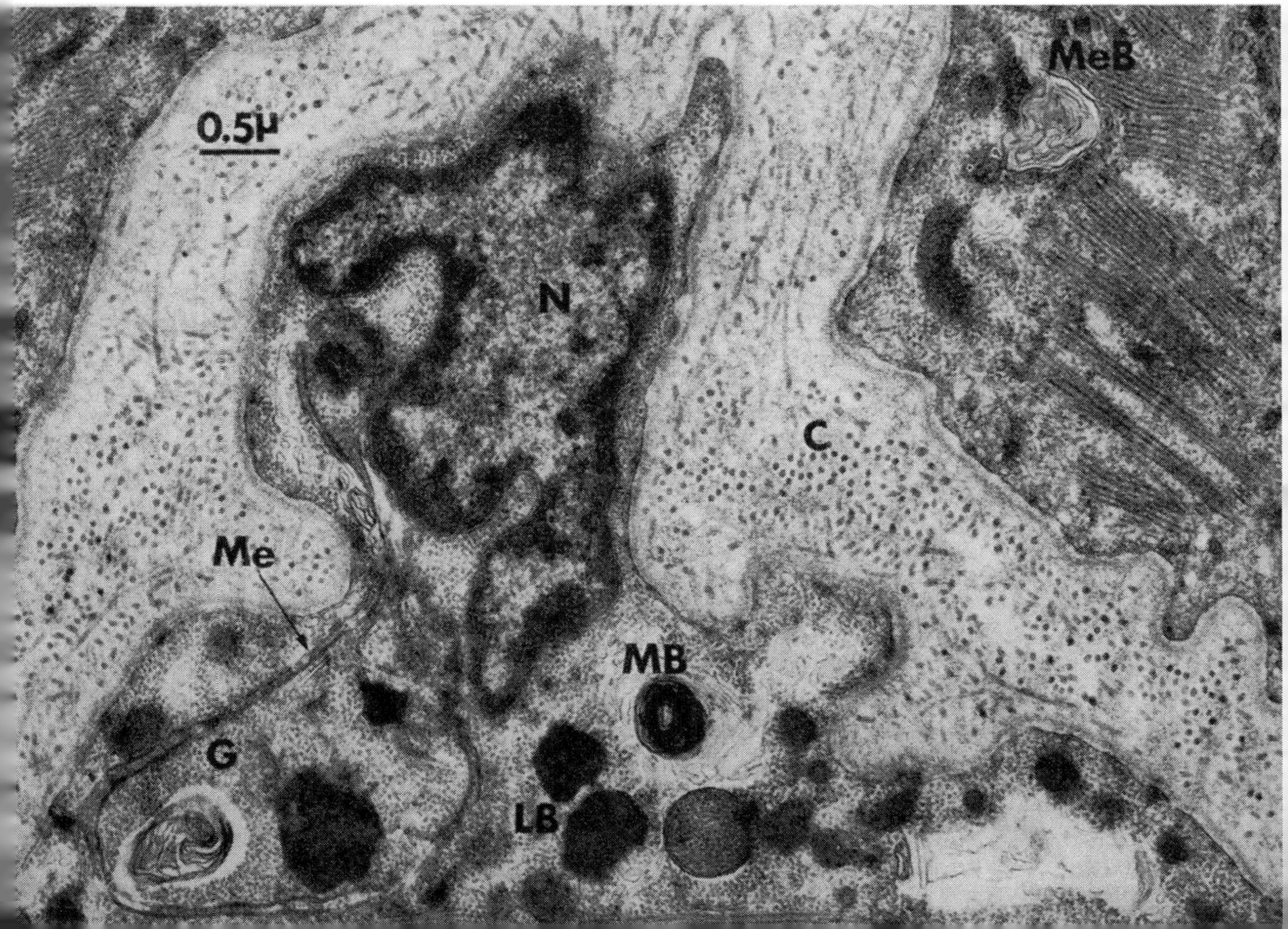
MeB
0.5μ
N
C
Me
MB
G
LB

PLATE 69. ATROPHIED MUSCLE FIBRE IN DENERVATION

The central fibre is undergoing degeneration. The nucleus lies in the middle of the muscle fibre and has a prominent nucleolus: the chromatin is distributed throughout the nucleus with an electron dense marginal zone. The myofibrils are disorganised with shortened and thickened Z-lines forming rods identical to those seen in nemaline myopathy. The sarcoplasm contains numerous small granules, some electron dense ovoid bodies and many vesicles. Displaced triads are seen throughout the muscle fibre. The plasma membrane is thicker than normal. At the top left is a fibroblast.

MAGNIFICATION 9,000 ×.

From a patient with alcoholic polyneuropathy.

F Fibroblast
Mf Myofibril
N Nucleus
Ro Rods
Tr Triads
Z Z-lines

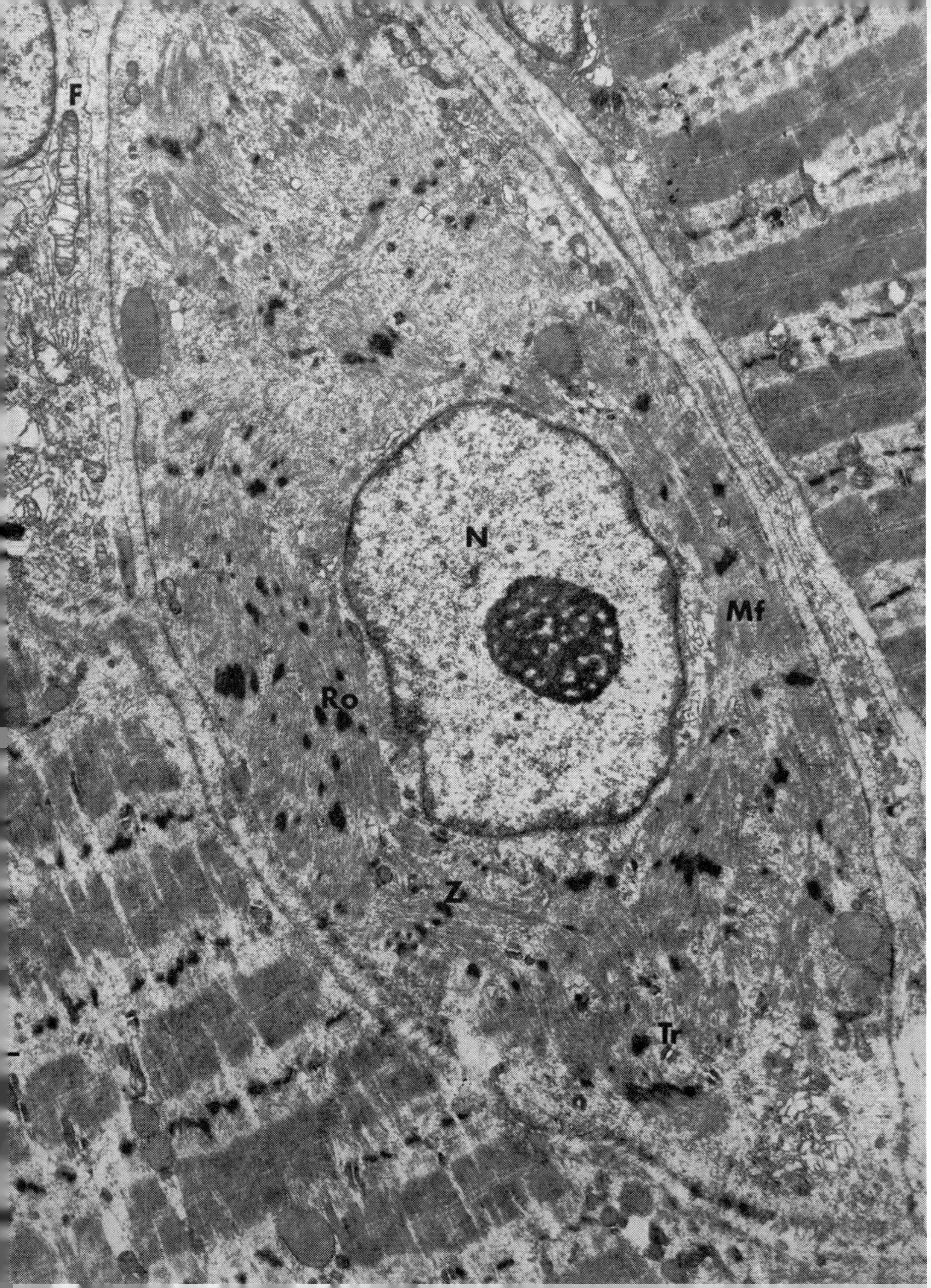
F
N
Mf
Ro
Z
Tr

PLATE 70. MUSCULAR DYSTROPHY (DUCHENNE TYPE)

UPPER. In the Duchenne type of muscular dystrophy as in other dystrophies the affected muscle fibres may show changes in all their components. The changes may be focal, however, and involve only one or two sarcomeres. The myofibrils at the top and bottom of the illustration are fairly well preserved, while the central ones show loss of filaments which is apparent in the I-bands of several sarcomeres, although remains of the Z-line can still be identified. The space between the affected myofibrils is increased. Triads may persist even if the related myofibrils and Z-lines show degenerative changes. Lipid bodies lie near the Z-lines and the mitochondria which are distended and their cristae broken.

MAGNIFICATION 19,000 ×.

LOWER. A striking feature of the Duchenne type of muscular dystrophy is the occurrence of a large amount of collagen around the muscle fibres. The fibroblasts also increase in number. Some have prominent rough endoplasmic reticulum. The nucleus of the muscle fibre has a distinct nucleolus: the nuclear chromatin is evenly dispersed except for a thin electron dense zone at the periphery. The Z-lines are somewhat distorted and slight changes are apparent in some of the I-bands.

MAGNIFICATION 9,000 ×.

A	A-band
C	Collagen
F	Fibroblast
I	I-band
LB	Lipid bodies
Mi	Mitochondria
N	Nucleus
Nu	Nucleolus
RER	Rough endoplasmic reticulum
Tr	Triads
V	Vesicles

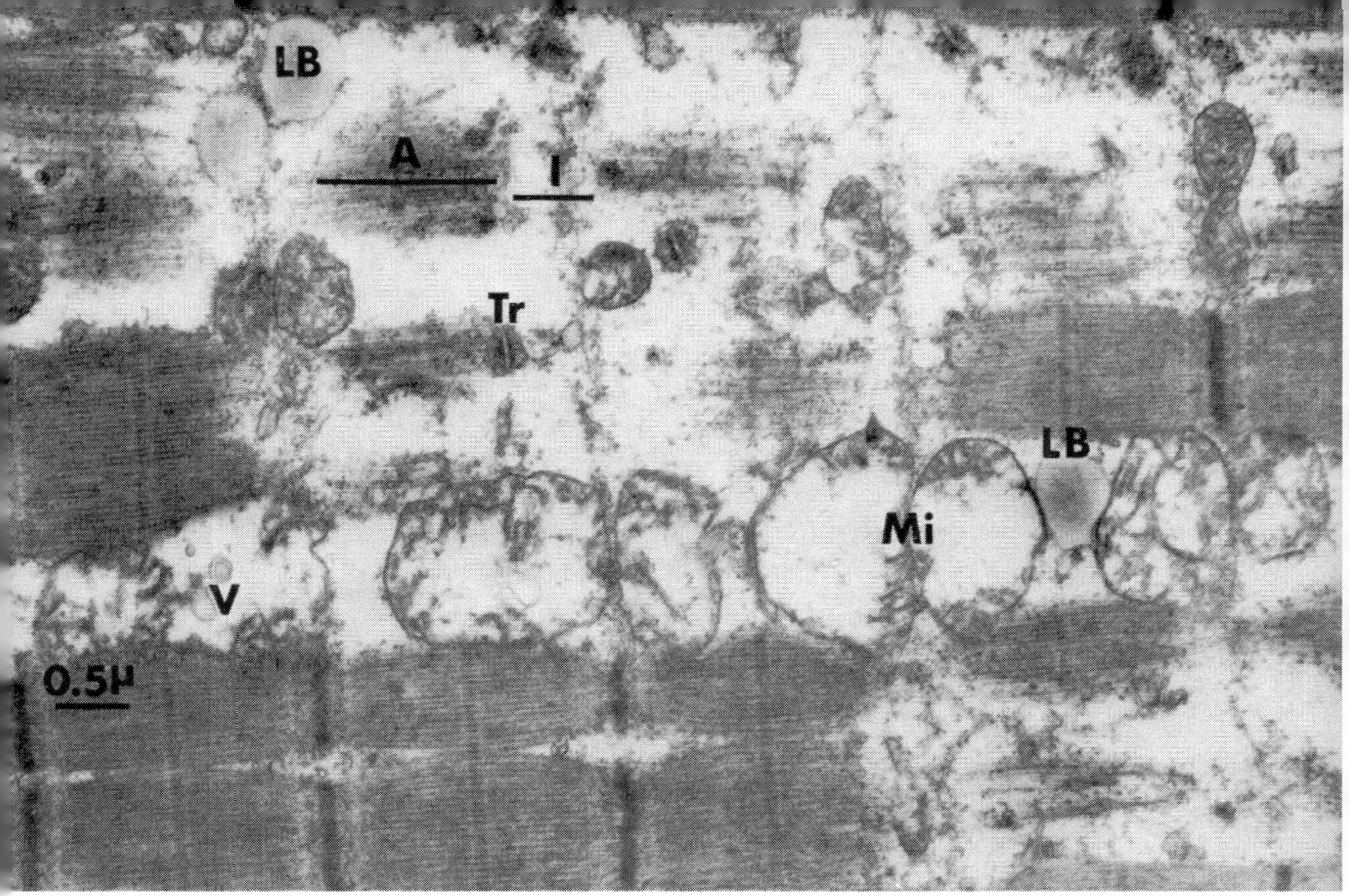
LB
A
I
Tr
LB
Mi
V
0.5μ

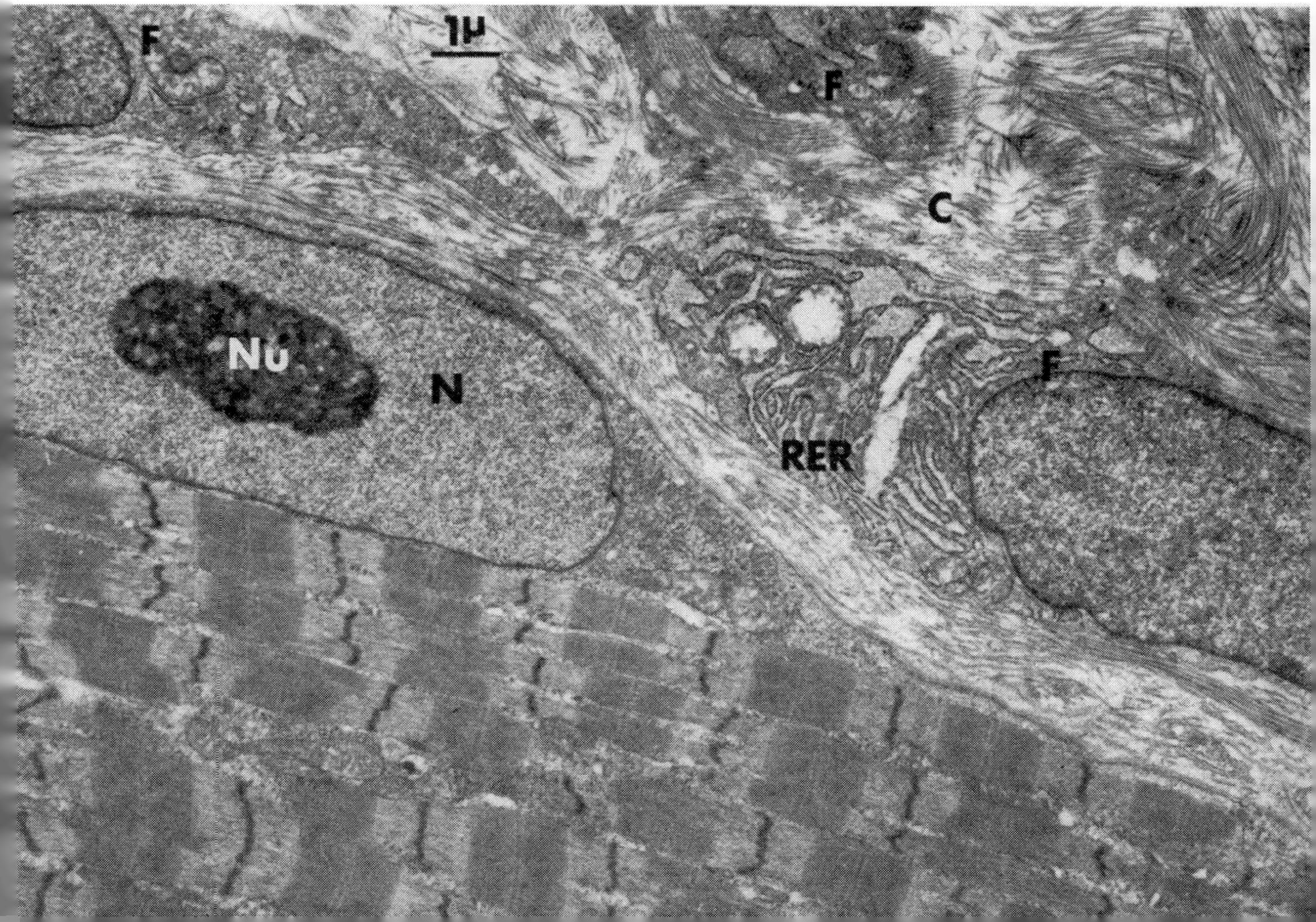
F
1μ
F
C
Nu
N
RER
F

PLATE 71. MUSCULAR DYSTROPHY
DOUBLE Z-LINES

An atrophying muscle fibre exhibits three nuclei in close proximity: two of them have a nucleolus. The chromatin is fairly evenly distributed throughout the nuclei with a rim of increased electron density around their margin. The myofibrils are irregularly distributed but the Z-lines and A-bands of some of them are in series. They present the striking anomaly of double Z-lines. Some of the Z-lines are thickened and distorted. An increase of glycogen granules is visible throughout the fibre: some lipid bodies occur amongst the myofibrils.

MAGNIFICATION 9,500 ×.

LB Lipid bodies
N Nucleus
Z Z-line

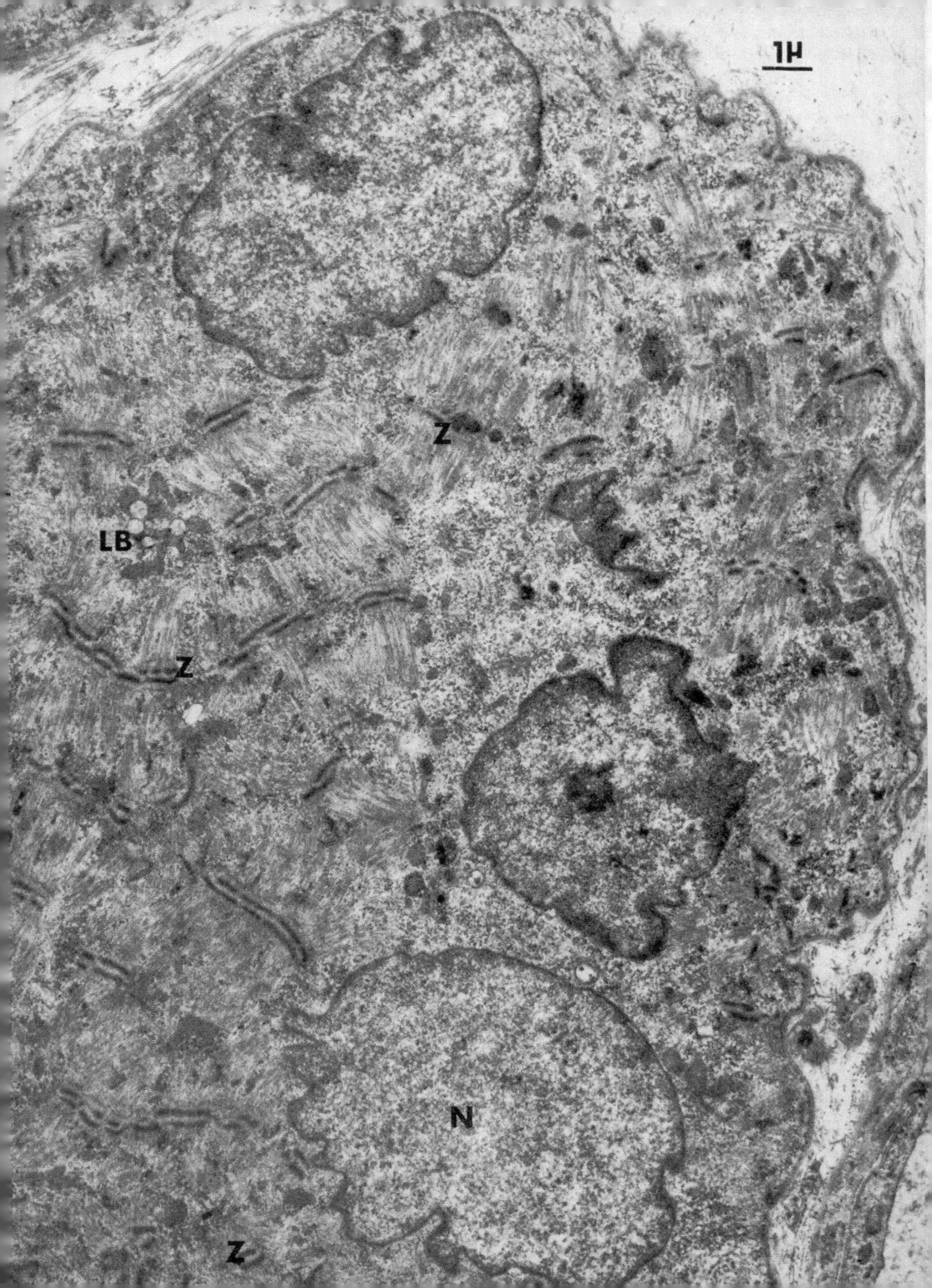
1μ
Z
LB
Z
N
Z

PLATE 72. MUSCULAR DYSTROPHY
ATROPHIED MUSCLE FIBRES

Several small atrophied muscle fibres are present and at the bottom left of the illustration is part of a ring fibre. Undulating, empty folds of basement membrane project at various points from the surface of the atrophied fibres whose myofibrils are disorganised. An increase of glycogen is seen in some of the fibres. Between the ring fibre and empty basement membrane folds lie processes of fibroblasts. Strands of collagen are scattered between the muscle fibres.

MAGNIFICATION 6,500 ×.

BM Basement membrane
C Collagen
F Fibroblast
G Glycogen
MF Muscle fibre
Z Z-line

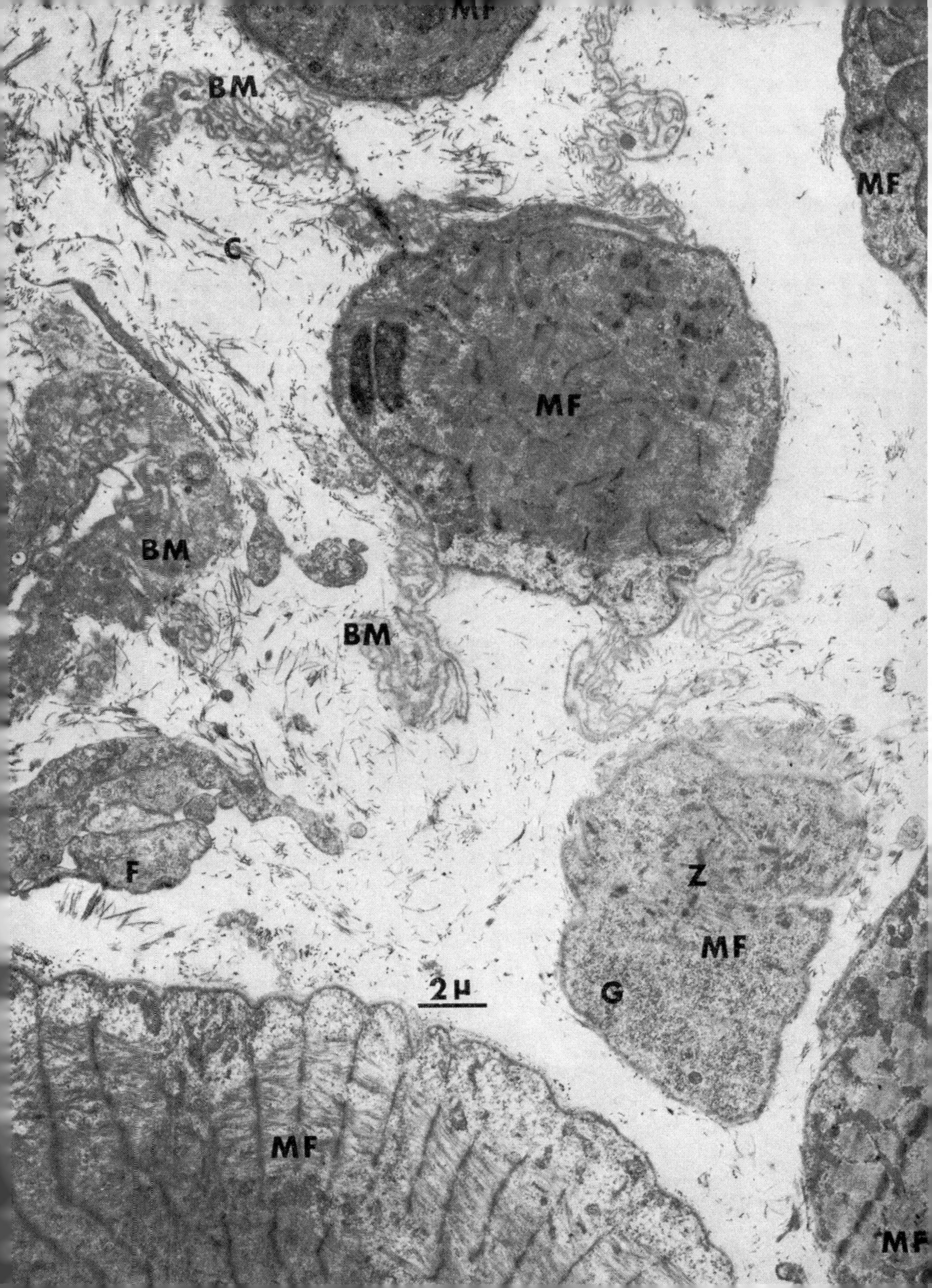

BM.
MF
C
MF
BM
BM
F
Z
MF
G
2 μ
MF
MF

PLATE 73. MUSCULAR DYSTROPHY
PHAGOCYTOSIS OF A DEGENERATING MUSCLE FIBRE

A degenerating muscle fibre is infiltrated by phagocytes, the cytoplasm of which is rich in ribosomes, polysomes (arrowed), vesicles, lipid bodies and mitochondria. In the phagocyte on the right occurs an inclusion of moderate electron density. Each phagocyte is bound by a well-defined plasma membrane. Degenerating myofilaments cut transversely and mitochondria whose cristae are not well defined lie between the plasma membranes of the phagocytes. The plasma membrane of the degenerating muscle fibre has disappeared but the wavy basement membrane persists. Collagen and part of a phagocyte whose cytoplasm is rich in polysomes, vesicles and lipid bodies lie between the degenerating muscle fibre and a normal fibre.

MAGNIFICATION 7,000 ×.

BM	Basement membrane	MF	Muscle fibre
DMF	Degenerating muscle fibre	Ph	Phagocyte
I	Inclusion	PM	Plasma membrane
LB	Lipid body	R	Ribosomes
Mit	Mitochondria	Ve	Vesicles
My	Myofilaments		

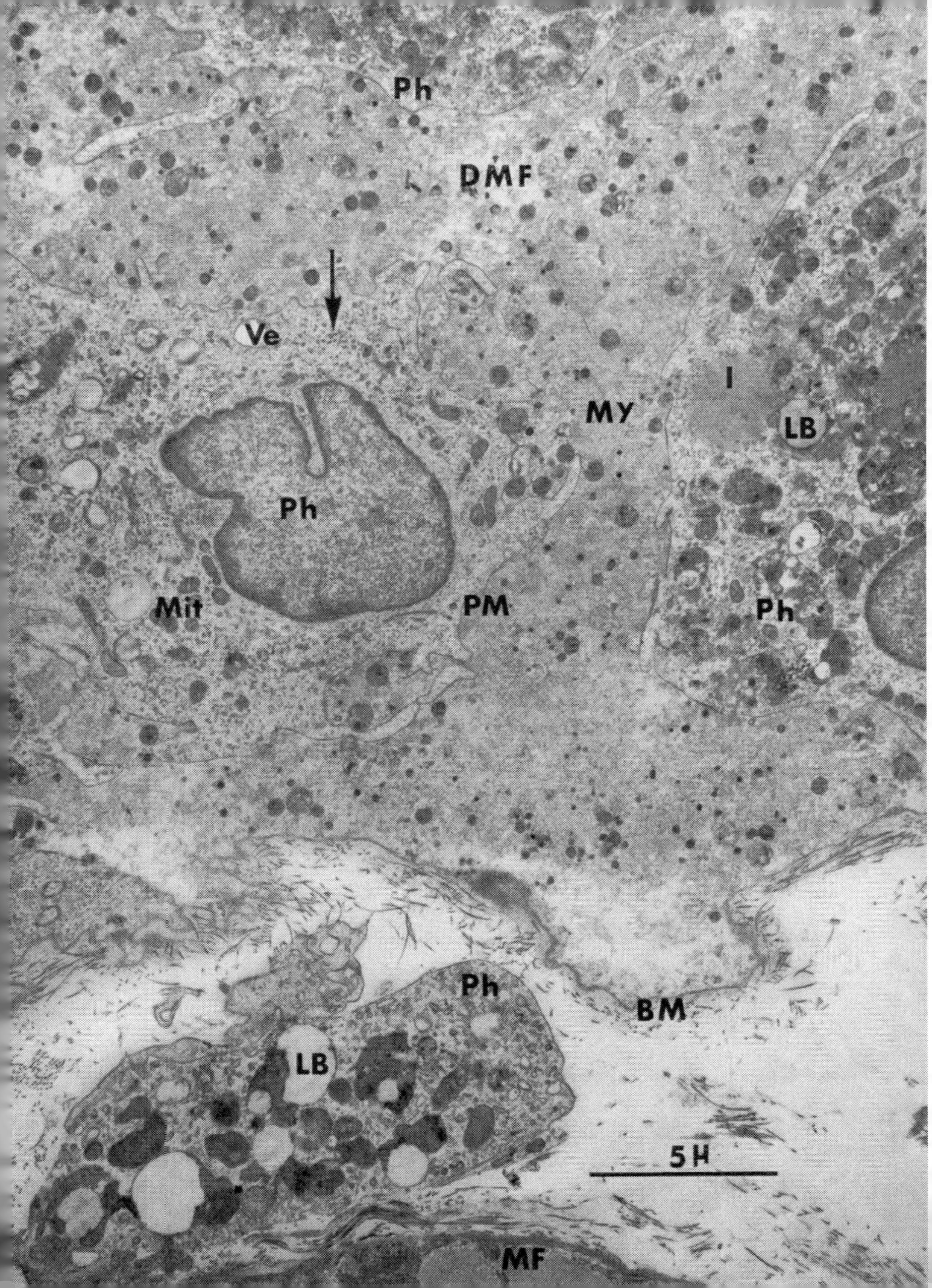

Ph
DMF
Ve
MY
I
LB
Ph
Mit
PM
Ph
Ph
BM
LB
5 μ
MF

PLATE 74. MUSCULAR DYSTROPHY
ELECTRON DENSE PARTICLES IN DEGENERATING MUSCLE FIBRES

UPPER. This atrophied fibre containing a cluster of nuclei around a lipid body presents also degenerate myofibrils with thickened Z-lines from which extend slender portions of myofilaments. It contains also groups of electron dense particles: one group is enclosed in a rectangle. Such particles were found infrequently and only in atrophied fibres.

MAGNIFICATION 13,000 ×.

LOWER LEFT. Higher magnification of the particles within the rectangle above shows that they are rounded, very electron dense and closely set. They are 350–400 Å in diameter.

MAGNIFICATION 125,000 ×.

LOWER RIGHT. In some fibres the hexagonal array of the particles is more evident (ringed).
The origin and the significance of these particles are unknown.
Similar particles have been reported as virus-like particles in myositis accompanying herpes zoster (see page 56).

MAGNIFICATION 58,000 ×.

All are from a patient with muscular dystrophy.

LB Lipid body
My Myofilaments
N Nuclei
Z Z-line

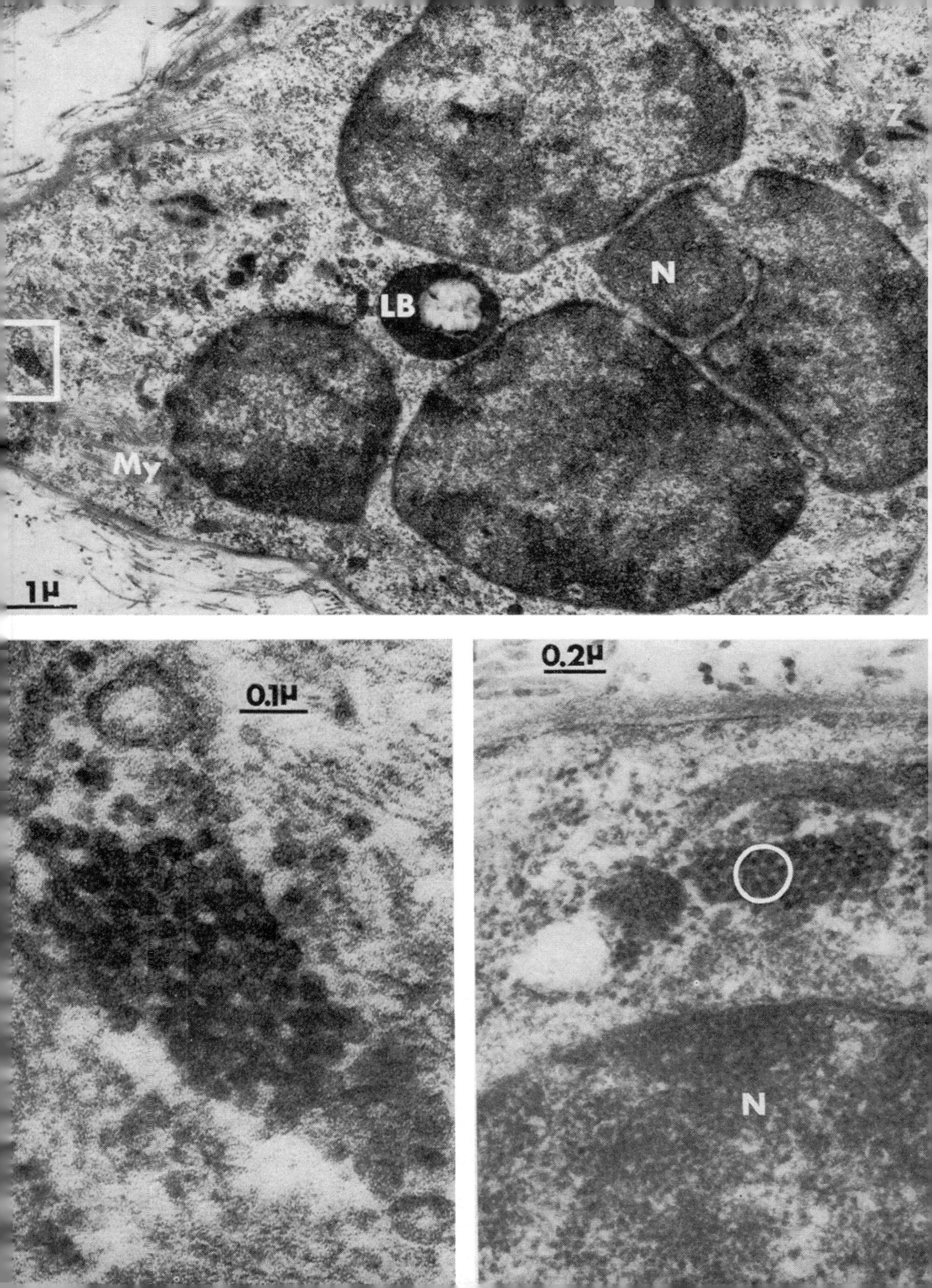

Z
N
LB
My
1μ
0.1μ
0.2μ
N

PLATE 75. POLYMYOSITIS
LEUCOCYTIC INFILTRATION

UPPER. Different types of leucocytes may occur around the blood vessels and between the muscle fibres in polymyositis. Top right lies a blood capillary containing a red blood corpuscle. Many organelles are present in the endothelial cell cytoplasm and in that of the pericytes present in the basement membrane which surrounds the capillary. The leucocytes lie in close proximity to one another and have a well-defined plasma membrane but have no basement membrane. The cytoplasm of those leucocytes having phagocytic properties contain bodies of various types and some of them are bound by membranes. Fibroblasts, their processes and surrounding collagen are present amongst the groups of leucocytes. The muscle cell adjacent to the cellular exudate contains a satellite cell within its basement membrane.

MAGNIFICATION 5,500 ×.

LOWER. Some leucocytes have a rounded nucleus and few electron dense bodies in their cytoplasm but it is difficult to classify them. The polymorphs have a lobed nucleus and their cytoplasm contains electron dense bodies of different size and shape. Strands of collagen occur between the groups of leucocytes.

MAGNIFICATION 5,000 ×.

C	Collagen	Ph	Phagocyte
F	Fibroblast	Poly	Polymorph
MF	Muscle fibre	RBC	Red blood corpuscle
Pe	Pericyte	S	Satellite cell

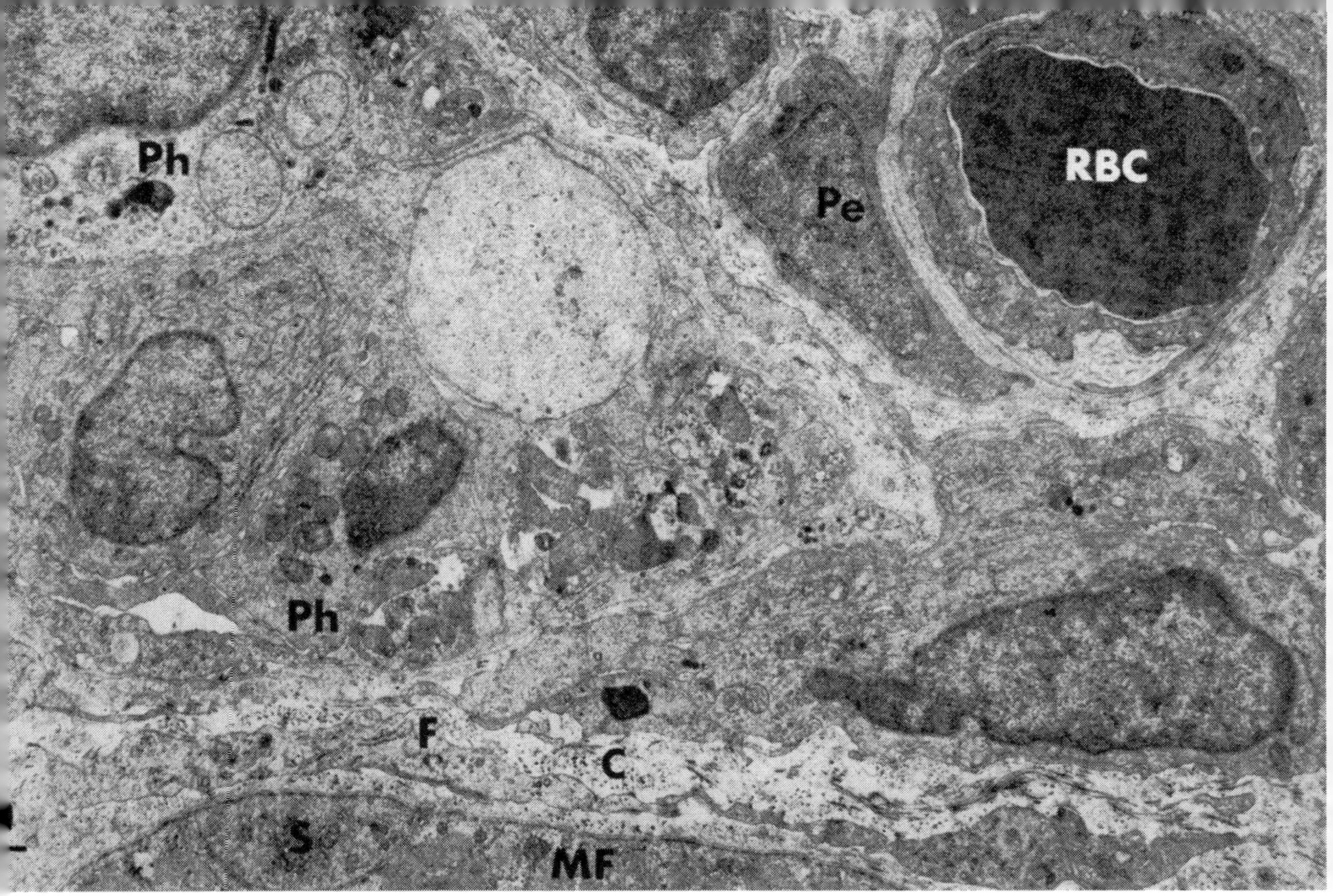
Ph
RBC
Pe
Ph
F
C
S
MF

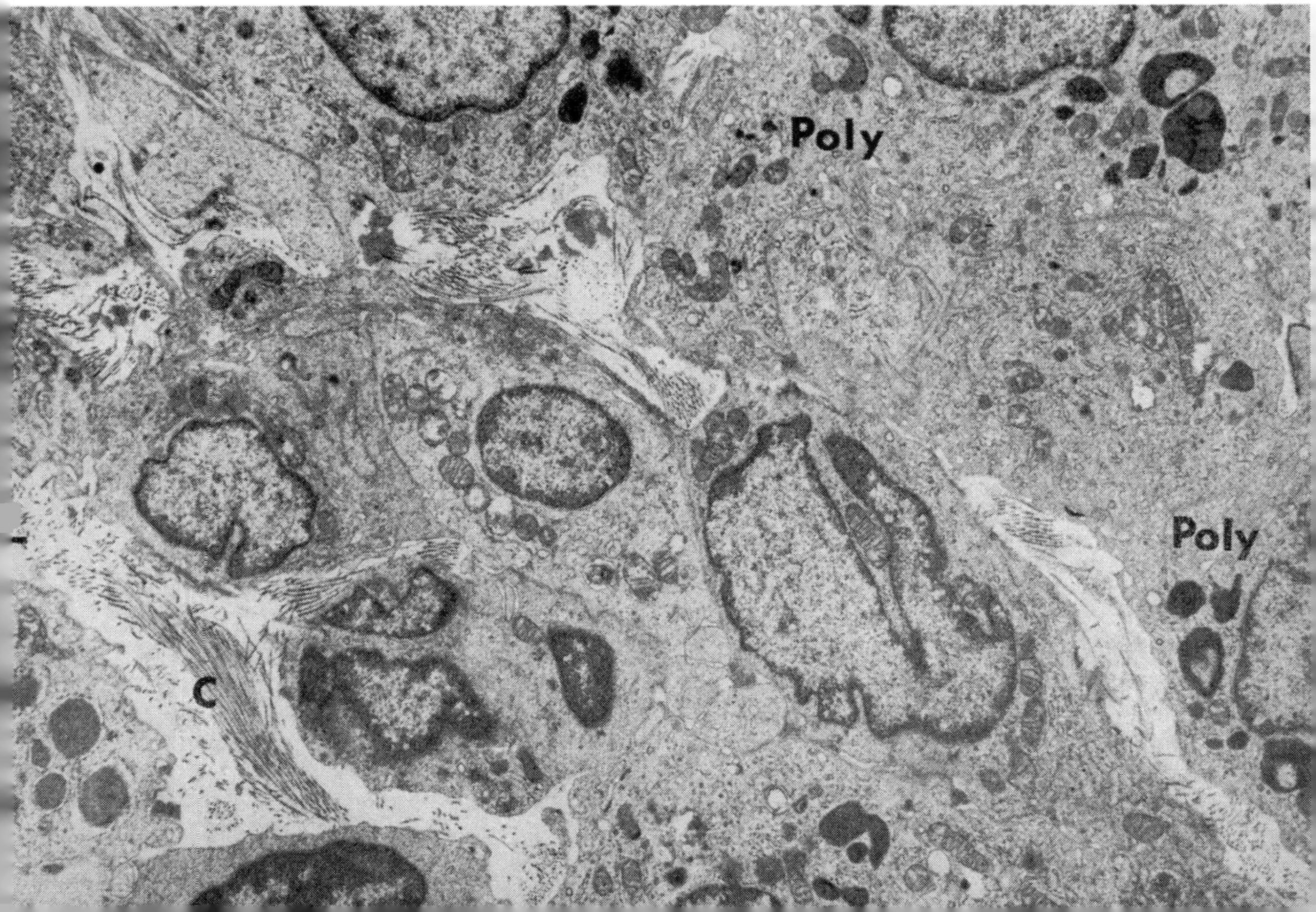
Poly
Poly
C

PLATE 76. POLYMYOSITIS
DEGENERATING MUSCLE FIBRE

Here is a degenerating muscle fibre with undulating margins and thickened plasma membrane which is frequently indented and has many vesicles immediately under it. The myofibrils are broken and widely separated from one another by accumulations of glycogen granules. Some myofibrils are cut transversely and others longitudinally. A few mitochondria and triads lie randomly in the fibre. Collagen and fibroblast processes lie between the degenerating muscle fibre and an adjacent muscle fibre whose plasma membrane also shows electron dense thickenings. Above the degenerating muscle fibre lies part of a phagocyte and a blood capillary with a prominent lumen. The endothelial cell cytoplasm contains numerous vesicles and some vacuoles. A pericyte lies between the basement membrane layers of the blood capillary.

MAGNIFICATION 14,000 ×.

BC	Blood capillary	Pe	Pericyte
BM	Basement membrane	Ph	Phagocyte
C	Collagen	PM	Plasma membrane
F	Fibroblast	Tr	Triad
G	Glycogen	TS	Transverse section
L	Lumen	V	Vesicles
LS	Longitudinal section	Va	Vacuole
Mi	Mitochondria	Z	Z-line

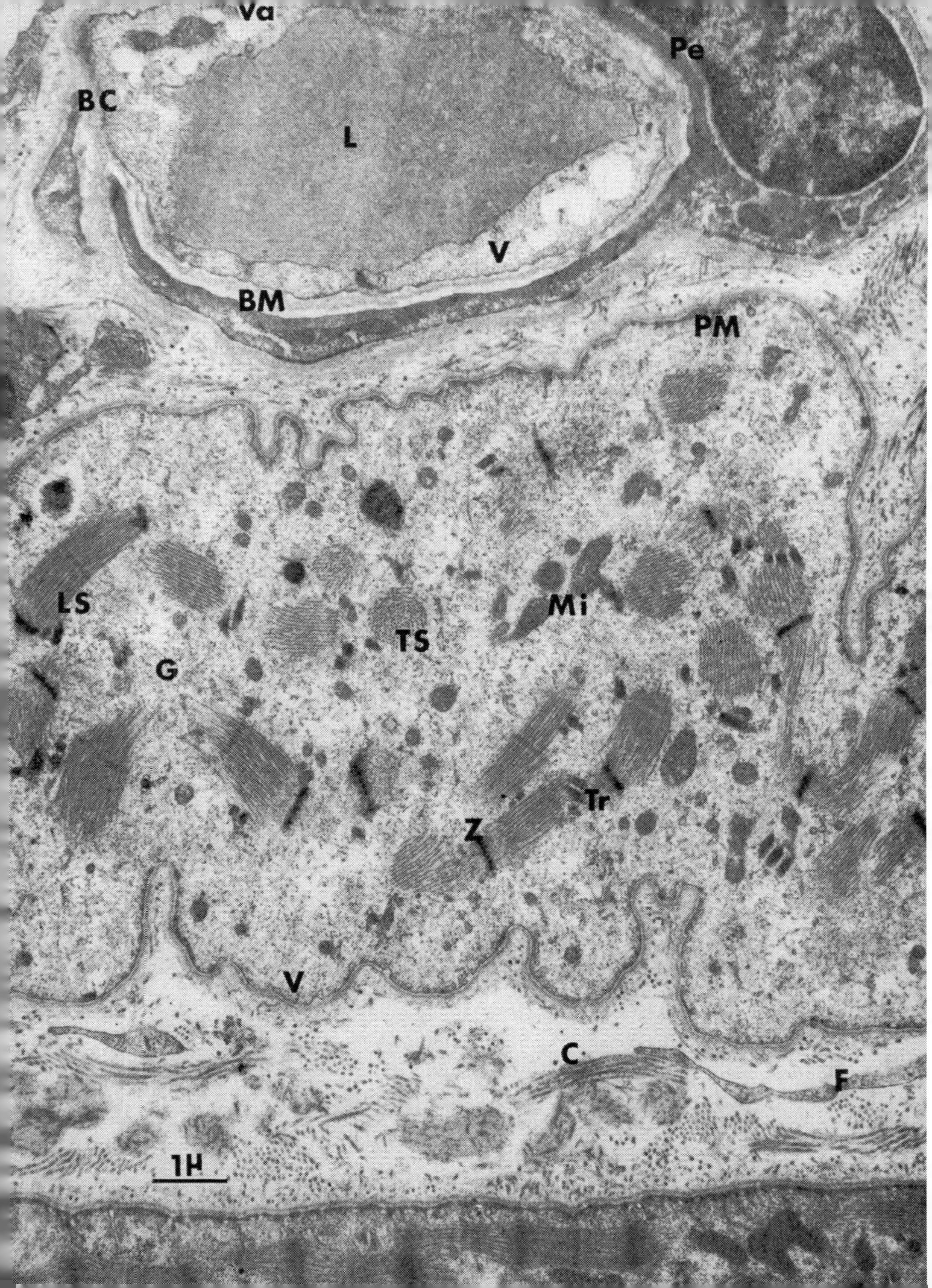
Va
Pe
BC
L
V
BM
PM
LS
Mi
TS
G
Tr
Z
V
C
F
1μ

PLATE 77. POLYMYOSITIS
RODS IN A DEGENERATING MUSCLE FIBRE

In a degenerating muscle fibre collections of electron dense rods occur near the nuclei and have the same features as nemaline rods. This section shows four nuclei in close proximity: they are granular in appearance with a more electron dense, peripheral rim of chromatin. The outer nuclear membrane of the uppermost nucleus is ballooned (arrowed). The fibre contains randomly disposed filaments, numerous vesicles and degenerating mitochondria. At the top of the illustration outside the muscle fibre lie phagocytes.

MAGNIFICATION 8,000 ×.

Fi	Filaments	Ph	Phagocyte
Mit	Mitochondria	Ro	Rods
N	Nucleus	V	Vesicles

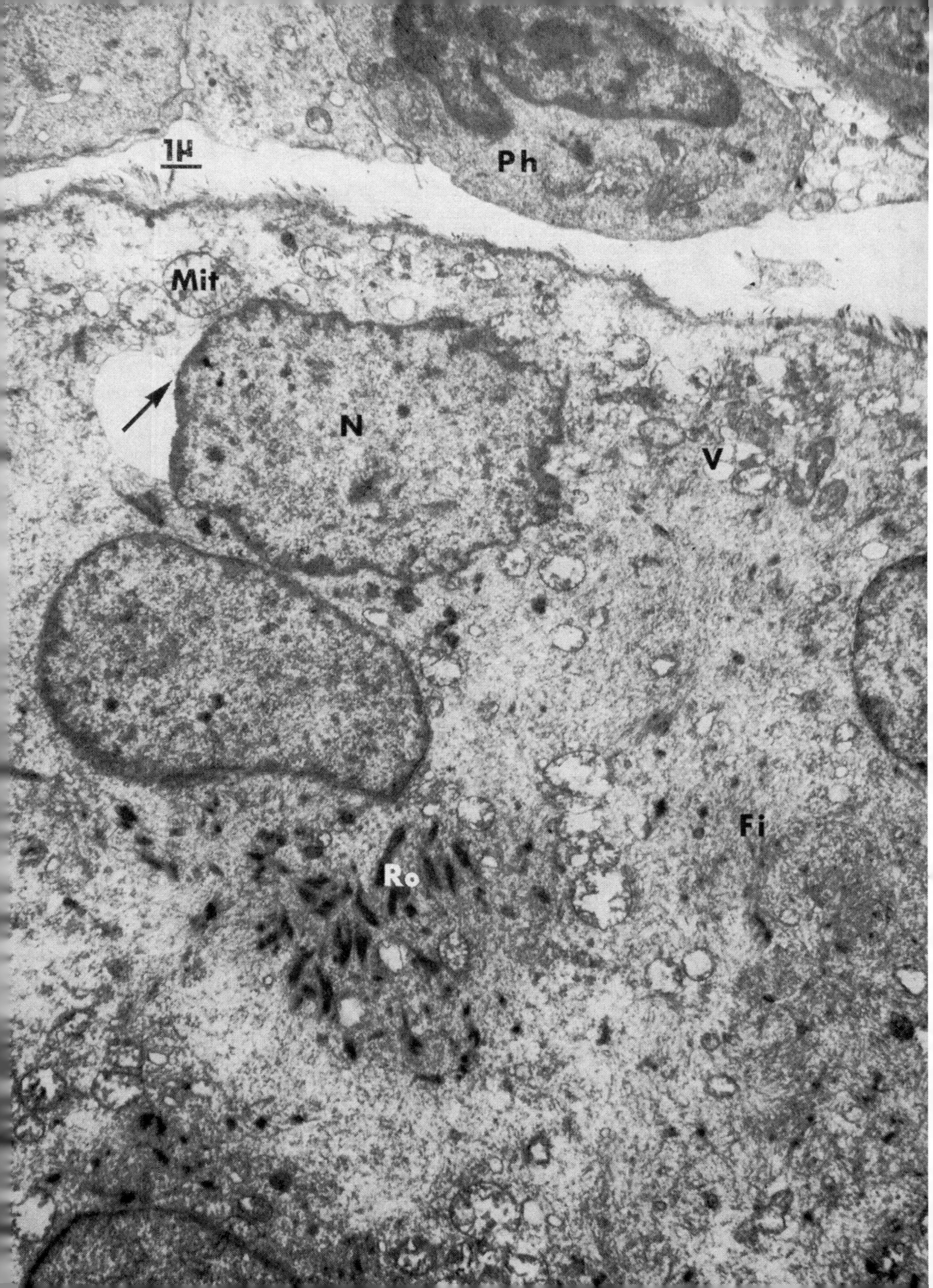

1μ
Ph
Mit
N
V
Fi
Ro

PLATE 78. STEROID MYOPATHY

UPPER. Membranous bodies occur in the muscle, both under the plasma membrane or between myofibrils. These bodies consist of concentric laminae formed of double membranes separated by a less dense electron zone. A clear space lies between the double membranes. Granular material occurs in the centre of these membranous bodies. A large amount of glycogen surrounds them.

MAGNIFICATION 50,000 ×.

LOWER. Higher magnification of the muscle shows that some of these concentric laminated bodies form part of a mitochondrion. It lies between a myofibril and a large amount of glycogen granules. The mitochondria are more electron dense than normal and the cristae are abnormal.

MAGNIFICATION 75,000 ×.

Both are from a patient receiving steroid therapy.

C Collagen
G Glycogen
Mf Myofibrils
Mi Mitochondria
MeB Membranous body

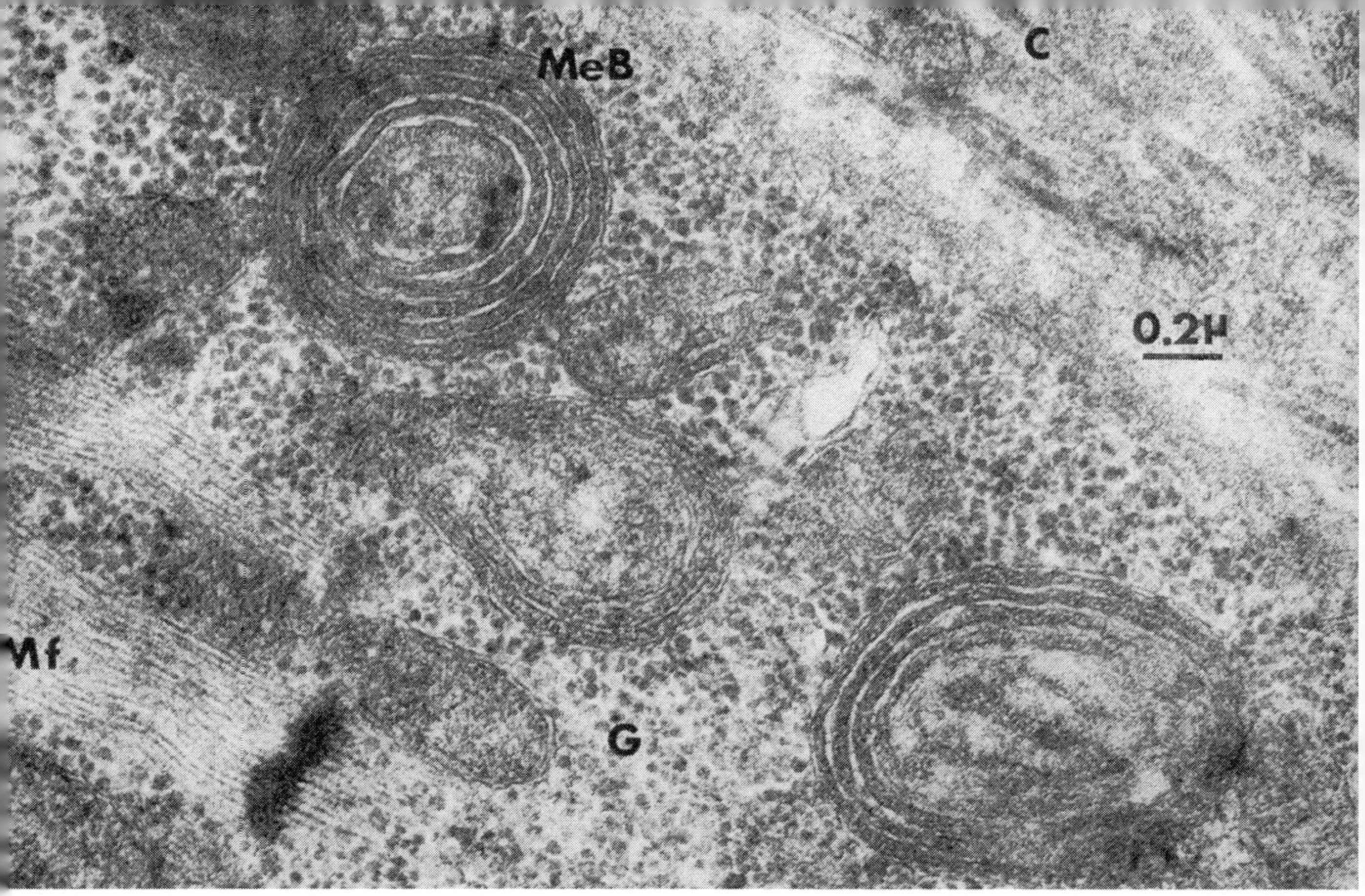

MeB
C
0.2μ
Mf
G

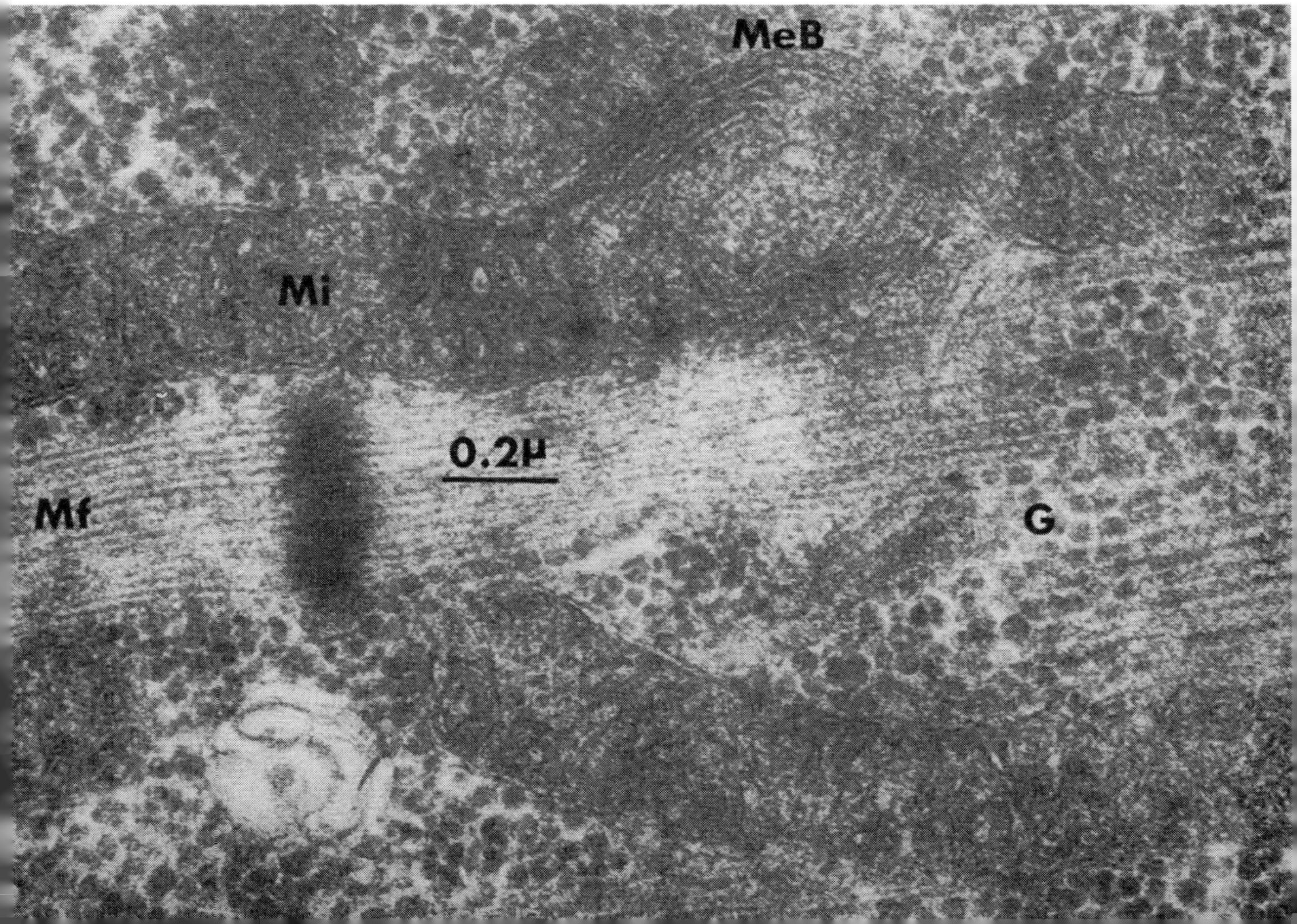

MeB
Mi
0.2μ
Mf
G

PLATE 79. VINCRISTINE NEUROMYOPATHY

UPPER. In this muscle fibre are large vacuoles containing tubules and membranes. The vacuoles lie between the myofibrils and in the neighbourhood of the mitochondria which show distensions and breaking down of the cristae. The origin of the vacuoles is far from clear.

MAGNIFICATION 22,000 ×.

LOWER LEFT. The T-system at the I- and A-band junctions are much more prominent than in normal muscle. The continuity of the T-tubules over several myofibrils can be traced. The electron dense lateral sacs of the sarcoplasmic reticulum which abut on the T-tubules to form the triads show a granular pattern. Glycogen granules abound between the myofibrils and around the triads.

MAGNIFICATION 66,000 ×.

LOWER RIGHT. Accumulations of lipid bodies of varying electron density which some authors regard as lipofuscin may be plentiful around the nuclei of the muscle fibre as is illustrated here.

MAGNIFICATION 15,000 ×.

All are from a patient treated with vincristine sulphate for malignant disease.

A	A-band	N	Nucleus
G	Glycogen	SR	Sarcoplasmic reticulum
I	I-band	T	T-system
LB	Lipid body	Tr	Triads
Me	Membranes	Va	Vacuole
Mi	Mitochondria	Z	Z-line

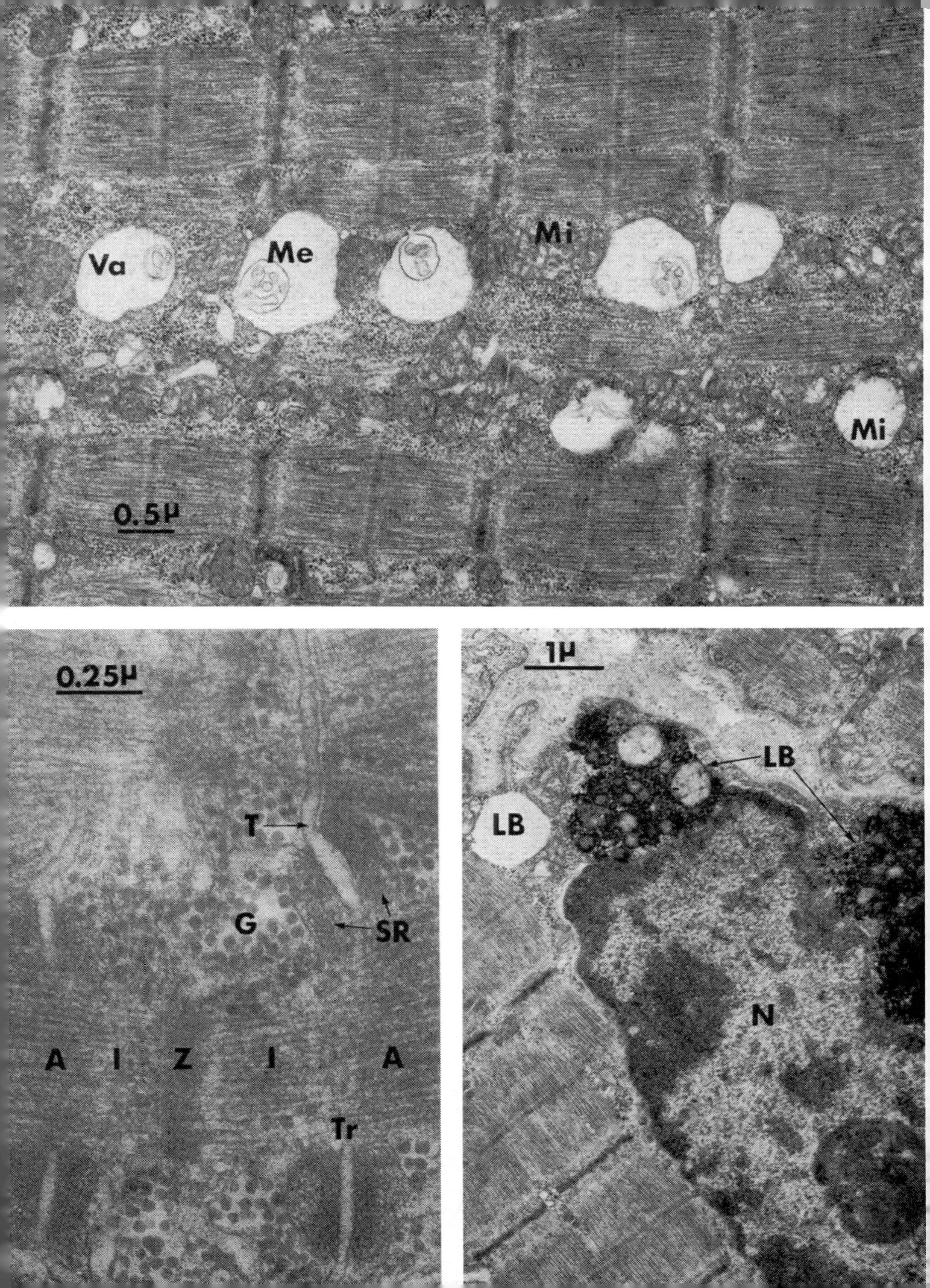
Va
Me
Mi
Mi
0.5μ
0.25μ
T
G
SR
A
I
Z
I
A
Tr
1μ
LB
LB
LB
N

PLATE 80. VINCRISTINE NEUROMYOPATHY

UPPER. Near the surface of a much indented muscle fibre are complex membranous bodies close to dense lipid bodies and a subsarcolemmal nucleus. The neighbouring mitochondria also show structural change.

MAGNIFICATION 34,000 ×.

From a patient treated with vincristine sulphate for malignant disease.

LOWER. Membranous bodies are much more frequent and more elaborate in the muscle of rats which have been intoxicated with vincristine. The membranous bodies often lie in close proximity to mitochondria and may arise in them.

MAGNIFICATION 44,000 ×.

From a rat treated with vincristine.

BM	Basement membrane	Mf	Myofibril
C	Collagen	MeB	Membranous body
LB	Lipid body	N	Nucleus

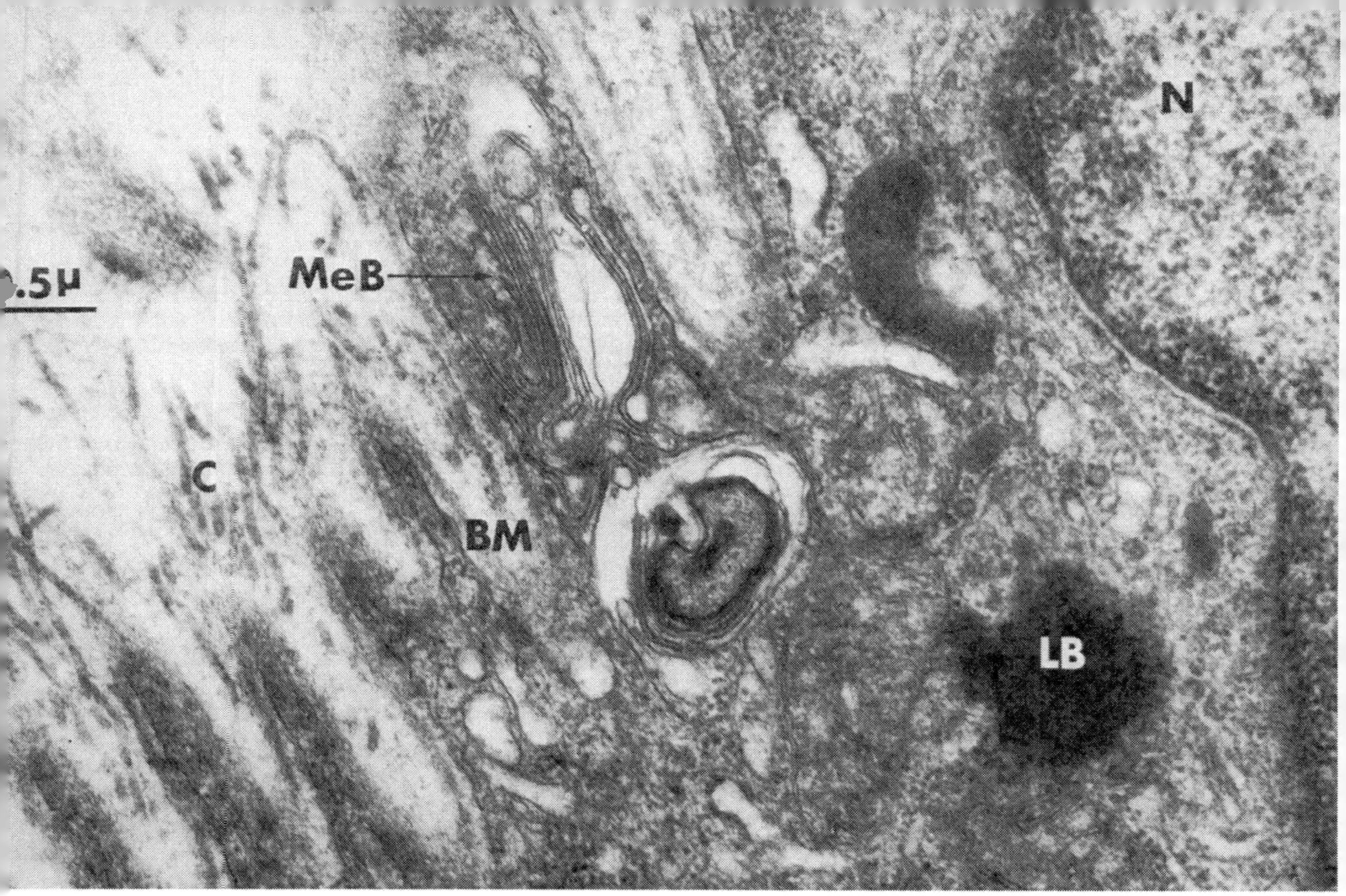

N
0.5μ
MeB
C
BM
LB

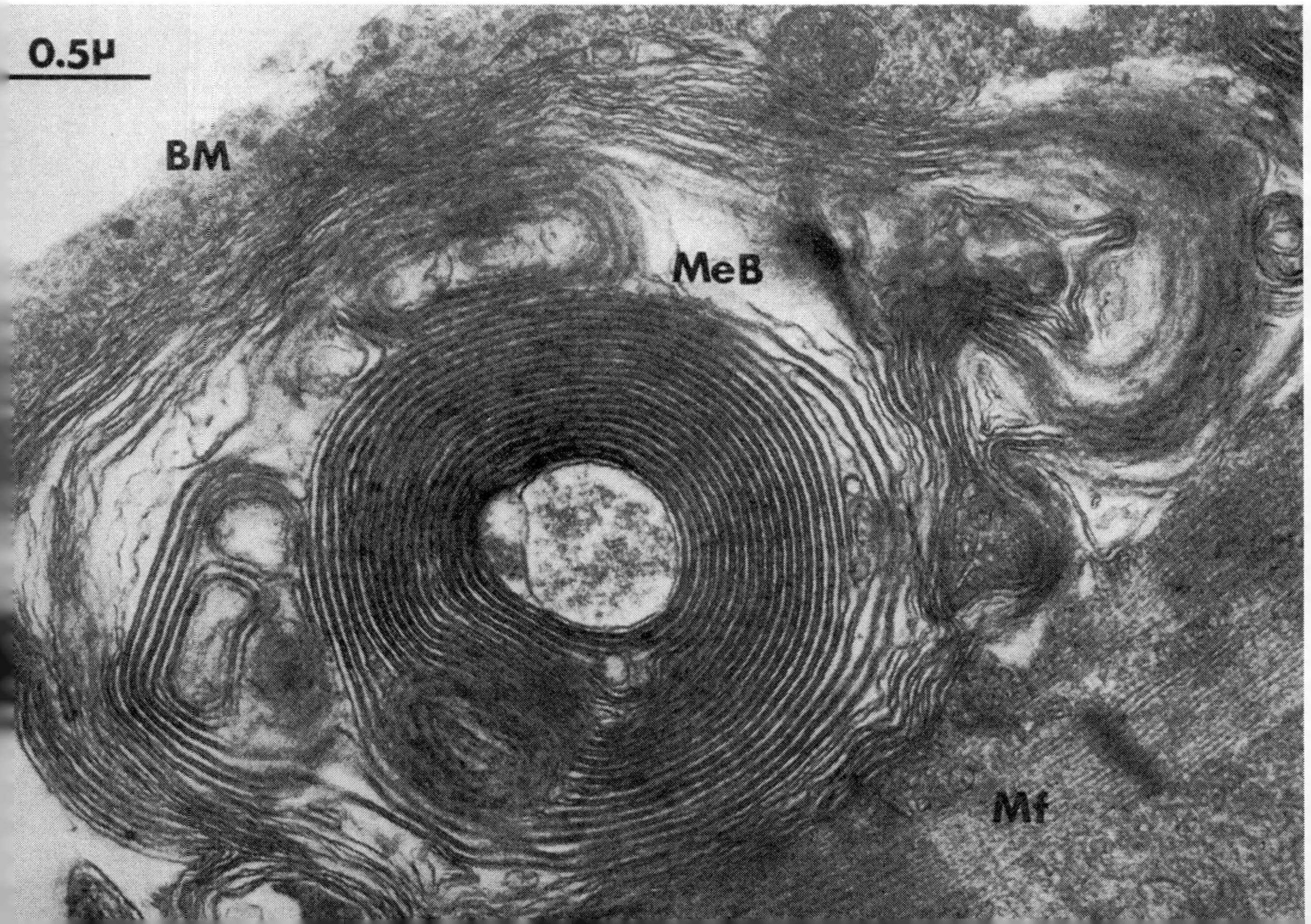

0.5μ
BM
MeB
Mf

PLATE 81. CHLOROQUINE MYOPATHY

UPPER. Very striking accumulations of mitochondria occur under the plasma membrane and between the myofibrils. The plasma membrane is thicker than normal and some myofibrils are disintegrating. An abundance of glycogen granules lie around the mitochondria.

MAGNIFICATION 16,000 ×.

LOWER. Degeneration of the myofibrils may be very advanced in some fibres which contain a large amount of granular material and vacuoles. Some of the vacuoles are large and clear, while others contain complex membranous or myelin bodies.

MAGNIFICATION 25,000 ×.

G	Glycogen	MB	Myelin body
Gr	Granules	PM	Plasma membrane
MeB	Membranous body	Va	Vacuoles
Mi	Mitochondria		

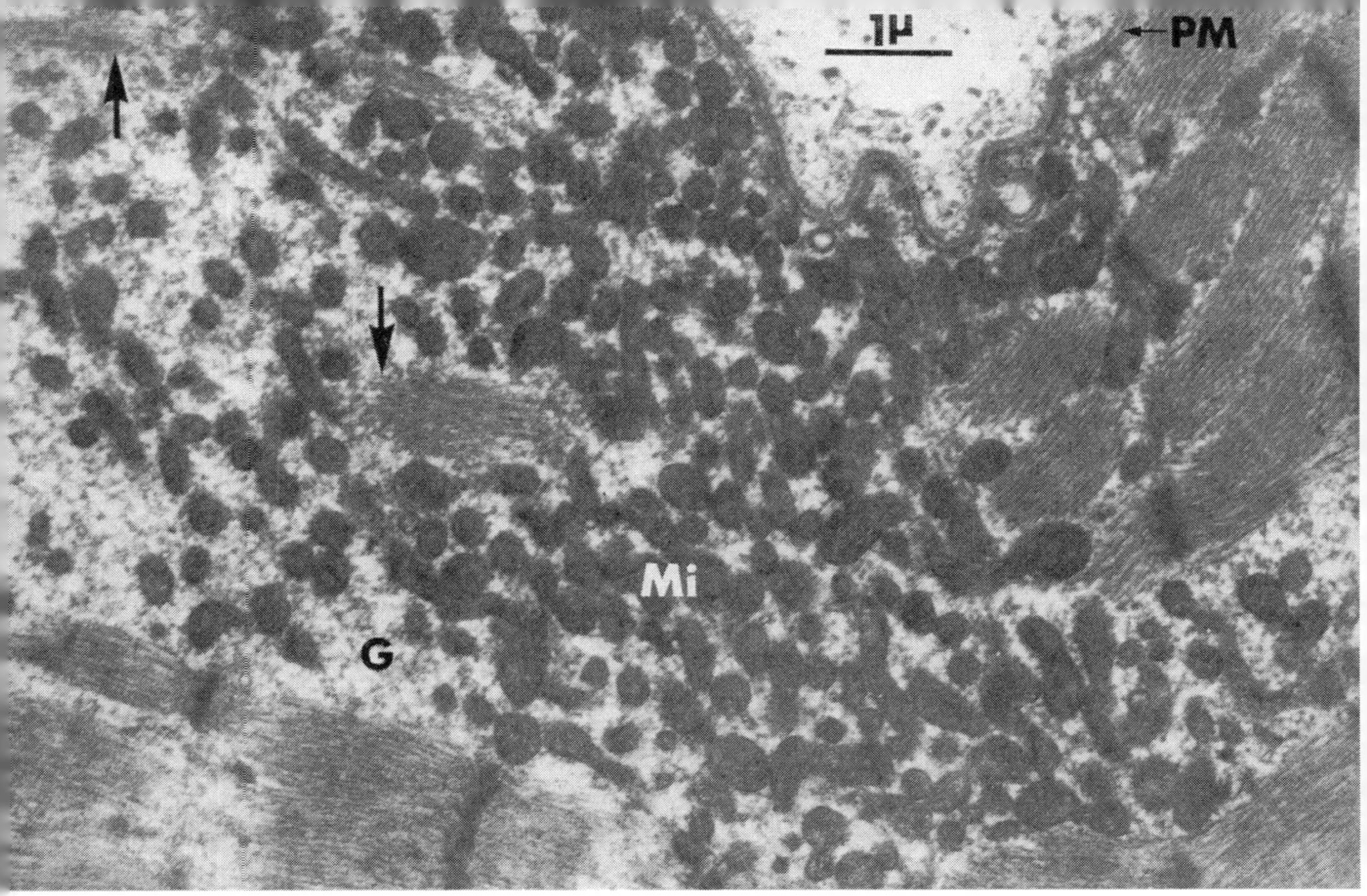
1µ
PM
Mi
G

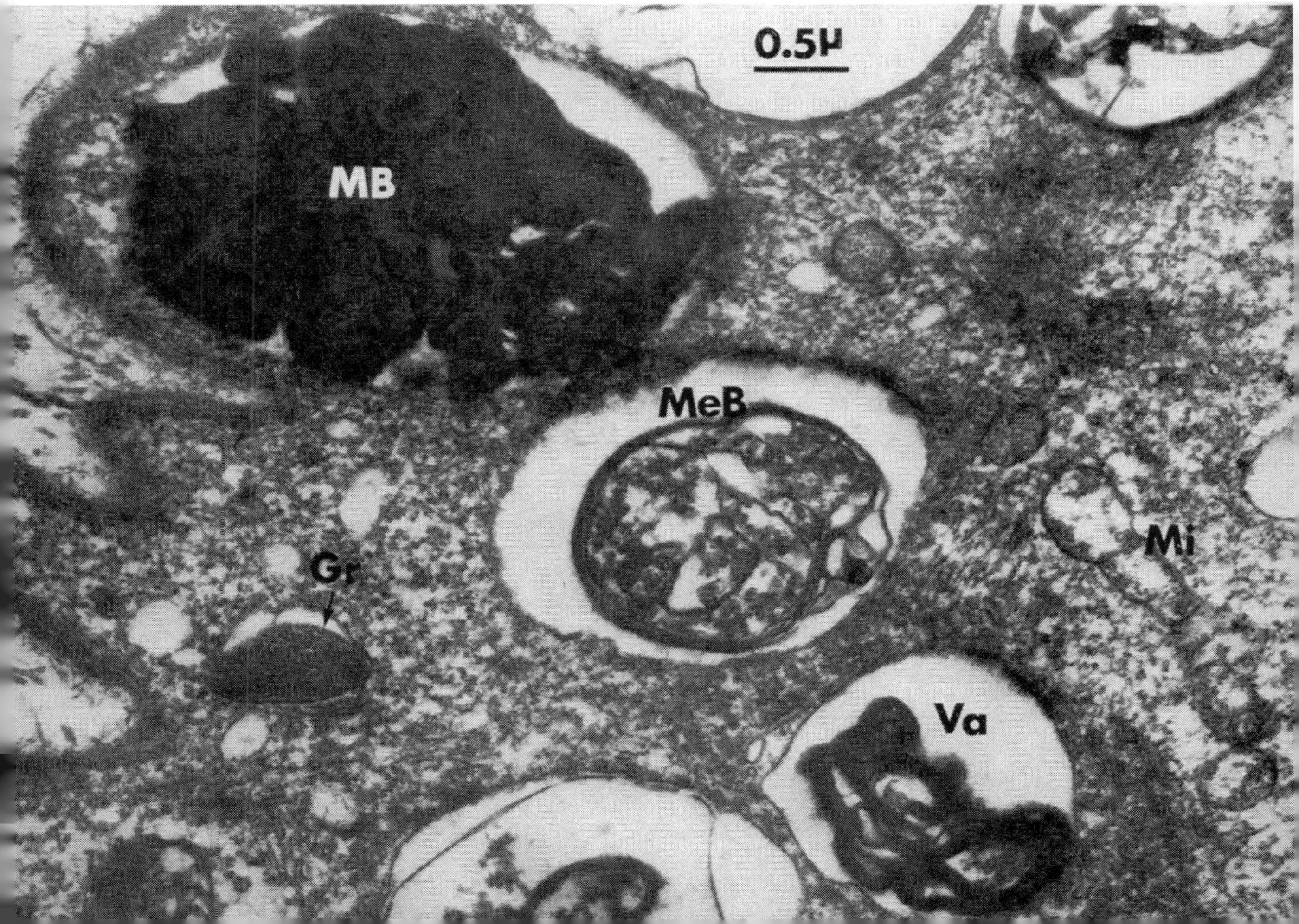
0.5µ
MB
MeB
Gr
Mi
Va

PLATE 82. CHLOROQUINE MYOPATHY

UPPER. Degenerating muscle fibres as illustrated are frequently found in this disease. The myofibrils of the upper fibre have largely disappeared and in the sarcoplasm are numerous glycogen granules and mitochondria. Electron dense, coagulated material lies at the edge of the fibre. The lower fibre has a vesicular nucleus and close to it are large vacuoles.

MAGNIFICATION 15,000 ×.

LOWER. This atrophied fibre presents granular material around the nucleus. The outer nuclear membrane is distended: the distension on the left has an electron dense mass attached to it: on the right is a larger distension which contains granules which are attached to one another and also to a larger electron dense mass. The appearances suggest that the dense material may result from the breaking down of the nucleus.

MAGNIFICATION 18,000 ×.

Both are from a patient with lupus erythematosus treated with chloroquine.

G Glycogen
Mf Myofibril
Mi Mitochondria
My Myofilaments
N Nucleus
Va Vacuoles

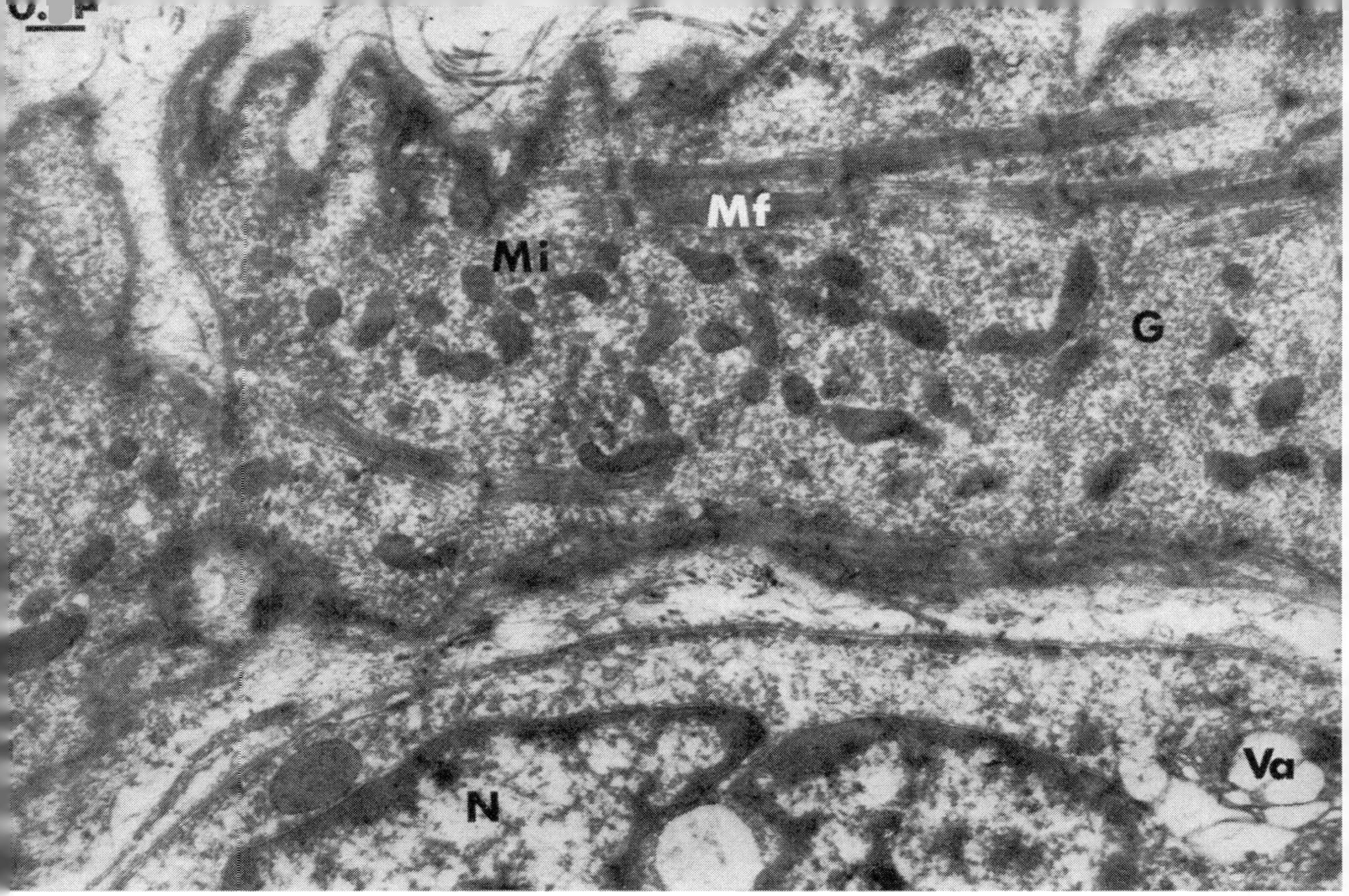
Mf
Mi
G
N
Va

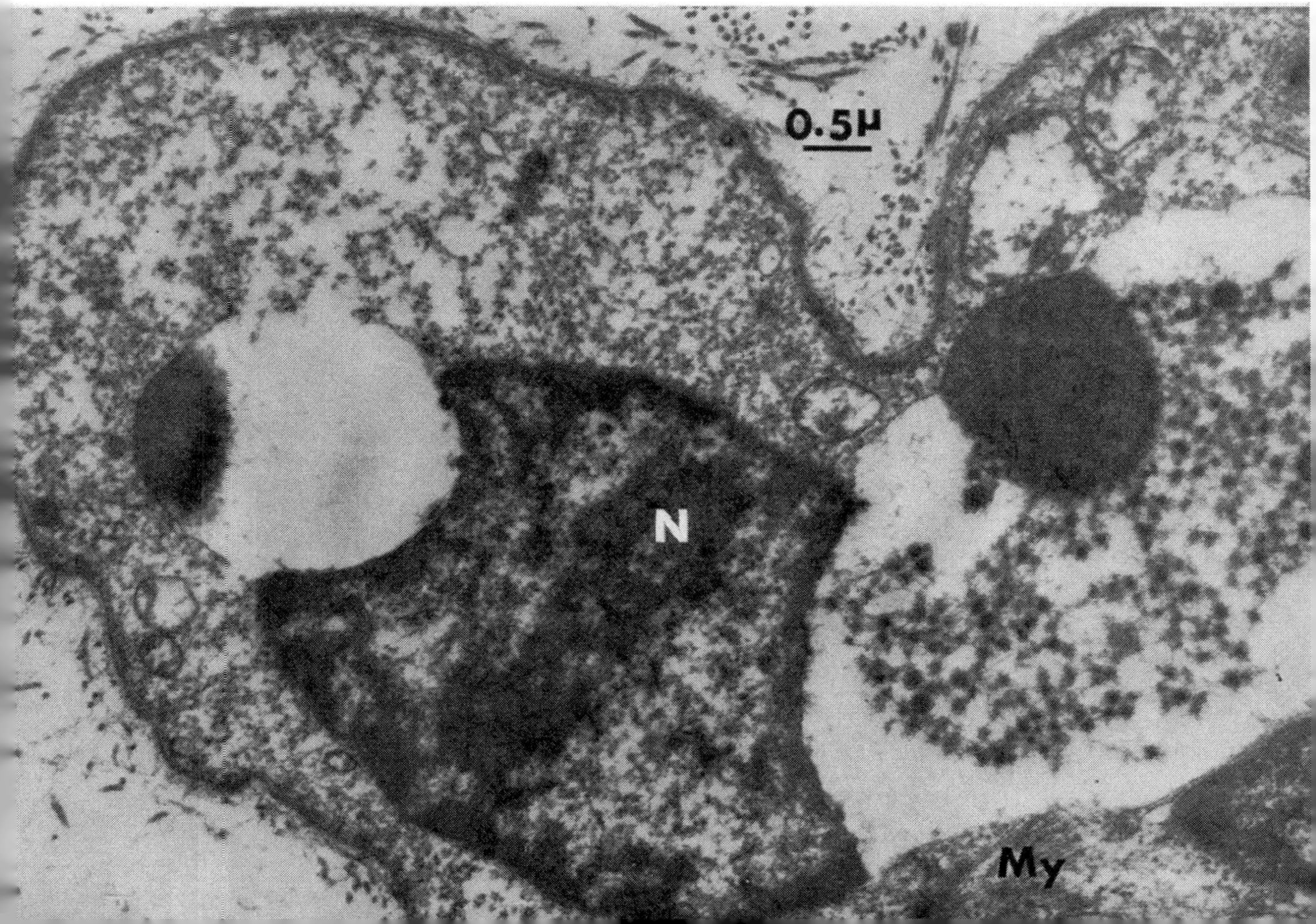
0.5μ
N
My

PLATE 83. VITAMIN E DEFICIENCY DEGENERATING MUSCLE FIBRES

UPPER. The myofibrils are disorganised, some lying obliquely and others transversely. Many clear vacuoles occur in the fibre; one of them contains membranous and granular material. Near the surface of the fibre are collections of parallel and concentric tubules. Those bordering the myofibrils have distensions measuring from 80 to 190 mμ in diameter: they contain granular material. Similar tubules lie adjacent to the fibre near collections of collagen and folds of basement membrane.

MAGNIFICATION 26,000 ×.

LOWER. A degenerating fibre with a crenated surface occupies the greater part of the illustration. The nucleus lies at the edge of the fibre and vesicles and electron dense bodies between the atrophying myofibrils. Collagen and fibroblast processes surround the fibre. Another degenerating muscle fibre above it has granular electron dense material at its edge and a loose fold of basement membrane around it.

MAGNIFICATION 16,000 ×.

BM	Basement membrane	N	Nucleus
C	Collagen	OS	Oblique section
DMF	Degenerating muscle fibre	Tu	Tubules
F	Fibroblast	TS	Transverse section
I	I-band	Va	Vacuoles
My	Myofilaments	Z	Z-line

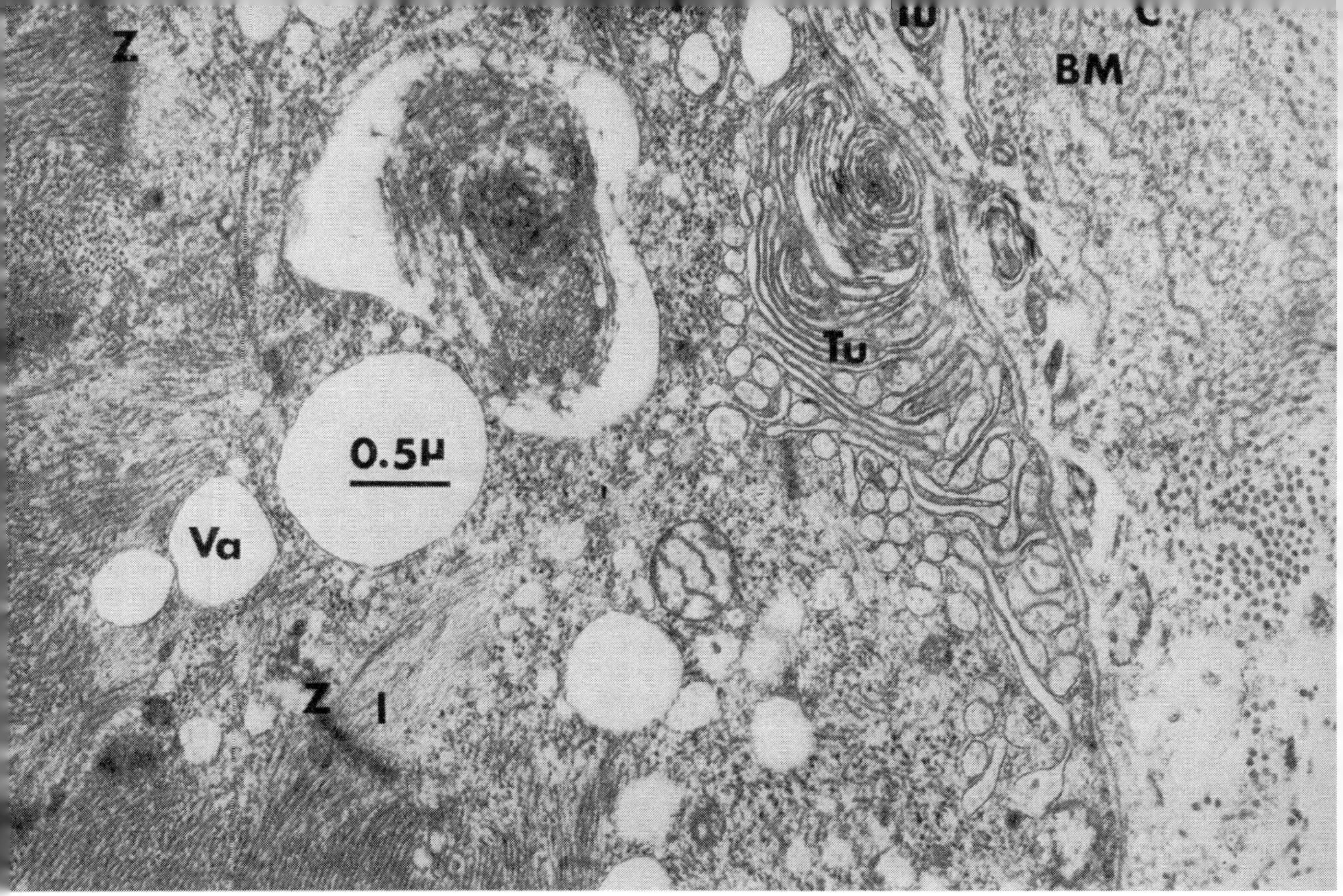
Z
BM
Tu
0.5μ
Va
Z
I

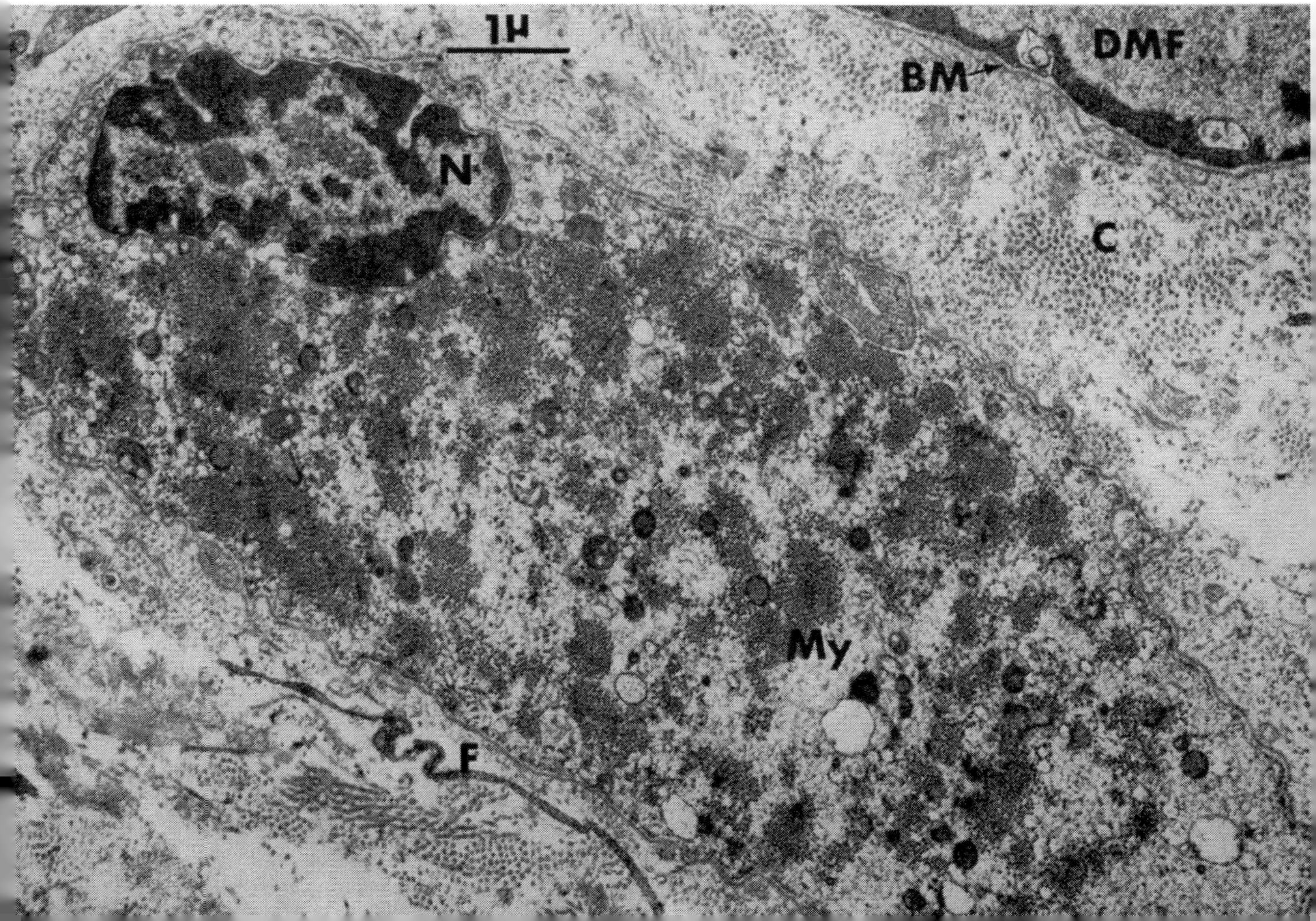
1μ
DMF
BM
N
C
My
F

PLATE 84. VITAMIN E DEFICIENCY
DEGENERATING MUSCLE FIBRES

UPPER. The plasma membrane has disappeared from the degenerating muscle fibre in the centre, but the basement membrane remains and at the lower left exhibits numerous folds. A prominent phagocyte lies within the fibre. To the right of this phagocyte are disintegrating myofibrils and a few mitochondria and to the left are processes of other phagocytes. Amongst the collagen below this degenerating fibre is another phagocyte with several pseudopodia. At the bottom of the illustration is a muscle fibre whose myofilaments are agglutinated into electron dense masses in which large vacuoles containing granules have appeared.

MAGNIFICATION 12,000 ×.

LOWER. Phagocytes lie in the neighbourhood of muscle fibres in advanced stages of degeneration. The basement membrane folds of the muscle fibres persist but the plasma membranes have disappeared. A few disintegrating myofilaments, electron dense bodies and vacuoles lie in one of the basement membrane tubes. A satellite cell is present within the basement membrane of a normal muscle fibre to the right.

MAGNIFICATION 10,000 ×.

BM	Basement membrane	N	Nucleus
Mi	Mitochondria	Ph	Phagocyte
My	Myofilaments	S	Satellite cell
MF	Muscle fibre	Va	Vacuole

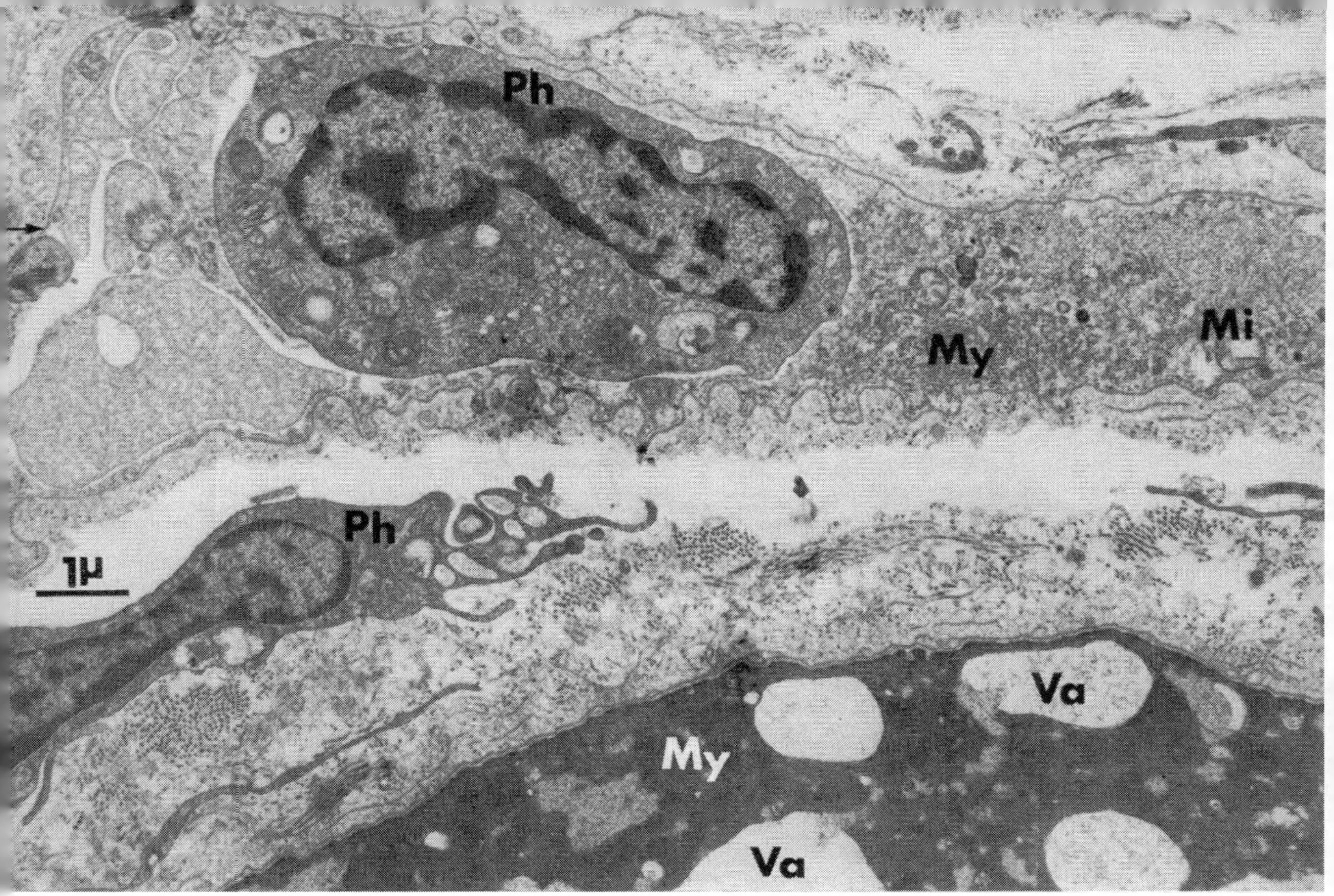
Ph
Mi
My
Ph
1µ
Va
My
Va

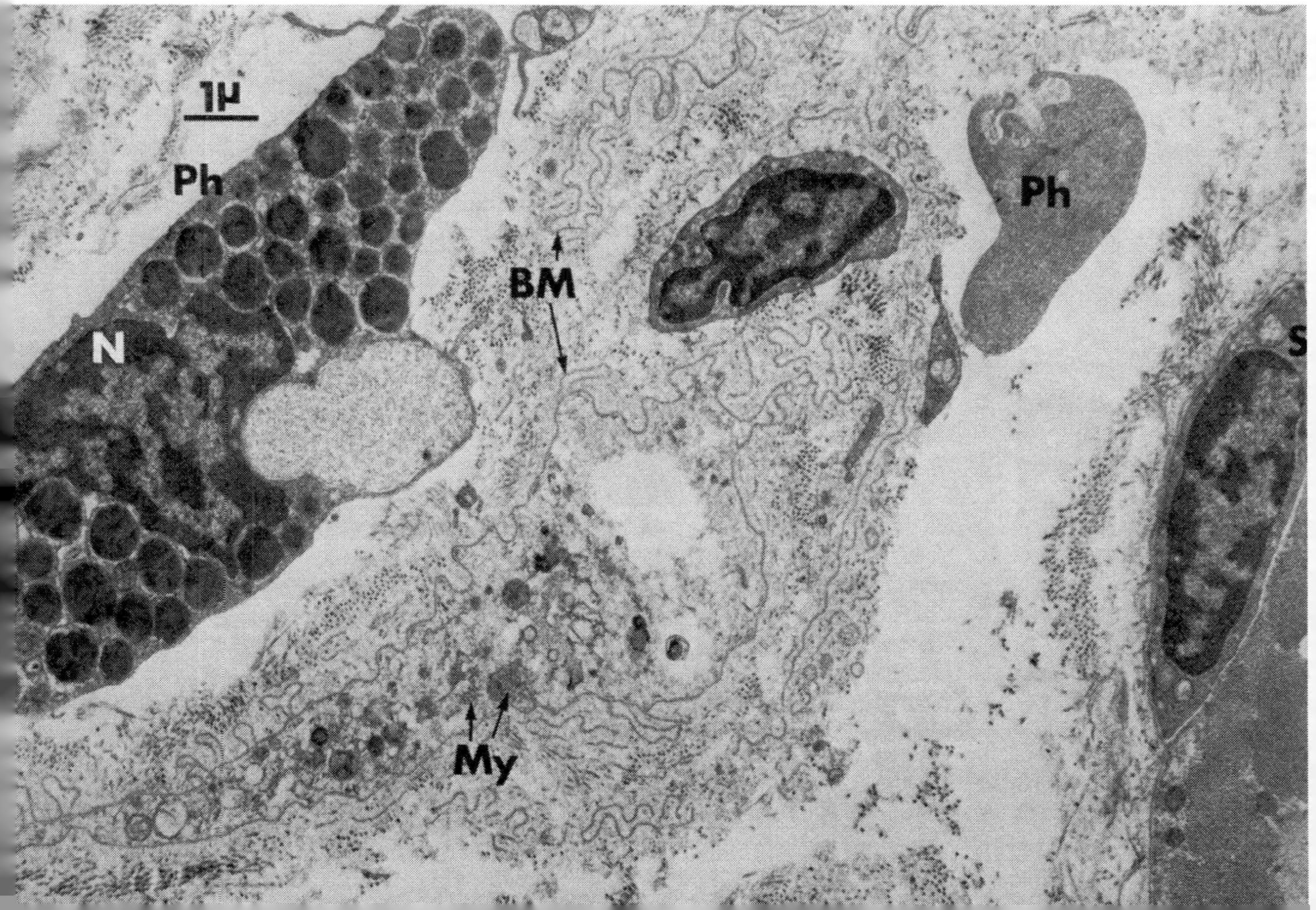
1µ
Ph
Ph
BM
N
S
My

References

Adal, M. N. (1969). The fine structure of the sensory region of cat muscle spindles. *J. Ultrastruct. Res.* **26**, 332–354.

Adams, R. D., Denny-Brown, D. and Pearson, C. M. (1953). *Diseases of Muscle. A Study in Pathology.* 1st ed. New York: Hoeber.

Adams, R. D., Denny-Brown, D. and Pearson, C. M. (1962). *Diseases of Muscle. A Study in Pathology.* 2nd ed. New York: Hoeber.

Afifi, A. K. (1969). Histology and cytology of muscle in Prader Willi syndrome. *Devl. Med. child Neurol.* **11**, 363–364.

Afifi, A. K., Aleu, F. P., Goodgold, J. and Mackay, B. (1966). Ultrastructure of atrophic muscle in amyotrophic lateral sclerosis. *Neurology, Minneap.* **16**, 475–481.

Afifi, A. K. and Bergman, R. A. (1969). Steroid myopathy. A study of the evolution of the muscle lesions in rabbits. *Johns Hopkins med. J.* **124**, 66–86.

Afifi, A. K., Bergman, R. A. and Harvey, J. C. (1968). Steroid myopathy. Clinical, histological and cytological observations. *Johns Hopkins med. J.* **123**, 158–174.

Afifi, A. K., Smith, J. W. and Zellweger, H. (1965). Congenital nonprogressive myopathy. Central core and nemaline myopathy in one family. *Neurology, Minneap.* **15**, 371–381.

Afifi, A. K. and Zellweger, H. (1969). Pathology of muscular hypotonia in the Prader Willi syndrome. Light and electron microscopic study. *J. neurol. Sci.* **9**, 49–61.

Afifi, A. K., Zellweger, H., McCormick, W. F. and Mergner, W. (1969). Congenital muscular dystrophy: light and electron microscopic observations. *J. Neurol. Neurosurg. Psychiat.* **32**, 273–280.

Agostini, B. and Noetzel, H. (1970). Morphological study of muscle fibres and motor end plates in tetanus. In *Proceedings. International Congress on Muscle Diseases, Milan 1969.* Ed. Walton, J. N., Canal, N. and Scarlato, G. Int. Congr. Ser. No. 199, pp. 123–127. Amsterdam: Excerpta medica.

Aguayo, A. J. and Hudgson, P. (1970). Observations on the short-term effects of chloroquine on skeletal muscle. An experimental study in rabbits. *J. neurol. Sci.* **11**, 301–325.

Aleu, F. P. and Afifi, A. K. (1964). Ultrastructure of muscle in myotonic dystrophy. Preliminary observations. *Am. J. Path.* **45**, 221–231.

Allbrook, D. (1962). An electron microscopic study of regenerating skeletal muscle. *J. Anat.* **96**, 137–152.

Allen, D. E., Johnson, A. G. and Woolf, A. L. (1969). The intramuscular nerve endings in dystrophia myotonica—a biopsy study by vital staining and electron microscopy. *J. Anat.* **105**, 1–26.

Allen, E. R. and Pepe, F. A. (1965). Ultrastructure of developing muscle cells in the chick embryo. *Am. J. Anat.* **116**, 115–147.

Anderson, P. J. and Song, S. K. (1966a). Experimental myositis. A cytochemical and electron microscopic study of drug-induced degeneration. *Proc. 5th Int. Congr. Neuropath.* Int. Congr. Ser. No. 100, pp. 687–693. Amsterdam: Excerpta medica.

Anderson, P. J. and Song, S. K. (1966b). Skeletal muscle necrosis secondary to calvacin. *J. Neuropath. exp. Neurol.* **25**, 149–150.

Anderson, P. J., Song, S. K. and Slotwiner, P. (1967). The fine structure of spheromembranous degeneration of skeletal muscle induced by vincristine. *J. Neuropath. exp. Neurol.* **26,** 15–24.

Andersson-Cedergren, E. (1959). Ultrastructure of motor end plate and sarcoplasmic components of mouse skeletal muscle fiber as revealed by three-dimensional reconstructions from serial sections. *J. Ultrastruct. Res.* Suppl. 1, 1–191.

Andrade, C. (1952). A peculiar form of peripheral neuropathy. Familial atypical generalised amyloidosis with special involvement of the peripheral nerves. *Brain,* **75,** 408–427.

André, J. (1959). Sur l'existence d'un état paracristallin du matériel chondriosomique de certains spermatozoïdes. *C.r. hebd. Séanc. Acad. Sci., Paris,* **249,** 1264–1266.

Asbøe-Hansen, G., Iversen, K. and Wichmann, R. (1952). Malignant exophthalmos: muscular changes and thyrotropin content in serum. *Acta endocr., Copenh.* **11,** 376–399.

Auber, J. and Couteaux, R. (1963). Ultrastructure de la strie Z dans les muscles de diptères. *J. Microsc.* **2,** 309–324.

Babel, J., Bischoff, A. and Spoendlin, H. (1970). *Ultrastructure of the Peripheral Nervous System and Sense Organs. Atlas of Normal and Pathological Anatomy.* Stuttgart: Georg Thieme.

Badurska, B., Fidziánska, A., Kamieniecka, Z., Prot, J. and Strugalska, H. (1969). Myotubular myopathy. *J. neurol. Sci.* **8,** 563–571.

Banerjee, A. K. and Mair, W. G. P. To be published.

Banker, B. Q. (1967). A phase and electron microscopic study of dystrophic muscle. I. The pathological changes in the two-week-old Bar Harbour 129 dystrophic mouse. *J. Neuropath. exp. Neurol.* **26,** 259–275.

Banker, B. Q. (1968). A phase and electron microscopic study of dystrophic muscle. II. The pathological changes in the newborn Bar Harbour 129 dystrophic mouse. *J. Neuropath. exp. Neurol.* **27,** 183–209.

Barker, D. (1948). The innervation of muscle-spindle. *Q. Jl microsc. Sci.* **89,** 143–186.

Barker, D., Stacey, M. J. and Adal, M. N. (1970). Fusimotor innervation in the cat. *Phil. Trans. R. Soc.* **B 258,** 315–346.

Barrnett, R. J. (1962). The fine structural localization of acetylcholinesterase at the myoneural junction. *J. Cell Biol.* **12,** 247–262.

Bataillon, E. (1891). Recherches anatomiques et expérimentales sur la metamorphose des amphibiens anoures. *Annls Univ. Lyon,* **2,** 1–123.

Batten, F. E. (1897). The muscle-spindle under pathological conditions. *Brain,* **20,** 138–179.

Battig, C. G. and Low, F. N. (1961). The ultrastructure of human cardiac muscle and its associated tissue space. *Am. J. Anat.* **108,** 199–229.

Bauer, W. C., Blumberg, J. M. and Zacks, S. I. (1962). Short and long-term ultrastructure changes in denervated mouse motor end plates. *Proc. 4th Int. Congr. Neuropath.* Vol. II, pp. 16–18. Stuttgart: Georg Thieme.

Beams, H. W. and Evans, T. C. (1953). Electron micrographs of motor end plates. *Proc. Soc. exp. Biol. Med.* **82,** 344–346.

Beckmann, R., Kloke, W. D. and Freund-Mölbert, E. R. G. (1970). Ultrastructural findings in 'carriers' of Duchenne muscular dystrophy. In *Proceedings. International Congress on Muscle Diseases, Milan, 1969.* Ed. Walton, J. N., Canal, N. and Scarlato, G. Int. Congr. Ser. No. 199, pp. 439–444. Amsterdam: Excerpta medica.

Bencosme, S. A., West, R. O., Kerr, J. W. and Wilson, D. L. (1966). Diabetic capillary angiopathy in human skeletal muscle. *Am. J. Med.* **40,** 67–77.

Bennett, H. S. (1955). Modern concepts of structure of striated muscle. *Am. J. phys. Med.* **34,** 46–67.

Bennett, H. S. and Porter, K. R. (1953). An electron microscope study of sectioned breast muscle of the domestic fowl. *Am. J. Anat.* **93,** 61–105.

Bergman, R. A. (1962). Observations on the morphogenesis of rat skeletal muscle. *Bull. Johns Hopkins Hosp.* **110,** 187–201.

Bergman, R. A., Afifi, A. K., Dunkle, L. M. and Johns, R. J. (1970). Muscle pathology in hypokalemic periodic paralysis with hyperthyroidism. *Johns Hopkins med. J.* **126,** 100–118.

Bergmann, S. B. and Mair, W. G. P. To be published.

Bergouignan, M., Vital, C. and Bataille, J. M. (1967). Les myopathies hypothyroïdiennes. Aspects cliniques et histopathologiques. *Presse méd.* **75,** 1551–1556.

Bethlem, J., Meijer, A. E. F. H., Schellens, J. P. M. and Vroom, J. J. (1968). Centronuclear myopathy. *Eur. Neurol.* **1,** 325–333.

Bethlem, J. and Meyjes, F. E. P. (1960). Congenital, non-progressive central core disease of Shy and Magee. *Psychiat. Neurol. Neurochir.* **63,** 246–251.

Bethlem, J., van Gool, J., Hülsmann, W. C. and Meijer, A. E. F. H. (1966). Familial non-progressive myopathy with muscle cramps after exercise. A new disease associated with cores in the muscle fibres. *Brain,* **89,** 569–588.

Bethlem, J., van Wijngaarden, G. K., Mumenthaler, M. and Meijer, A. E. F. H. (1970). Centronuclear myopathy with type I fiber atrophy and 'myotubes'. *Archs Neurol., Chicago,* **23,** 70–73.

Biczyskowa, W., Fidziánska, A. and Jedrzejowska, H. (1969). Light and electron microscopic study of the muscles in hypokalemic periodic paralysis. *Acta neuropathol.* **12,** 329–338.

Birks, R., Huxley, H. E. and Katz, B. (1960). The fine structure of the neuromuscular junction of the frog. *J. Physiol., Lond.* **150,** 134–144.

Birks, R., Katz, B. and Miledi, R. (1959). Dissociation of the 'surface membrane complex' in atrophic muscle fibres. *Nature, Lond.* **184,** 1507–1508.

Birks, R., Katz, B. and Miledi, R. (1960). Physiological and structural changes at the amphibian myoneural junction, in the course of nerve degeneration. *J. Physiol., Lond.* **150,** 145–168.

Blaxter, K. L. (1969). Myopathies in animals. In *Disorders of Voluntary Muscle.* Ed. Walton, J. N. 2nd ed., pp. 733–762. London: Churchill.

Bordiuk, J. M., Legato, M. J., Lovelace, R. E. and Blumenthal, S. (1970). Pompe's disease. Electromyographic, electron microscopic and cardiovascular aspects. *Archs Neurol., Chicago,* **23,** 113–119.

Borgström, B., Nordén, Å. and Ståhl, E. (1971). Primary (?) bile acid deficiency in a patient with malabsorption syndrome. *Acta Pediat. Scand.* **60,** 379–380.

Boyd, I. A. (1962). The structure and innervation of the nuclear bag muscle fibre system and the nuclear chain muscle fibre system in mammalian muscle spindles. *Phil. Trans. R. Soc.* **B 245,** 81–136.

Bradley, W. G. (1969). Ultrastructural changes in adynamia episodica hereditaria and normokalaemic familial periodic paralysis. *Brain,* **92,** 379–390.

Bradley, W. G. (1970). The neuromyopathy of vincristine in the guinea pig. An electrophysiological and pathological study. *J. neurol. Sci.* **10,** 133–162.

Bradley, W. G., Hudgson, P., Gardner-Medwin, D. and Walton, J. N. (1969). Myopathy associated with abnormal lipid metabolism in skeletal muscle. *Lancet*, **1**, 495–498.

Bradley, W. G., Lassman, L. P., Pearce, G. W. and Walton, J. N. (1970). The neuromyopathy of vincristine in man. Clinical, electrophysiological and pathological studies. *J. neurol. Sci.* **10**, 107–131.

Brandt, D. E. and Leeson, C. R. (1966). Structural differences of fast and slow fibres in human extra-ocular muscle. *Am. J. Ophthal.* **62**, 478–487.

Brody, I. A. and Dudley, A. W. (1969). Thyrotoxic hypokalemic periodic paralysis. Muscle morphology and functional assay of sarcoplasmic reticulum. *Archs Neurol., Chicago*, **21**, 1–6.

Brooke, M. H. and Kaiser, K. K. (1970). Muscle fibre types: How many and what kind? *Archs Neurol., Chicago*, **23**, 369–379.

Brownell, B., Hughes, J. T., Goldby, F. S. and Woods, H. F. (1969). McArdle's myopathy. A report of a case with observations on the muscle ultrastructure. *J. neurol. Sci.* **9**, 515–526.

Bruni, C. B. and Paluello, F. M. (1970). A biochemical and ultrastructural study of liver, muscle, heart and kidney in type II glycogenosis. *Virchows Arch., Abt. B Zellpath.* **4**, 196–207.

Bubenzer, H. J. (1966). Die dünnen und die dicken Muskelfasern des Zwerchfells der Ratte. *Z. Zellforsch. mikrosk. Anat.* **69**, 520–550.

Bullard, H. H. (1912). On the interstitial granules and fat droplets of striated muscle. *Am. J. Anat.* **14**, 1–46.

Burch, G. E., Sohal, R. S., Colcolough, H. L. and Sun, S. C. (1968). Virus-like particles in skeletal muscle of a heat stroke victim. *Archs envir. Hlth*, **17**, 984–985.

Burdette, W. J. and Ashford, T. P. (1965). Structural changes in the human myocardium following hypoxia. *J. thorac. cardiovasc. Surg.* **50**, 210–220.

Buscaino, G. A., De Giacomo, P. and Mazzarella, L. (1970). Two cases of so-called 'mitochondrial myopathy'. Preliminary report. In *Proceedings. International Congress on Muscle Diseases, Milan, 1969*. Ed. Walton, J. N., Canal, N. and Scarlato, G. Int. Congr. Ser. No. 199, pp. 112–115. Amsterdam: Excerpta medica.

Buzzard, E. F. and Greenfield, J. G. (1921). *Pathology of the Nervous System*. London: Constable.

Caesar, R., Edwards, G. A. and Ruska, H. (1958). Electron microscopy of the impulse conducting system of the sheep heart. *Z. Zellforsch. mikrosk. Anat.* **48**, 698–719.

Campbell, M. J., Rebeiz, J. J. and Walton, J. N. (1969). Myotubular, centronuclear or peri-centronuclear myopathy? *J. neurol Sci.* **8**, 425–443.

Cancilla, P. A. and Zimmerman, H. M. (1965). The fine structure of a cerebellar hemangioblastoma. *J. Neuropath. exp. Neurol.* **24**, 621–628.

Cape, C. A., Johnson, W. W. and Pitner, S. E. (1970). Nemaline structures in polymyositis. A nonspecific pathological reaction of skeletal muscle. *Neurology, Minneap.* **20**, 494–502.

Cardiff, D. R. (1966). A histochemical and electron microscope study of skeletal muscle in a case of Pompe's disease (glycogenosis II). *Pediatrics, N.Y.* **37**, 249–259.

Castaigne, P., Laplane, D., Escourolle, E., Fardeau, M., Poirier, J. and Tuhpin, J. C. (1970). Étude anatomoclinique, ultrastructurale, histoenzymatique d'un cas de paramyotonie d'Eulenburg. Communication to *II Journ. int. Path. Neuro-musculaire, Marseille.*

Caulfield, J. B. (1966). Electron microscopic observations on the dystrophic hamster muscle. *In* Experimental primary myopathies and their relationship to human muscle diseases. Ed. Bajusz, E. *Ann. N.Y. Acad. Sci.* **138,** 151–159.

Caulfield, J. B., Rebeiz, J. and Adams, R. D. (1968). Viral involvement of human muscle. *J. Path. Bact.* **96,** 232–234.

Cazzato, G. and Walton, J. N. (1968). The pathology of the muscle spindle. A study of biopsy material in various muscular and neuromuscular diseases. *J. neurol. Sci.* **7,** 15–70.

Chalmers, R. A., Johnson, M., Pallis, C. and Watts, R. W. E. (1969). Xanthinuria with myopathy. *Q. Jl Med.* **38,** 493–512.

Cheng, K. and Breinin, G. M. (1966). A comparison of the fibre structure of extra-ocular and interosseous muscles in the monkey. *Invest. ophthal.* **5,** 535–549.

Cheng, K. and Breinin, G. M. (1965). Fine structure of nerve endings in extra-ocular muscle. *Archs Ophthal. N.Y.* **74,** 822–834.

Cheville, N. F. (1966). The pathology of vitamin E deficiency in the chick. *Path. Vet. (Basel)*, **3,** 208–225.

Chou, S. M. (1967a). 'Megaconial' mitochondria observed in a case of chronic polymyositis. *Neurology, Minneap.* **17,** 309.

Chou, S. M. (1967b). Myxovirus-like structures in a case of chronic polymyositis. *Science, N.Y.* **158,** 1453–1455.

Chou, S. M. (1968). Myxovirus-like structures and accompanying nuclear changes in chronic polymyositis. *Archs Path.* **86,** 649–658.

Chou, S. M. (1969). 'Megaconial' mitochondria observed in a case of chronic polymyositis. *Acta neuropath.* **12,** 68–89.

Chou, S. M. and Gutmann, L. (1970). Picornavirus-like crystals in subacute polymyositis. *Neurology, Minneap.* **20,** 205–213.

Church, J. C. T. (1969). Satellite cells and myogenesis; a study in the fruit-bat web. *J. Anat.* **105,** 419–438.

Church, J. C. T., Noronha, R. J. X. and Allbrook, D. B. (1966). Satellite cells and skeletal muscle regeneration. *Br. J. Surg.* **53,** 638–642.

Coërs, C. (1967). Structure and organization of the myoneural junction. *Int. Rev. Cytol.* **22,** 239–267.

Coërs, C. and de Harven, E. (1962). La microscopie electronique de la jonction neuromusculaire humaine. *Proc. 4th Int. Congr. Neuropath.* Vol. II, pp. 7–16. Stuttgart: Georg Thieme.

Conen, P. E. and Bell, C. D. (1970). Study of satellite cells in mature and fetal muscle and rhabdomyosarcoma. In *Regeneration of Striated Muscle and Myogenesis*. Ed. Mauro A., Shafiq, S. A., and Milhorat, A. T. Int. Congr. Ser. No. 218, pp. 194–211. Amsterdam: Excerpta medica.

Conen, P. E., Murphy, E. G. and Donohue, W. L. (1963). Light and electron microscopic studies of 'myogranules' in a child with hypotonia and muscle weakness. *Canad. med. Ass. J.* **89,** 983–986.

Cooper, S. and Daniel, P. M. (1949). Muscle spindles in human extrinsic eye muscles. *Brain,* **72,** 1–24.

Cooper, S. and Daniel, P. M. (1963). Muscle spindles in man; their morphology in the lumbricals and the deep muscle of the neck. *Brain,* **86,** 563–586.

Cornog, J. L. and Gonatas, N. K. (1967). Ultrastructure of rhabdomyoma. *J. Ultrastruct. Res.* **20,** 433–450.

Couteaux, R. (1941). Recherches sur l'histogénèse du muscle strié des mammifères et la formation des plaques motrices. *Bull. Biol. Fr. Belg.* **75,** 101–239.

D'Agostino, A. N. (1963). An electron microscopic study of skeletal and cardiac muscle of the rat poisoned by plasmocid. *Lab. Invest.* **12,** 1060–1071.

D'Agostino, A. N. (1964). An electron microscopy study of cardiac necrosis produced by 9 α-fluorocortisol and sodium phosphate. *Am. J. Path.* **45,** 633–644.

D'Agostino, A. N. and Chiga, M. (1966a). Cortisone myopathy in rabbits. A light and electron microscopic study. *Neurology, Minneap.* **16,** 257–263.

D'Agostino, A. N. and Chiga, M. (1966b). Morphologic changes in cardiac and skeletal muscle induced by corticosteroids. *In* Experimental primary myopathies and their relationship to human muscle diseases. Ed. Bajusz, E. *Ann. N.Y. Acad. Sci.* **138,** 73–81.

D'Agostino, A. N., Ziter, F. A. and Bray, P. F. (1967). Hereditary myopathy with abnormal muscle mitochondria. *Trans. Am. neurol. Ass.* **92,** 222–224.

D'Agostino, A. N., Ziter, F. A., Ralliston, M. L. and Bray, P. F. (1968). Familial myopathy with abnormal muscle mitochondria. *Archs Neurol., Chicago,* **18,** 388–401.

Daniel, P. M. and Strich, S. J. (1964). Abnormalities in the muscle spindles in dystrophia myotonica. *Neurology, Minneap.* **14,** 310–316.

De Duve, C. (1969). The lysosomes in retrospect. In *Lysosomes in Biology and Pathology.* Ed. Dingle, J. T. and Fell, H. B. Vol. I, pp. 3–40. Amsterdam: North Holland.

De Harven, E. and Coërs, C. (1959). Electron microscopy study of the human neuromuscular junction. *J. biophys. biochem. Cytol.* **6,** 7–10.

De Recondo, J. (1970a). Amyotrophie de Charcot-Marie-Tooth. Étude ultrastructurale du nerf sensitif et de la jonction myo-neurale. *Proc. 6th Int. Congr. Neuropath.* pp. 721–722. Paris: Masson.

De Recondo, J. (1970b). Amyotrophie de Charcot-Marie-Tooth. Étude ultrastructurale du muscle squelettique. *Proc. 6th Int. Congr. Neuropath.* pp. 1072–1073. Paris: Masson.

De Recondo, J., Fardeau, M. and Lapresle, J. (1966). Étude au microscope électronique des lésions musculaires d'atrophie neurogène par atteinte de la corne antérieure (observées dans huit cas de sclérose latérale amyotrophique). *Revue neurol.* **114,** 169–192.

Dessouky, D. A. and Hibbs, R. G. (1965). An electron microscope study of the development of the somatic muscle of the chick embryo. *Am. J. Anat.* **116,** 523–565.

Dietert, S. E. (1965). The demonstration of different types of muscle fibres in human extra-ocular muscle by electron microscopy and cholinesterase staining. *Invest. Ophthal.* **4,** 51–63.

Dos Remedios, C. G. (1970). Structural studies on the M-line striated muscle and a proposed function. *J. Anat.* **106,** 195.

Douglas, R. M., Fewing, J. D., Casley-Smith, J. R. and West, R. F. (1966). Recurrent rhabdomyolysis precipitated by alcohol: a case report with physiological and electron microscope studies of skeletal muscle. *Australas. Ann. Med.* **15,** 251–261.

Draper, M. H. and Hodge, A. J. (1949). Studies on muscle with the electron microscope. I. The ultrastructure of toad muscle. *Aust. J. exp. Biol. med. Sci.* **27,** 465–503.

Duane, D. D. and Engel, A. G. (1970). Emetine myopathy. *Neurology, Minneap.* **20,** 733–739.

Dubowitz, V, and Pearse, A. G. E. (1960a). Reciprocal relationship of phosphorylase and oxidative enzymes in skeletal muscle. *Nature, Lond.* **185,** 701–702.

Dubowitz, V. and Pearse, A. G. E. (1960b). Oxidative enzymes and phosphorylase in central-core disease of muscle. *Lancet,* **2,** 23–24.

Dubowitz, V. and Pearse, A. G. E. (1960c). A comparative histochemical study of oxidative enzyme and phosphorylase activity in skeletal muscle. *Histochemie,* **2,** 105–117.

Dubowitz, V. and Pearse, A. G. E. (1961). Enzymic activity of normal and dystrophic human muscle: a histochemical study. *J. Path. Bact.* **81,** 365–378.

Dubowitz, V. and Platts, M. (1965). Central core disease of muscle with focal wasting. *J. Neurol. Neurosurg. Psychiat.* **28,** 432–437.

Dubowitz, V. and Roy, S. (1970). Central core disease of muscle: clinical, histochemical and electron microscopic studies of an affected mother and child. *Brain,* **93,** 133–146.

Dunkle, L. M., Diggs, C. H., Bergman, R. A. and Johns, R. J. (1970). A light and electron microscopy study of a second case of hypokalemic periodic paralysis with hyperthyroidism. *Johns Hopkins med. J.* **126,** 225–236.

Edwards, W. (1970). Ultrastructural changes in the human motor end plate in myasthenia gravis. *Proc. 6th Int. Congr. Neuropath.* pp. 751–752. Paris: Masson.

Engel, A. G. (1965). Electron microscopic observations in metabolic myopathies (three types of hypokalemic periodic paralysis, thyroid myopathy and steroid-induced myopathy). *J. Neuropath. exp. Neurol.* **24,** 141–142.

Engel, A. G. (1966a). Late onset rod myopathy (a new syndrome?): light and electron microscopic observations in two cases. *Proc. Staff Meet. Mayo Clin.* **41,** 713–741.

Engel, A. G. (1966b). Electron microscopic observations in thyrotoxic and corticosteroid-induced myopathies. *Proc. Staff Meet. Mayo Clin.* **41,** 785–796.

Engel, A. G. (1966c). Electron microscopy observations in primary hypokalemic and thyrotoxic periodic paralyses. *Proc. Staff Meet. Mayo Clin.* **41,** 797–808.

Engel, A. G. (1967). Pathological reactions of the Z-disc. In *Exploratory Concepts in Muscular Dystrophy and Related Disorders.* Ed. Milhorat, A. T. Int. Congr. Ser. No. 147, pp. 398–412. Amsterdam: Excerpta medica.

Engel, A. G. (1970a). Acid maltase deficiency in adults: studies in four cases of a syndrome which may mimic muscular dystrophy or other myopathies. *Brain,* **93,** 599–616.

Engel, A. G. (1970b). Acid maltase deficiency in adult life. Morphological and biochemical data in three cases of a syndrome simulating other myopathies. In *Proceedings. International Congress on Muscle Diseases, Milan, 1969.* Ed. Walton, J. N., Canal, N. and Scarlato, G. Int. Congr. Ser. No. 199, pp. 236–245. Amsterdam: Excerpta medica.

Engel, A. G. and Dale, A. J. D. (1968). Autophagic glycogenosis of late onset with mitochondrial abnormalities: light and electron microscopic observations. *Proc. Staff Meet. Mayo Clin.* **43,** 233–279.

Engel, A. G. and Gomez, M. R. (1966). Congenital myopathy associated with multifocal degeneration of muscle fibres. *Trans. Am. neurol. Ass.* **91,** 222–223.

Engel, A. G. and Gomez, M. R. (1967). Nemaline (Z disk) myopathy: observations on the origin, structure and solubility properties of the nemaline structures. *J. Neuropath. exp. Neurol.* **26,** 601–619.

Engel, A. G. and Macdonald, R. D. (1970). Ultrastructural reactions in muscle disease and their light-microscopic correlates. In *Proceedings. International Congress on Muscle Diseases, Milan, 1969.* Ed. Walton, J. N., Canal, N. and Scarlato, G. Int. Congr. Ser. No. 199, pp. 71–89. Amsterdam: Excerpta medica.

Engel, W. K. (1961). Muscle target fibres, a newly recognized sign of denervation. *Nature, Lond.* **191,** 389–390.

Engel, W. K. (1962). The essentiality of histo- and cytochemical studies of skeletal muscle in the investigation of neuromuscular disease. *Neurology, Minneap.* **12,** 778–794.

Engel, W. K. (1964). Mitochondrial aggregates in muscle disease. *J. Histochem. Cytochem.* **12,** 46–48.

Engel, W. K. (1967). A critique of congenital myopathies and other disorders. In *Exploratory Concepts in Muscular Dystrophy and Related Disorders*. Ed. Milhorat, A. T. Int. Congr. Ser. No. 147, pp. 27–40. Amsterdam: Excerpta medica.

Engel, W. K. (1970). Selective and nonselective susceptibility of muscle fibre types. A new approach to human neuromuscular diseases. *Archs Neurol., Chicago.* **22,** 97–117.

Engel, W. K., Bishop, D. W. and Cunningham, G. G. (1970). Tubular aggregates in type II muscle fibres: ultrastructural and histochemical correlation. *J. Ultrastruct. Res.* **31,** 507–525.

Engel, W. K., Foster, J. B., Hughes, B. P., Huxley, H. E. and Mahler, R. (1961). Central core disease—an investigation of a rare muscle cell abnormality. *Brain,* **84,** 167–185.

Engel, W. K. and Resnick, J. S. (1966). Late-onset rod myopathy: a newly recognized, acquired and progressive disease. *Neurology, Minneap.* **16,** 308–309.

Engel, W. K., Wanko, T. and Fenichel, G. M. (1964). Nemaline myopathy. A second case. *Archs Neurol., Chicago.* **11,** 22–39.

Ezerman, E. B. and Ishikawa, H. (1967). Differentiation of the sarcoplasmic reticulum and T system in developing chick skeletal muscle in vitro. *J. Cell Biol.* **35,** 405–420.

Fardeau, M. (1965). Présence de nombreux microtubules dans les fibres musculaires squelettiques au cours de l'atrophie neurogène par atteinte périphérique. *C.r. Séanc. Soc. Biol.* **159,** 302–303.

Fardeau, M. (1969a). Ultrastructure des fibres musculaires squelettiques. *Presse méd.* **77,** 1341–1344; 1563–1566.

Fardeau, M. (1969b). Étude d'une nouvelle observation de 'nemaline myopathy'. II. Données ultrastructurales. *Acta neuropath.* **13,** 250–266.

Fardeau, M. (1970). Ultrastructural lesions in progressive muscular dystrophies. A critical study of their specificity. In *Proceedings. International Congress on Muscle Diseases, Milan, 1969*. Ed. Walton, J. N., Canal, N. and Scarlato, G. Int. Congr. Ser. No. 199, pp. 98–108. Amsterdam: Excerpta medica.

Fardeau, M. and Engel, W. K. (1970). Relation entre la morphologie des plaques motrices et le type des fibres musculaires squelettiques (chez le cobaye). In *Proc. 6th Int. Congr. Neuropath.* pp. 740–741. Paris: Masson.

Fardeau, M. and Godet-Guillain, J. (1970). Étude ultrastructurale des plaques motrices du muscle squelettique humain et de leurs modifications pathologiques. In *Proc. 6th Int. Congr. Neuropath.* pp. 746–747. Paris: Masson.

Fardeau, M., Lapresle, J. and Milhaud, M. (1965). Contribution a l'étude des lésions élémentaires du muscle squelettique: ultrastructure des masses sarcoplasmiques laterales (observées dans un cas de dystrophie myotonique). *C.r. Séanc. Soc. Biol.* **159,** 15–17.

Fawcett, D. W. (1966). *An Atlas of Fine Structure. The Cell: its Organelles and Inclusions.* Philadelphia: Saunders.

Fawcett, D. W. (1968). The sporadic occurrence in cardiac muscle of anomalous Z-bands exhibiting a periodic structure suggestive of tropomyosin. *J. Cell Biol.* **36,** 266–270.

Fawcett, D. W. and McNutt, N. S. (1969). The ultrastructure of the cat myocardium. I. Ventricular papillary muscle. *J. Cell Biol.* **42,** 1–45.

Fernando, N. V. P. and Movat, H. Z. (1964). The fine structure of the terminal vascular bed. III. The capillaries. *Exp. molec. Path.* **3,** 87–97.

Fischman, D. A. (1967). An electron microscope study of myofibril formation in embryonic chick skeletal muscle. *J. Cell Biol.* **32,** 557–575.

Fisher, E. R., Cohn, R. E. and Danowski, T. S. (1966). Ultrastructural observations of

skeletal muscle in myopathy and neuropathy with special reference to muscular dystrophy. *Lab. Invest.* **15,** 778–793.
Fisher, E. R. and Danowski, T. S. (1969). Mitochondrial myopathy. *Am. J. clin. Path.* **51,** 619–630.
Forssmann, W. G. and Girardier, L. (1970). A study of the T-system in rat heart. *J. Cell Biol.* **44,** 1–19.
Franke, W. W. and Schinko, W. (1969). Nuclear shape in muscle cells. *J. Cell Biol.* **42,** 326–331.
Franzini-Armstrong, C. and Porter, K. R. (1964a). Sarcolemmal invaginations and the T-system in fish skeletal muscle. *Nature, Lond.* **202,** 355–357.
Franzini-Armstrong, C. and Porter, K. R. (1964b). Sarcolemmal invaginations constituting the T-system in fish muscle fibres. *J. Cell Biol.* **22,** 675–696.
Freund-Mölber, E. R. G., Jontofson, R., Ketelsen, U. P. and Beckmann, R. (1970). Ultrastructural study of experimental cortisol myopathy. In *Proceedings. International Congress on Muscle Diseases, Milan, 1969.* Ed. Walton, J. N., Canal, N. and Scarlato, G. Int. Congr. Ser. No. 199, pp. 497–502. Amsterdam: Excerpta medica.
Galavazi, G. and te Lintel Hekkert, T. J. (1968). Identification of ribosomes and their polysomal configurations in sections of skeletal muscle of the adult rat. In *Electron-microscopy. Abstracts 4th European Regional Conference on Electron Microscopy.* pp. 301–302. Rome: Tipographia Poliglotta Vaticana.
Gambetti, P., Mellman, W. J. and Gonatas, N. K. (1969). Familial spongy degeneration of the central nervous system (van Bogaert–Bertrand disease). An ultrastructural study. *Acta neuropath.* **12,** 103–115.
Garancis, J. C. (1968). Type II glycogenosis. Biochemical and electron microscopic study. *Am. J. Med.* **44,** 289–300.
Garcin, R., Lapresle, J. and Hewitt, J. (1967). Déterminations musculaires au cours d'une maladie de Behçet (ou grande aftose de Touraine). Étude clinique; documents histologiques et ultra-structuraux concernant la biopsie musculaire. *Revue neurol.* **117,** 345–361.
Garcin, R., Legrain, M., Rondot, P. and Fardeau, M. (1966). Étude clinique et métabolique d'une observation de paramyotonie congénitale d'Eulenburg. Documents ultrastructuraux concernant la biopsie musculaire. *Revue neurol.* **115,** 295–311.
Garcin, R., Rondot, P. and Fardeau, M. (1964). Sur les accidents neuro-musculaires et en particulier sur une 'myopathie vacuolaire' observés au cours d'un traitement prolongé par la chloroquine. *Revue neurol.* **111,** 177–195.
Gauthier, G. F. (1969). On the relationship of ultrastructural and cytochemical features to color in mammalian skeletal muscle. *Z. Zellforsch. mikrosk. Anat.* **95,** 462–482.
Gauthier, G. F. and Padykula, H. A. (1966). Cytological studies of fiber types in skeletal muscle. A comparative study of the mammalian diaphragm. *J. Cell Biol.* **28,** 333–354.
Godet-Guillain, J. and Fardeau, M. (1970). Hypothyroid myopathy. Histological and ultrastructural study of an atrophic form. In *Proceedings. International Congress on Muscle Diseases, Milan, 1969.* Ed. Walton, J. N., Canal, N. and Scarlato, G. Int. Congr. Ser. No. 199, pp. 512–515. Amsterdam: Excerpta medica.
Golding, D. N., Murray, S. M., Pearce, G. W. and Thompson, M. (1961). Corticosteroid myopathy. *Ann. phys. Med.* **6,** 171–177.
Gonatas, N. K. (1966). The fine structure of the rod-like bodies in nemaline myopathy and their relation to the Z-discs. *J. Neuropath. exp. Neurol.* **25,** 409–421.
Gonatas, N. K. (1967). A generalized disorder of nervous system, skeletal muscle and

heart resembling Refsum's disease and Hurler's Syndrome. II. Ultrastructure. *Am. J. Med.* **42,** 169–178.

Gonatas, N. K., Perez, M. C., Shy, G. M. and Evangelista, I. (1965). Central 'core' disease of skeletal muscle. Ultrastructural and cytochemical observations in two cases. *Am. J. Path.* **47,** 503–524.

Gonatas, N. K. and Shy, G. M. (1966). Childhood myopathies with abnormal mitochondria. *Proc. 5th Int. Congr. Neuropath., Zurich, 1965.* Int. Congr. Ser. No. 100. pp. 606–611. Amsterdam: Excerpta medica.

Gonatas, N. K., Shy, G. M. and Godfrey, E. H. (1966). Nemaline myopathy. The origin of nemaline structures. *New Engl. J. Med.* **274,** 535–539.

Grabow, J. D. and Chou, S. M. (1968). Thyrotrophin hormone deficiency with a peripheral neuropathy. *Archs Neurol., Chicago.* **19,** 284–291.

Greenfield, J. G., Cornman, T. and Shy, G. M. (1958). The prognostic value of the muscle biopsy in the 'floppy infant'. *Brain,* **81,** 461–484.

Greenfield, J. G., Shy, G. M., Alvord, E. C. and Berg, L. (1957). *An Atlas of Muscle Pathology in Neuromuscular Diseases.* Edinburgh: Livingstone.

Gröschel-Stewart, U. (1971). Comparative studies of human smooth and striated muscle myosins. *Biochim. biophys. Acta,* **229,** 322–334.

Gruener, R., McArdle, B., Ryman, B. E. and Weller, R. O. (1968). Contracture of phosphorylase deficient muscle. *J. Neurol. Neurosurg. Psychiat.* **31,** 268–283.

Grünbaum, A. S. (1897). Note on muscle-spindles in pseudo-hypertrophic paralysis. *Brain,* **20,** 365–367.

Gruner, J. E. (1961). La structure fine du fuseau neuromusculaire humain. *Revue neurol.* **104,** 490–507.

Gruner, J. E. (1963). Sur quelques anomalies mitochondriales observées au cours d'affections musculaires variées. *C.r. Séanc. Soc. Biol.* **157,** 181–182.

Gruner, J. E. (1966). Amomalies du réticulum sarcoplasmique et prolifération de tubules dans le muscle d'une paralysie périodique familiale. *C.r. Séanc. Soc. Biol.* **160,** 193–195.

Gruner, J. E. and Porte, A. (1959). Les lésions musculaires de la paralysie périodique familiale. *Revue neurol.* **101,** 501–523.

Gubbay, S. S., Walton, J. N. and Pearce, G. W. (1966). Clinical and pathological study of a case of congenital muscular dystrophy. *J. Neurol. Neurosurg. Psychiat.* **29,** 500–508.

Guth, L. and Samaha, F. J. (1969). Qualitative differences between actomyosin ATPase of slow and fast mammalian muscle. *Expl. Neurol.* **25,** 138–152.

Gutmann, E., Tuček, S. and Hanzlíková, V. (1969). Changes in the choline acetyltransferase and cholinesterase activities in the levator ani muscle of rats following castration. *Physiologia bohemoslov.* **18,** 195–203.

Hanson, J. and Huxley, H. E. (1953). Structural basis of the cross-striations in muscle. *Nature, Lond.* **172,** 530–532.

Hanson, J. and Huxley, H. E. (1957). Quantitative studies on the structure of the cross-striated myofibrils. II. Investigations by biochemical techniques. *Biochim. biophys. Acta,* **23,** 250–260.

Hanson, J. and Lowy, J. (1963). The structure of F-actin and of actin filaments isolated from muscle. *J. molec. Biol.* **6,** 46–60.

Hasselbach, W. and Schneider, G. (1951). Der L-Myosin und Aktingehalt des Kaninchenmuskels. *Biochem. Z.* **321,** 462–475.

Hausmanowa-Petrusewicz, I., Askanas, W., Badurska, B., Emeryk, B., Fidziánska, A.,

Garbalínska, W., Hetnarska, L., Jedrzejowska, H., Kamieniecka, Z., Niebrój-Dobosz, I., Prot, J. and Sawicka, E. (1968). Infantile and juvenile spinal muscular atrophy. *J. neurol. Sci.* **6**, 269–287.

Hayward, M. and Mair, W. G. P. (1970). The ultrastructure of ring fibres in dystrophic muscle. *Acta neuropath.* **16**, 161–172.

Heffernan, L. P., Rewcastle, N. B. and Humphrey, J. G. (1968). The spectrum of rod myopathies. *Archs Neurol., Chicago*, **18**, 529–542.

Henriksson, F. K.-G., Nordén, Å. and Mair, W. G. P. To be published.

Henson, R. A., Russell, D. S. and Wilkinson, M. (1954). Carcinomatous neuropathy and myopathy: a clinical and pathological study. *Brain*, **77**, 82–121.

Hers, H. G. and van Hoof, F. (1968). Glycogen-storage diseases. Type II and type VI glycogenosis. In *Carbohydrate Metabolism and its Disorders*. Ed. Dickens, F., Randle, P. J. and Whelan, W. J. Vol. II, pp. 152–168. New York: Academic Press.

Hess, A. (1960). The structure of extrafusal muscle fibres in the frog and their innervation studied by cholinesterase technique. *Am. J. Anat.* **107**, 129–151.

Hess, A. (1961). Structural differences of fast and slow extrafusal muscle fibres and their nerve endings in chickens. *J. Physiol., Lond.* **157**, 221–231.

Hess, A. (1962). Structural differences of fast and slow extrafusal muscle fibres and their nerve endings. *Proc. 4th Int. Congr. Neuropath.* Vol. II, pp. 3–4. Stuttgart: Georg Thieme.

Hess, A. (1965). The sarcoplasmic reticulum, the T-system and the motor terminals of slow and twitch muscle fibres in the gaster snake. *J. Cell Biol.* **26**, 467–476.

Hess, A. and Pilar, G. (1963). Slow fibres in the extraocular muscle of the cat. *J. Physiol., Lond.* **169**, 780–798.

Hess, A. and Rosner, S. (1970). The satellite cell bud and myoblast in denervated mammalian muscle fibers. *Am. J. Anat.* **129**, 21–39.

Heuson-Stiennon, J. A. (1965). Morphogenèse de la cellule musculaire striée etudiée au microscope électronique. I. Formation des structures fibrillaires. *J. microsc.* **4**, 657–678.

Hibbs, R. G. (1956). Electron microscopy of developing cardiac muscle in chick embryos. *Am. J. Anat.* **99**, 17–52.

Hibbs, R. G., Ferrans, V. F., Black. W. C., Weilbaecher, D. G., Walsh, J. J. and Burch, G. E. (1965). Alcoholic cardiomyopathy. An electron microscopic study. *Am. Heart J.* **69**, 766–779.

Hirano, H. (1967). Ultrastructural study on the morphogenesis of the neuromuscular junction in the skeletal muscle of the chick. *Z. Zellforsch. mikrosk. Anat.* **79**, 198–208.

Hirschl, S. (1969). Electron microscopic analysis of human amyloid. *J. Ultrastruct. Res.* **29**, 281–292.

Hodge, A. J. (1960). Ultrastructure of the muscle fiber. *Res. Publs Ass. Res. nerv. ment Dis.* **38**, 31–51.

Hodge, A. J., Huxley, H. E. and Spiro, D. (1954). Electron microscope studies on ultrathin sections of muscle. *J. exp. Med.* **99**, 201–206.

Howes, E. L., Price, H. M. and Blumberg, J. M. (1964). The effects of a diet producing lipochrome pigment (ceroid) on the ultrastructure of skeletal muscle in the rat. *Am. J. Path.* **45**, 599–631.

Howes, E. L., Price, H. M., Pearson, C. M. and Blumberg, J. M. (1966). Hypokalemic periodic paralysis. Electronmicroscopic changes in the sarcoplasm. *Neurology, Minneap.* **16**, 242–256.

Hudgson, P. (1968). Ultrastructural changes in dystrophic muscle. In *Proceedings. 4th Symposium on Research in Muscular Dystrophy*. pp. 207–222. London: Pitman.

Hudgson, P. (1970). The value of electron microscopy in muscle biopsies. *Proc. R. Soc. Med.* **63,** 470–474.
Hudgson, P., Gardner-Medwin, D., Fulthorpe, J. L. and Walton, J. N. (1967). Nemaline myopathy. *Neurology Minneap.* **17,** 1125–1142.
Hudgson, P., Gardner-Medwin, D., Worsfold, M., Pennington, R. J. T. and Walton, J. N. (1968). Adult myopathy from glycogen storage disease due to acid maltase deficiency. *Brain,* **91,** 435–462.
Hudgson, P., Jenkison, M. and Larson, P. F. (1970). An ultrastructural study of chick embryo and human foetal muscle. In *Proceedings. International Congress on Muscle Diseases, Milan, 1969.* Ed. Walton, J. N., Canal, N. and Scarlato, G. Int. Congr. Ser. No. 199, pp. 90–97. Amsterdam: Excerpta medica.
Hudgson, P. and Pearce, G. W. (1969). Ultramicroscopic studies of diseased muscle. In *Disorders of Voluntary Muscle.* Ed. Walton, J. N. pp. 277–317. London: Churchill.
Hudgson, P., Pearce, G. W. and Walton, J. N. (1967). Pre-clinical muscular dystrophy: histopathological changes observed on muscle biopsy. *Brain,* **90,** 565–576.
Hudson, A. J., Cholod, E. J. and Haust, M. D. (1970). Familial hyperparathyroid myopathy. In *Proceedings. International Congress on Muscle Diseases, Milan, 1969.* Ed. Walton, J. N., Canal, N. and Scarlato, G. Int. Congr. Ser. No. 199, pp. 526–530. Amsterdam: Excerpta medica.
Hug, G., Garancis, J. C., Schubert, W. K. and Kaplan, S. (1966). Glycogen storage disease, types II, III, VIII and IX. A biochemical and electron microscopic analysis. *Am. J. Dis. Childh.* **111,** 457–474.
Hughes, J. T. and Brownell, B. (1969). Ultrastructure of muscle in Werdnig-Hoffmann's disease. *J. neurol. Sci.* **8,** 363–379.
Hülsmann, W. C., Bethlem, J., Meijer, A. E. F. H., Fleury, P. and Schellens, J. P. M. (1967). Myopathy with abnormal structure and function of muscle mitochondria. *J. Neurol. Neurosurg. Psychiat.* **30,** 519–525.
Humphrey, J. G. and Rewcastle, N. B. (1963). Vacuolar myopathy. A clinical and electron microscopic study. *Trans. Am. neurol. Ass.* **88,** 225–226.
Hurwitz, L. J., Carson, N. A. J., Allen, I. V. and Chopra, J. S. (1969). Congenital ophthalmoplegia, floppy baby syndrome, myopathy and amino-aciduria. Report of a family. *J. Neurol. Neurosurg. Psychiat.* **32,** 495–508.
Hurwitz, L. J., Carson, N. A. J., Allen, I. V., Fannin, T. F., Lyttle, J. A. and Neill, D. W. (1967). Clinical, biochemical and histopathological findings in a family with muscular dystrophy. *Brain,* **90,** 799–816.
Huxley, A. F. (1957a). Muscle structure and theories of contraction. *Prog. Biophys. biophys. Chem.* **7,** 255–318.
Huxley, A. F. (1957b). Local activation of striated muscle from the frog and the crab. *J. Physiol., Lond.* **135,** 17–18P.
Huxley, A. F. and Niedergerke, R. (1954). Structural changes in muscle during contraction. Interference microscopy of living muscle fibres. *Nature, Lond.* **173,** 971–973.
Huxley, A. F. and Straub, R. W. (1958). Local activation and interfibrillary structures in striated muscle. *J. Physiol., Lond.* **143,** 40–41P.
Huxley, A. F. and Taylor, R. E. (1958). Local activation of striated muscle fibres. *J. Physiol., Lond.* **144,** 426–441.
Huxley, H. E. (1953). Electron microscope studies of the organisation of the filaments in striated muscle. *Biochim. biophys. Acta,* **12,** 387–394.

Huxley, H. E. (1957). The double array of filaments in cross striated muscle. *J. biophys. biochem. Cytol.* **3**, 631–648.
Huxley, H. E. (1960). Muscle cells. In *The Cell. Biochemistry, Physiology, Morphology.* Ed. Brachet, J. and Mirsky, A. E. Vol. IV. Specialised cells. pp. 365–481. New York: Academic Press.
Huxley, H. E. (1963). Electron microscope studies on the structure of natural and synthetic protein filaments from striated muscle. *J. molec. Biol.* **7**, 281–308.
Huxley, H. E. (1964). Evidence for continuity between the central elements of the triads and extracellular space in frog sartorius muscle. *Nature, Lond.* **202**, 1067–1071.
Huxley, H. E. and Brown, W. (1967). The low-angle X-ray diagram of vertebrate striated muscle and its behaviour during contraction and rigor. *J. molec. Biol.* **30**, 383–434.
Huxley, H. E. and Hanson, J. (1954). Changes in the cross-striations of muscle during contraction and stretch and their structural interpretation. *Nature, Lond.* **173**, 973–976.
Huxley, H. E. and Hanson, J. (1957). Quantitative studies on the structure of cross-striated myofibrils. I. Investigations by interference microscopy. *Biochim. biophys. Acta.* **23**, 229–249.
Ichikawa, A. and Okajima, H. (1969). Fine structural changes in response to total denervation of the rat lumbrical muscle. *J. Electron Microsc., Tokyo*, **18**, 217.
Ionescu, V., Radu, H. and Nicolescu, P. (1970). Electron microscopic study in Steinert's disease. In *Proc. 7th Int. Conf. Electron Microsc.* Ed. Favard, P. pp. 813–814. Paris: Société Française de Microscopie Electronique.
Isch, F., Juif, J. G., Sacrez, R. and Thiébaut, F. (1966). Glycogénose musculaire à forme myopathique par déficit en maltase acid. *Pédiatrie*, **21**, 71–86.
Ishikawa, H. (1965). The fine structure of myo-tendon junction in some mammalian skeletal muscles. *Archvm histol. jap.* **25**, 257–296.
Ishikawa, H. (1966). Electron microscopic observations of satellite cells with special reference to the development of mammalian skeletal muscles. *Z. Anat. EntwGesch.* **125**, 43–63.
Ishikawa, H. (1968). Formation of elaborate networks of T-system tubules in cultured skeletal muscle with special reference to the T-system formation. *J. Cell. Biol.* **38**, 51–66.
Ishikawa, H. (1970). Satellite cells in developing muscle and tissue culture. In *Regeneration of Striated Muscle and Myogenesis.* Ed. Mauro, A., Shafiq, S. A. and Milhorat, A. T. Int. Congr. Ser. No. 218, pp. 167–179. Amsterdam: Excerpta medica.
Ishikawa, H., Bishoff, R. and Holtzer, H. (1968). Mitosis and intermediate-sized filaments in developing skeletal muscle. *J. Cell. Biol.* **38**, 538–555.
Iversen, K., Asbøe-Hansen, G. and Carlsen, F. (1953). Electron microscopy of certain muscle lesions in patients with pituitary-thyroid disorders. *Acta endocr., Copenh.* **14**, 177–180.
Iwayama, T. (1968). Electron microscope observation on neuromuscular junction after denervation. *J. Electron Microsc., Tokyo*, **17**, 354.
Iwayama, T. and Ohta, M. (1969). Ultrastructure of neuromuscular junction in myasthenic patients. *J. Electron Microsc., Tokyo*, **18**, 215.
Jaffurs, W. J., Herman, R. H., McDowell, M. K. and Blumberg, J. M. (1963). Hyperkalemic paralysis (adynamia episodica hereditaria): ultrastructural studies of muscles in two cases. *Metabolism*, **12**, 740–750.
Jamieson, J. D. and Palade, G. E. (1964). Specific granules in atrial muscle cells. *J. Cell. Biol.* **23**, 151–172.

Jerusalem, F. (1970). Bioptische Befunde des T-systems und tubuläre Strukturkomplexe bei neoplasticher Cortisonmyopathie. *Acta neuropath.* **14**, 338–344.

Jerusalem, F. and Schick, G. (1970). Die Frühphase der Regeneration der denervierten Muskels. Tierexperimentalle elektronenmikroskopische und autoradiographische Befunde. *Proc. 6th Int. Congr. Neuropath.* pp. 1068–1069. Paris: Masson.

Johnson, M. and Pearse, A. G. E. (1968). The cytochemistry and electron microscopy of congenital muscular dystrophy in the hamster. In *Proceedings. 4th Symposium on Research in Muscular Dystrophy*. pp. 171–187. London: Pitman.

Kakulas, B. A. (1969). Experimental myopathies. In *Disorders of Voluntary Muscle.* Ed. Walton, J. N. pp. 363–384. London: Churchill.

Karlsson, U. and Andersson-Cedergren, E. (1966). Motor myoneural junctions on frog intrafusal muscle fibre. *J. Ultrastruct. Res.* **14**, 191–211.

Karlsson, U. and Andersson-Cedergren, E. (1968). Small leptomeric organelles in intrafusal muscle fibres of the frog as revealed by electron microscopy. *J. Ultrastruct. Res.* **23**, 417–426.

Karlsson, U., Andersson-Cedergren, E. and Ottoson, D. (1966). Cellular organization of the frog muscle spindle as revealed by serial sections for electron microscopy. *J. Ultrastruct. Res.* **14**, 1–35.

Karpati, G., Carpenter, S. and Nelson, R. F. (1970). Type I muscle fibre atrophy and central nuclei. A rare familial neuromuscular disease. *J. neurol. Sci.* **10**, 489–500.

Katz, B. (1961). The terminations of the afferent nerve fibre in the muscle spindle of the frog. *Phil. Trans. R. Soc.* **B 243**, 221–240.

Kelly, D. E. (1967). Models of muscle Z-band fine structure based on a looping filament configuration. *J. Cell. Biol.* **34**, 827–840.

Kelly, A. M. and Zacks, S. I. (1969). The histogenesis of rat intercostal muscle. *J. Cell. Biol.* **42**, 135–153.

Kinoshita, M. and Cadman, T. E. (1968). Myotubular myopathy. *Archs. Neurol., Chicago*, **18**, 265–271.

Kisch, B., Grey, C. E. and Kelsch, J. J. (1948). Electron histology of the heart. *Expl Med. Surg.* **6**, 346–365.

Klinkerfuss, G. H. (1967). An electron microscopic study of myotonic dystrophy. *Archs Neurol., Chicago*, **16**, 181–193.

Klinkerfuss, G., Bleisch, V., Dioso, M. M. and Perkoff, G. T. (1967). A spectrum of myopathy associated with alcoholism. II. Light and electron microscopic observations. *Ann. intern. Med.* **67**, 493–510.

Knappeis, G. G. and Carlsen, F. (1962). The ultrastructure of the Z-disc in skeletal muscle. *J. Cell. Biol.* **13**, 323–335.

Knappeis, G. G. and Carlsen, F. (1968). The ultrastructure of the M-line in skeletal muscle. *J. Cell. Biol.* **38**, 202–211.

Kniffen, J. C. and Quick, D. T. (1970). Carbohydrate abnormalities in amyotrophic lateral sclerosis. In *Proceedings. International Congress on Muscle Diseases, Milan, 1969.* Ed. Walton, J. N., Canal, N. and Scarlato, G. Int. Congr. Ser. No. 199, pp. 345–349. Amsterdam: Excerpta medica.

Kolin, I. S. (1967). Nemaline myopathy. A fatal case. *Am. J. Dis. Childh.* **114**, 95–100.

Konigsberg, I. R. (1965). Aspects of cytodifferentiation of skeletal muscle. In *Organogenesis.* Ed. De Haan, R. L. and Ursprung, H. pp. 337–358. New York: Holt, Rinehart and Winston.

Krüger, P. (1929). Über einen möglichen Zusammenhang zwischen Struktur, Funktion und chemischer Beschaffenheit der Muskeln. *Biol. Zbl.* **49,** 616–622.

Krüger, P. (1949). Die Innervation der tetanischen und tonischen Fasern der quergestreiften Skelettmuskulatur der Wirbeltiere. *Anat. Anz.* **97,** 169–175.

Kugelberg, E. and Edström, L. (1968). Differential histochemical effects of muscle contractions on phosphorylase and glycogen in various types of fibres: relation to fatigue. *J. Neurol. Neurosurg. Psychiat.* **31,** 415–423.

Laguens, R. (1963). Satellite cells of skeletal muscle fibres in human progressive muscular dystrophy. *Virchows Arch. path. Anat. Physiol.* **336,** 564–569.

Lancet. (1969). A syndrome of vitamin E deficiency? *Lancet,* **1,** 405–406.

Landon, D. N. (1966a). Electron microscopy of muscle spindles. In *Control and Innervation of Skeletal Muscle.* Ed. Andrew, B. L. pp. 96–111. Dundee: Thomson.

Landon, D. N. (1966b). The fine structure of the annulospiral sensory nerve ending in the muscle spindles of the rat. *J. Physiol., Lond.* **185,** 6–7P.

Landon. D. N. (1970). The influence of fixation upon the fibre structure of the Z-disc of rat striated muscle. *J. Cell. Sci.* **6,** 257–276.

Lapresle, J. and Fardeau, M. (1968). Les désorganisations spatiales des myofibrilles, des sarcomères et des myofilaments dans les zones péripheriques de fibres musculaires pathologiques étudiés en microscope électronique. *Acta neuropath.* **10,** 105–116.

Lapresle, J., Fardeau, M. and Milhaud, M. (1964). Sur un type particulier d'alterations de la structure myofibrillaire recontrées dans cinq cas de dystrophie musculaire progressive. *C.r. Séanc. Soc. Biol.* **158,** 1807–1808.

Lapresle, J., Fardeau, M. and Milhaud, M. (1966). Étude des ultrastructures dans les dystrophies musculaires progressives. *Proc. 5th Int. Congr Neuropath.* pp. 602–603. Amsterdam: Excerpta medica.

Lapresle, J. and Milhaud, M. (1964). Pathologie du fuseau neuro-musculaire. *Revue neurol.* **110,** 97–122.

Larson, P. F., Hudgson, P. and Walton, J. N. (1969). Morphological relationship of polyribosomes and myosin filaments in developing and regenerating skeletal muscle. *Nature, Lond.* **222,** 1168–1169.

Larson, P. F., Jenkison, M. and Hudgson, P. (1970). The morphological development of chick embryo skeletal muscle grown in tissue culture as studied by electron microscopy. *J. neurol. Sci.* **10,** 384–405.

Leak, L. V. and Burke, J. F. (1964). The ultrastructure of human embryonic myocardium. *Anat. Rec.* **149,** 623–649.

Lee, J. C. (1963). Observations on lamellated structures and their formation in denervated skeletal muscle. *Jl R. microsc. Soc.* **82,** 17–22.

Lee, J. C. and Altschul, R. (1963). Electron microscopy of the nuclei of denervated skeletal muscle. *Z. Zellforsch. mikrosk. Anat.* **61,** 168–182.

Lehrer, G. M. (1960). The fine structure of the neuromuscular junction. *Res. Publs Ass. Res. nerv. ment. Dis.* **38,** 52-69.

Lehrer, G. M. (1962). The electronmicroscopic localization of cholinesterase in synaptic structures. *Proc. 4th Int. Congr. Neuropath.* Vol. II, pp. 20-21. Stuttgart: Georg Thieme.

Lentz, T. L. (1969). Development of neuromuscular junction. I. Cytological and cytochemical studies on the neuromuscular junction of differentiating muscle in the regenerating limb of the newt *triturus.* *J. Cell. Biol.* **42,** 431–443.

Lentz, T. L. (1970). Development of the neuromuscular junction. II. Cytological and cytochemical studies on the neuromuscular junction of differentiating muscle in the regenerating limb of the newt *triturus*, *J. Cell. Biol.* **47**, 423–436.

Linder, E. (1957). Die submikroskopische Morphologie der Herzmuskels. *Z. Zellforsch. mikrosk. Anat.* **45**, 702–746.

Lindsey, J. R., Hopkins, I. J. and Clark, D. B. (1966). Pathology of nemaline myopathy. Studies of two adult cases including an autopsy. *Bull. Johns Hopkins Hosp.* **119**, 378–406.

Luft, R., Ikkos, D., Palmieri, G., Ernster, L. and Afzelius, B. (1962). A case of severe hypermetabolism of nonthyroid origin with a defect in the maintenance of mitochondrial respiratory control: a correlated clinical, biochemical and morphological study. *J. clin. Invest.* **41**, 1776–1804.

McArdle, B. (1969). Metabolic and endocrine myopathies. In *Disorders of Voluntary Muscle*. Ed. Walton, J. N. pp. 607–638. London: Churchill.

Macdonald, R. D. and Engel, A. G. (1969). The cytoplasmic body: another structural anomaly of the Z disc. *Acta neuropath.* **14**, 99–107.

Macdonald, R. D. and Engel, A. G. (1970). Experimental chloroquine myopathy. *J. Neuropath. exp. Neurol.* **29**, 479–499.

Macdonald, R. D., Rewcastle, N. B. and Humphrey, J. G. (1968). Myopathy of hyperkalemic periodic paralysis. An electron microscopic study. *Archs Neurol., Chicago,* **19**, 274–283.

Macdonald, R. D., Rewcastle, N. B. and Humphrey, J. G. (1969). Myopathy of hypokalemic periodic paralysis. An electron microscopic study. *Archs Neurol., Chicago,* **20**, 565–585.

McNutt, N. S. (1970). Ultrastructure of intercellular junctions in adult and developing cardiac muscle. *Am. J. Cardiol.* **25**, 169–183.

McNutt, N. S. and Fawcett, D. W. (1969). The ultrastructure of the cat myocardium. II. Atrial muscle. *J. Cell. Biol.* **42**, 46–67.

Mahoudeau, D., Gruner, J., Dubrisay, J., Aullas, M. and Kaplan, G. (1961). Maladie de Steinert. Étude histologique de trois cas au microscope électronique. *Presse méd.* **69**, 1722–1724.

Mair, W. G. P. (1965). Electron microscopic findings in biopsies from various myopathies. In *Proceedings. 3rd Symposium on Research in Muscular Dystrophy*. pp. 164–180. London: Pitman.

Manasek, F. J. (1968). Mitosis in developing cardiac muscle. *J. Cell. Biol.* **37**, 191–196.

Manasek, F. J. (1970). Histogenesis of the embryonic myocardium. *Am. J. Cardiol.* **25**, 149–168.

Mastaglia, F. L., McCollum, J. P. K., Larson, P. F. and Hudgson, P. (1970). Steroid myopathy complicating McArdle's disease. *J. Neurol. Neurosurg. Psychiat.* **33**, 111–120.

Mastaglia, F. L., Papadimitriou, J. M. and Kakulas, B. A. (1969a). Regeneration in Duchenne muscular dystrophy. A histological, electron microscopic and histochemical study. *Proc. Aust. Ass. Neurol.* **6**, 93–106.

Mastaglia, F. L., Papadimitriou, J. M. and Kakulas, B. A. (1969b). Restricted forms of muscular dystrophy: a study of 11 cases. *Proc. Aust. Ass. Neurol.* **6**, 107–121.

Mastaglia, F. L., Papadimitriou, J. M. and Kakulas, B. A. (1970). Regeneration of muscle in Duchenne muscular dystrophy: an electron microscopy study. *J. neurol. Sci.* **11**, 425–444.

Mastaglia, F. L. and Walton, J. N. (1970). Coxsackie virus-like particles in skeletal muscle from a case of polymyositis. *J. neurol. Sci.* **11**, 593–599.

Mauro, A. (1961). Satellite cell of skeletal muscle fibres. *J. biophys. biochem. Cytol.* **9,** 493–495.

Mauro, A., Shafiq, S. A. and Milhorat, A. T. (eds.) (1970). Regeneration of striated muscle and myogenesis. Int. Congr. Ser. No. 218. Amsterdam: Excerpta medica.

Merrillees, N. C. R. (1960). The fine structure of muscle spindles in the lumbrical muscles of the rat. *J. biophys. biochem. Cytol.* **7,** 725–742.

Michalowsky, R. and Kudejko, J. (1966). Electron microscopic observations on skeletal muscle in diffuse scleroderma. *Br. J. Derm.* **78,** 24–28.

Miledi, R. and Slater, C. R. (1969). Electron-microscopic structure of denervated skeletal muscle. *Proc. R. Soc.* **B 174,** 253–269.

Miledi, R. and Slater, C. R. (1970). On the degeneration of rat neuromuscular junctions after nerve section. *J. Physiol., Lond.* **207,** 507–528.

Milhaud, M., Fardeau, M. and Lapresle, J. (1964). Contribution à l'étude des lésions elementaires du muscle squelettique: ultrastructure des fibres annulaires (observées dans la dystrophie myotonique). *C.r. Séanc. Soc. Biol.* **158,** 2274–2275.

Milhorat, A. T. and Goldstone, L. (1969). Muscular dystrophy of Duchenne type in females. In *Progress in Neuro-genetics.* Ed. Barbeau, A. and Brunette, J. R. Int. Congr. Ser. No. 175, pp. 148–152. Amsterdam: Excerpta medica.

Milhorat, A. T., Shafiq, S. A. and Goldstone, L. (1966). Changes in muscle structure in dystrophic patients, carriers and normal siblings seen by electron microscopy: correlation with levels of serum creatino-phosphokinase (CPK). *Ann. N.Y. Acad. Sci.* **138,** 246–292.

Miller, F., de Harven, E. and Palade, G. E. (1966). The structure of eosinophil leukocyte granules in rodents and in man. *J. Cell. Biol.* **31,** 349–362.

Miller, A. and Tregear, R. T. (1970). Evidence concerning crossbridge attachment during muscle contraction. *Nature, Lond.* **226,** 1060–1061.

Mintz, G., González-Angulo, A. and Fraga, A. (1968). Ultrastructure of muscle in polymyositis. *Am. J. Med.* **44,** 216–224.

Mitin, K. S., Knyazeva, G. D., Kuzin, M. I., Sekamova, S. M. and Bykov, G. P. (1969). Changes of the ultrastructure in skeletal muscles in myasthenia gravis. (In Russian.) *Zh. nevropat. Psikhiat.* **69,** 801–807.

Mölbert, E. (1960). Das elektronenmikroskopische Bild des Skelettmuskels bei Dystrophia musculorum progressiva Erb. *Naturwissenschaften,* **47,** 186–187.

Monticone, G. F. and Gabella, G. (1969). Studio istochimico ed ultrastrutturale della distrofia miotonica. *Acta neurol.* **24,** 638–639.

Monticone, G. F., Gabella, G. and Bergamini, L. (1970). Ultrastructural and histochemical changes in some human myopathies. In *Proceedings. International Congress on Muscle Diseases, Milan, 1969.* Ed. Walton, J. N., Canal, N. and Scarlato, G. Int. Congr. Ser. No. 199, pp. 44–52. Amsterdam: Excerpta medica.

Morgan-Hughes, J. A., Anderson, R. McD. and Mair, W. G. P. To be published.

Morgan-Hughes, J. A., LeQuesne, P. M. and Mair, W. G. P. To be published.

Morgan-Hughes, J. A., Mair, W. G. P. and Lascelles, P. T. (1970). A disorder of skeletal muscle associated with tubular aggregates. *Brain,* **93,** 873–880.

Mrozek, K., Strugalska, M. and Fidziánska, A. (1970). A sporadic case of central core disease. *J. neurol. Sci.* **10,** 339–348.

Muir, A. R., Kanji, A. H. M. and Allbrook, D. (1965). The structure of the satellite cells in skeletal muscle. *J. Anat.* **99,** 435–444.

Mukuno, K. (1966). The fine structure of the human extraocular muscles. I. A 'laminated structure' in the muscle fibres. (In Japanese.) *J. Electron Microsc., Tokyo,* **15,** 227–236.

Mukuno, K. (1968a). The fine structure of the human extraocular muscles. Report 2. The classification of muscle fibres. *Jap. J. Ophthal.* **12,** 111–122.

Mukuno, K. (1968b). Fine structure of the human extraocular muscles. Part 3. Neuromuscular junctions in the normal human extraocular muscles. (In Japanese.) *Acta Soc. ophthal., jap.* **72,** 104–121.

Mukuno, K. (1969). Electron microscopic studies on the human extraocular muscles under pathologic conditions. Part I. Rod formation in normal and diseased muscles (polymyositis and ocular myasthenia). *Jap. J. Ophthal.* **13,** 35–51.

Munsat, T. L., Thompson, L. R. and Coleman, R. F. (1969). Centronuclear ('myotubular') myopathy. *Archs Neurol., Chicago,* **20,** 120–131.

Murata, F. and Ogata, T. (1969). The ultrastructure of neuromuscular junction of human red, white and intermediate striated fibres. *Tohoku J. exp. Med.* **99,** 289–301.

Muscatello, U., Margreth, A. and Aloisi, M. (1965). On the differential response of sarcoplasm and myoplasm to denervation in frog muscle. *J. Cell. Biol.* **27,** 1–24.

Mussini, I., Di Mauro, S. and Angelini, C. (1970). Early ultrastructural and biochemical changes in muscle in dystrophia myotonica. *J. neurol. Sci.* **10,** 585–604.

Mussini, I., Di Mauro, S. and Margreth, A. (1968). Hypertrophy and proliferative changes of the SR in periodic paralysis. In *Abstracts. 4th European Regional Conference on Electron Microscopy.* pp. 309–310. Rome: Tipographia Poliglotta Vaticana.

Naccarato, R., Maschio, G., Sirigu, F., Previato, G., Rizzo, A., Mioni, G. and Bazzato, G. (1970). The muscle in diabetes mellitus. A histologic (light and electron microscope) and biochemical study by means of needle biopsy. *Virchows Arch., Abt. B. Zellpath.* **4,** 283–293.

Nakashima, N., Tamura, Z., Okamoto, S. and Goto, H. (1970). Inclusion bodies in human neuromuscular disorder. *Archs Neurol., Chicago,* **22,** 270–278.

Namba, T., Nakamura, T., Takahashi, A. and Grob, D. (1968). Motor nerve endings in extraocular muscle fibres. *J. comp. Neurol.* **134,** 385–396.

Nelson, D. A. and Benson, E. S. (1963). On the structural continuities of the transverse tubular system of rabbit and human myocardial cells. *J. Cell Biol.* **16,** 297–313.

Neustein, H. B. (1969). Fine structure of skeletal muscle in type III glycogenosis. *Archs Path.* **88,** 130–136.

Norris, F. H., Dramov, B., Calder, C. D. and Johnson, S. G. (1969). Virus-like particles in myositis accompanying herpes zoster. *Archs Neurol., Chicago,* **21,** 25–31.

Norris, F. H. and Panner, B. J. (1966). Hypothyroid myopathy. Clinical, electromyographical and ultrastructural observations. *Archs Neurol., Chicago,* **14,** 574–589.

Norris, F. H., Panner, B. J. and Stormont, J. M. (1968). Thyrotoxic periodic paralysis. Metabolic and ultrastructural studies. *Archs Neurol., Chicago,* **19,** 88–98.

Ochoa, J. and Mair, W. G. P. (1968). The ultrastructure of normal foetal muscle and foetal muscle from known dystrophic carriers. In *Proceedings. 4th Symposium on Research in Muscular Dystrophy.* pp. 223–239. London: Pitman.

Odor, D. L., Patel, A. N. and Pearce, L. A. (1967). Familial hypokalemic periodic paralysis with permanent myopathy. A clinical and ultrastructural study. *J. Neuropath. exp. Neurol.* **26,** 98–114.

Ogata, T. and Murata, F. (1969a). Fine structure of motor endplate in red, white and intermediate fibres of mammalian fast muscle. *Tohoku J. exp. Med.* **98,** 107–115.

Ogata, T. and Murata, F. (1969b). Cytological features of three fiber types in human striated muscle. *Tohoku J. exp. Med.* **99,** 225–245.

Ortiz De Zarate, J. C. and Maruffo, A. (1970). The descending ocular myopathy of early childhood. Myotubular or centronuclear myopathy. *Eur. Neurol.* **3,** 1–12.

Padykula, H. and Gauthier, G. F. (1967). Morphological and cytochemical characteristics of fiber types in normal mammalian skeletal muscle. In *Exploratory Concepts in Muscular Dystrophy and Related Disorders.* Ed. Milhorat, A. T. Int. Congr. Ser. No. 147, pp. 117–128. Amsterdam: Excerpta medica.

Padykula, H. A. and Gauthier, G. F. (1970). The ultrastructure of neuromuscular junctions of mammalian red, white and intermediate skeletal muscle fibres. *J. Cell. Biol.* **46,** 27–41.

Page, S. (1964). The organization of the sarcoplasmic reticulum in frog muscle. *J. Physiol., Lond.* **175,** 10–11P.

Page, S. G. (1965). A comparison of the fine structures of frog slow and twitch muscle fibres. *J. Cell. Biol.* **26,** 477–497.

Palade, G. E. (1954). Electron microscope observations of interneuronal and neuromuscular synapses. *Anat. Rec.* **118,** 335–336.

Palade, G. E. (1956). A small particulate component of the cytoplasm. In *Proc. Int. Conf. Electron Microsc.* pp. 417–423. London: Royal Microscopical Society.

Palmeiro, J., Behrend, R. Ch. and Wechsler, W. (1966). Elektronenmikroskopische Befunde an der Skeletmuskulatur bei Polymyositis. *Acta neuropath.* **7,** 26–43.

Paluello, F. H., Bruni, C. B. and Spiele, H. (1967). Type III A glycogenosis: a biochemical and ultrastructural study. *Virchows Arch. path. Anat. Physiol.* **343,** 164–176.

Papadimitriou, J. M., Mastaglia, F. L. and Kakulas, B. A. (1969). The natural history of Duchenne muscular dystrophy—an ultrastructural study. *Proc. Aust. Ass. Neurol.* **6,** 87–92.

Patel, A. N., Lalitha, V. S. and Dastur, D. K. (1968). The spindle in normal and pathological muscle. An assessment of the histological changes. *Brain,* **91,** 737–750.

Peachey, L. D. (1966). Fine structure of two fiber types in cat extra-ocular muscles. *J. Cell. Biol.* **31,** 84A.

Peachey, L. D. and Huxley, A. F. (1962). Structural identification of twitch and slow striated muscle fibres of the frog. *J. Cell. Biol.* **13,** 177–180.

Pearce, G. W. (1963). Electron microscopy in the study of muscular dystrophy. In *Muscular Dystrophy in Man and Animals.* Ed. Bourne, G. H. and Golarz, M. N. pp. 159–175. Basel: Karger.

Pearce, G. W. (1964). Tissue culture and electron microscopy in muscle disease. In *Disorders of Voluntary Muscle.* Ed. Walton, J. N. pp. 220–254. London: Churchill.

Pearce, G. W. (1966). Electron microscopy in the study of muscular dystrophy. *In* Experimental primary myopathies and their relationship to human muscle diseases. Ed. Bajusz, E. *Ann. N.Y. Acad. Sci.* **138,** 138–150.

Pearce, G. W., Adamson, D. G. and Salter, R. H. (1968). The pathology of muscle glycogenosis. In *Proceedings. 4th Symposium on Research in Muscular Dystrophy.* pp. 188–206. London: Pitman.

Pearse, A. G. E. and Johnson, M. (1970). Histochemistry in the study of normal and diseased muscle, with special reference to myopathy with tubular aggregates. In *Proceedings. International Congress on Muscle Diseases.* Ed. Walton, J. N., Canal, N. and Scarlato, G. Int. Congr. Ser. No. 199, pp. 25–32. Amsterdam: Excerpta medica.

Pellegrino, C. and Franzini, C. (1963). An electron microscope study of denervation atrophy in red and white skeletal muscle fibers. *J. Cell. Biol.* **17,** 327–349.

Perry, S. V. (1952). The bound nucleotide of the isolated myofibril. *Biochem. J.* **51,** 495–499.

Perry, S. V. (1967). The structure and interactions of myosin. *Prog. Biophys. biophys. Chem.* **17,** 325–381.

Perry, S. V. and Corsi, A. (1958). Extraction of proteins other than myosin from the isolated rabbit myofibril. *Biochem. J.* **68,** 5–12.

Peter, J. B., Stempel, K. and Armstrong, J. (1970). Biochemistry and electron microscopy of mitochondria in muscular and neuromuscular diseases. In *Proceedings. International Congress on Muscle Diseases.* Ed. Walton, J. N., Canal, N. and Scarlato, G. Int. Congr. Ser. No. 199, pp. 228–235. Amsterdam: Excerpta medica.

Pilar, G. and Hess, A. (1966). Differences in internal structure and nerve terminals of the slow and twitch muscle fibres in the cat superior oblique. *Anat. Rec.* **154,** 243–251.

Poche, R. and Ohm, H. G. (1963). Lichtmikroskopische, histochemische und elektronenmikroskopische Untersuchungen der Herzmuskels von Menschen nach induziertem Herzstillstand. *Arch. Kreislaufforsch.* **41,** 86–135.

Policard, A., Collet, A., Martin, J. C. and Pregermain, S. (1961). Études inframicroscopiques sur les processus d'alvéolite. *Presse méd.* **69,** 1709–1712.

Price, H. M. (1969). Ultrastructure of the skeletal muscle fibre. In *Disorders of Voluntary Muscle.* Ed. Walton, J. N. 2nd ed. pp. 29–56. London: Churchill.

Price, H. M., Gordon, G. B., Munsat, T. L. and Pearson, C. M. (1967). Myopathy with atypical mitochondria in type I skeletal muscle fibres. A histochemical and ultrastructural study. *J. Neuropath. exp. Neurol.* **26,** 475–497.

Price, H. M., Gordon, G. B., Pearson, C. M., Munsat, T. L. and Blumberg, J. M. (1965). New evidence for excessive accumulation of Z-band material in nemaline myopathy. *Proc. natn. Acad. Sci. U.S.A.* **54,** 1398–1406.

Price, H. M., Howes, E. L. and Blumberg, J. M. (1964a). Ultrastructural alterations in skeletal muscle fibers injured by cold. I. The acute degenerative changes. *Lab. Invest.* **13,** 1264–1278.

Price, H. M., Howes, E. L. and Blumberg, J. M. (1964b). Ultrastructural alterations in skeletal muscle fibres injured by cold. II. Cells of the sarcolemmal tube: observations on 'discontinuous' regeneration and myofibril formation. *Lab. Invest.* **13,** 1279–1302.

Price, H. M., Pease, D. C. and Pearson, C. M. (1962). Selective actin filament and Z-band degeneration induced by plasmocid. An electron microscopic study. *Lab. Invest.* **11,** 549–562.

Prineas, J. (1969a). Triorthocresyl phosphate myopathy. *Archs Neurol., Chicago,* **21,** 150–156.

Prineas, J. (1969b). The pathogenesis of dying-back polyneuropathies. Part I. An ultrastructural study of experimental tri-ortho-cresyl phosphate intoxication in cat. *J. Neuropath. exp. Neurol.* **28,** 571–597.

Prineas, J. (1969c). The pathogenesis of dying-back polyneuropathies. Part II. An ultrastructural study of experimental acrylamide intoxication in cat. *J. Neuropath. exp. Neurol.* **28,** 598–621.

Prineas, J., Hall, R., Barwick, D. D. and Watson, A. J. (1968). Myopathy associated with pigmentation following adrenalectomy for Cushing's syndrome. *Q. Jl Med.* **37,** 63–77.

Prineas, J. and Ng, R. C. Y. (1967). Ultrastructural features of intracellular lipid in normal human muscle. *Neurology, Minneap.* **17,** 1092–1098.

Przybylski, R. J. and Blumberg, J. M. (1966). Ultrastructural aspects of myogenesis in the chick. *Lab. Invest.* **15,** 836–863.

Radu, H., Pendefunda, G., Blücher, G., Radu, A., Darko, Z. and Gödri, I. (1970).

Comparative and correlative study of the myotonias. In *Proceedings. International Congress on Muscle Diseases*. Ed. Walton, J. N., Canal, N. and Scarlato, G. Int. Congr. Ser. No. 199, pp. 332–336. Amsterdam: Excerpta medica.
Ramsey, H. J. (1967). Altered synaptic terminals in cortex near tumor. *Am. J. Path.* **51,** 1093–1109.
Reedy, M. K. (1964). Discussion on the structure of actin filaments and the origin of the axial periodicity in the I-substance of vertebrate striated muscle. *Proc. R. Soc.* **B 160,** 458–460.
Reger, J. F. (1954). Electron microscopy of motor end-plate in intercostal muscle of the rat. *Anat. Rec.* **118,** 344.
Reger, J. F. (1955). Electron microscopy of the motor end-plate in rat intercostal muscle. *Anat. Rec.* **122,** 1–15.
Reger, J. F. (1959). Studies on the fine structure of normal and denervated neuromuscular junctions from mouse gastrocnemius. *J. Ultrastruct. Res.* **2,** 269–282.
Reger, J. F. and Craig, A. S. (1968). Studies on the fine structure of muscle fibers and associated satellite cells in hypertrophic human deltoid muscle. *Anat. Rec.* **162,** 483–500.
Resnick, J. S. and Engel, W. K. (1967). Target fibers—structural and cytochemical characteristics and their relationship to neurogenic muscle diseases and fiber types. In *Exploratory Concepts in Muscular Dystrophy and Related Disorders*. Ed. Milhorat, A. T. Int. Congr. Ser. No. 147, pp. 255–267. Amsterdam: Excerpta medica.
Revel, J. P. (1962). The sarcoplasmic reticulum of the bat cricothyroid muscle. *J. Cell. Biol.* **12,** 571–588.
Rewcastle, N. B. and Humphrey, J. G. (1965). Vacuolar myopathy: clinical, histochemical and microscopic study. *Archs Neurol., Chicago*, **12,** 570–582.
Reznik, M. and Engel, W. K. (1970). Ultrastructural and histochemical correlations of experimental muscle regeneration. *J. neurol. Sci.* **11,** 167–185.
Richter, G. W. and Kellner, A. (1963). Hypertrophy of the human heart at the level of fine structure. An analysis and two postulates. *J. Cell. Biol.* **18,** 195–206.
Rigdon, R. H. (1966). Hereditary myopathy in white Pekin duck. *In* Experimental primary myopathies and their relationship to human muscle diseases. Ed. Bajusz, E. *Ann. N.Y. Acad. Sci.* **138,** 28–48.
Riske-Neilsen, E. and Harmsen, A. In press.
Ritter, R. A. (1967). Effects of cortisone on the structure and strength of skeletal muscle. *Archs Neurol., Chicago*, **17,** 403–413.
Robertson, J. D. (1954). The ultrastructure of a reptilian myoneural junction. *J. appl. Phys.* **25,** 1466–1467.
Robertson, J. D. (1960). Electron microscopy of the motor end plate and the neuromuscular spindle. *Am. J. phys. Med.* **39,** 1–43.
Rose, A. L., Walton, J. N. and Pearce, G. W. (1967). Polymyositis: an ultramicroscopic study of muscle biopsy material. *J. neurol. Sci.* **5,** 457–472.
Rosenbluth, J. (1969). Sarcoplasmic reticulum of an unusual fast-acting crustacean muscle. *J. Cell. Biol.* **42,** 534–547.
Ross, M. H., Pappas, G. D. and Harman, P. J. (1958). A comparison of normal and dystrophic muscle in the mouse by means of electron microscopy. *Anat. Rec.* **130,** 365–366.
Ross, M. H., Pappas, G. D. and Harman, P. J. (1960). Alterations in muscle fine structure in hereditary muscular dystrophy of mice. *Lab. Invest.* **9,** 388–403.
Roth, R. G., Graziani, L. J., Terry, R. D. and Scheinberg, L. C. (1964). Ultrastructural

studies of muscle in progressive muscular atrophy (Kugelberg–Welander syndrome). *Neurology, Minneap.* **14,** 266.

Roth, R. G., Graziani, L. J., Terry, R. D. and Scheinberg, L. C. (1965). Muscle fine structure in the Kugelberg–Welander syndrome (chronic spinal muscular atrophy). *J. Neuropath. exp. Neurol.* **24,** 444–454.

Roy, S. and Dubowitz, V. (1970). Carrier detection in Duchenne muscular dystrophy. A comparative study of electron microscopy, light microscopy and serum enzymes. *J. neurol. Sci.* **11,** 65–79.

Roy, S., Dubowitz, V. and Wolman, L. (1971). Ultrastructure of muscle in infantile spinal muscular atrophy. *J. neurol. Sci.* **12,** 219–232.

Rumery, R. E. and Hampton, J. C. (1959). Microscopic and submicroscopic observations on skeletal muscle from vitamin E-deficient rats. *Anat. Rec.* **133,** 1–11.

Rumpelt, H. J. and Schmalbruch, H. (1969). Zur Morphologie der Bauelemente von Muskelspindeln bei Mensch und Ratte. *Z. Zellforsch. mikrosk. Anat.* **102,** 601–630.

Ruska, H. (1954). Elektronenmikroskopischen Beitrag zur Histologie der Skelettmuskel kleiner Säugetiere. *Z. Naturf.* **9b,** 358–371.

Ruska, H. and Edwards, G. A. (1957). A new cytoplasmic pattern in striated muscle fibers and its relation to growth. *Growth,* **21,** 73–88.

Salter, R. H., Adamson, D. G. and Pearce, G. W. (1967). McArdle's syndrome (myophosphorylase deficiency). A study of a family. *Q. Jl Med.,* **36,** 565–578.

Samaha, F. J. (1967). Human striated muscle myofibrils and actomyosin. *Neurology, Minneap.* **17,** 1152–1158.

Samaha, F. J. and Gergely, J. (1965). Ca^{++} uptake and ATPase of human sarcoplasmic reticulum. *J. clin. Invest.* **44,** 1425–1431.

Samaha, F. J. and Gergely, J. (1969). Biochemical abnormalities of the sarcoplasmic reticulum in muscular dystrophy. *New Engl. J. Med.* **280,** 184–188.

Samaha, F. J., Guth, L. and Albers, R. W. (1970). Phenotypic differences between the actomyosin ATPase of the three fiber types of mammalian skeletal muscle. *Expl Neurol.* **26,** 120–125.

Samaha, F. J., Schroeder, J. M., Rebeiz, J. and Adams, R. D. (1967). Studies on myotonia. Biochemical and electron microscopic studies on myotonia congenita and myotonia dystrophica. *Archs Neurol., Chicago,* **17,** 22–33.

Santa, T. (1969). Fine structure of the human skeletal muscle in myopathy. *Archs Neurol., Chicago,* **20,** 479–489.

Sato, T. and Tsubaki, T. (1968). Electron microscopic studies on the muscle of neuromuscular disease. (In Japanese.) *Clin. Neurol., Tokyo,* **8,** 3–12.

Schellens, J. P. M. and Ossentjuk, E. (1969). Mitochondrial ultrastructure with crystalloid inclusions in an unusual type of human myopathy. *Virchows Arch., Abt. B Zellpath.* **4,** 21–29.

Schiaffino, S., Hanzlíková, V. and Pierobon, S. (1970). Relations between structure and function in rat skeletal muscle fibres. *J. Cell. Biol.* **47,** 107–119.

Schimrigk, K., Mertens, H. G., Ricker, K., Führ, J., Eyer, P. and Pette, D. (1967). McArdle-Syndrom (Myopathie bei fehlender Muskelphosphorylase). *Klin. Wschr.* **45,** 1–17.

Schmalbruch, H. (1967). Kristalloide in menschlichen Skelettmuskelfasern. *Naturwissenschaften,* **54,** 519.

Schmalbruch, H. (1968). Lyse und Regeneration von Fibrillen in der normalen menschlichen Skelettmuskulatur. *Virchows Arch. path. Anat. Physiol.* **344,** 159–171.

Schotland, D. L. (1968). Ultrastructural abnormalities in myotonic dystrophy including an unusual T system alteration. *J. Neuropath. exp. Neurol.* **27,** 109–110.

Schotland, D. L. (1969). An electron microscopic study of target fibers, target-like fibers and related abnormalities in human muscle. *J. Neuropath. exp. Neurol.* **28,** 214–228.

Schotland, D. L. (1970). An electron microscopic investigation of myotonic dystrophy. *J. Neuropath. exp. Neurol.* **29,** 241–253.

Schotland, D. L., Spiro, D. and Carmel, P. (1966). Ultrastructural studies of ring fibers in human muscle disease. *J. Neuropath. exp. Neurol.* **25,** 431–442.

Schotland, D. L., Spiro, D., Rowland, L. P. and Carmel, P. (1965). Ultrastructural studies of muscle in McArdle's disease (deficiency of muscle phosphorylase). *J. Neuropath. exp. Neurol.* **24,** 629–644.

Schrodt, G. R. and Walker, S. M. (1966). Ultrastructure of membranes in denervation atrophy. *Am. J. Path.* **49,** 33–51.

Schroeder, J. M. (1970). Sarcolemmal indentations resembling junctional folds in myotonic dystrophy. In *Proceedings. International Congress on Muscle Diseases.* Ed. Walton, J. N., Canal, N. and Scarlato, G. Int. Congr. Ser. No. 199, pp. 109–111. Amsterdam: Excerpta medica.

Schroeder, J. M. and Adams, R. D. (1968). The ultrastructural morphology of the muscle fiber in myotonic dystrophy. *Acta neuropath.* **10,** 218–241.

Schroeder, J. M. and Kuhn, E. (1968). Zur Ultrastruktur der Muskelfaser bei der experimentallen 'Myotonie' mit 20, 25—Diazacholesterin. *Virchows Arch. path. Anat. Physiol.* **344,** 181–195.

Schutta, H. S. and Armitage, J. L. (1969). Thyrotoxic hypokalemic periodic paralysis. A fine structure study. *J. Neuropath. exp. Neurol.* **28,** 321–336.

Schutta, H. S., Kelly, A. M. and Zacks, S. I. (1969). Necrosis and regeneration of muscle in paroxysmal idiopathic myoglobinuria: electron microscopic observations. *Brain,* **92,** 191–202.

Seitelberger, F. and Stockinger, L. (1965). Bioptischerbefunde bei paroxysmaler Lähmung. *Proc. 8th Int. Congr. Neurol.* Vol. II. *Neuromuscular Diseases,* pp. 607–610. Vienna: Wiener Medizinische Akademie.

Seitelberger, F., Wanko, T. and Gavin, M. A. (1961). The muscle fiber in central core disease. Histochemical and electron microscopic observations. *Acta neuropath.* **1,** 223–237.

Serratrice, G., Roux, H., Aquaron, R., Gambarelli, D., Baret, R. and Recordier, A. M. (1970). Myopathy associated with arthropathic psoriasis. In *Proceedings. International Congress on Muscle Diseases.* Ed. Walton, J. N., Canal, N. and Scarlato G. Int. Congr. Ser. No. 199, pp. 642–644. Amsterdam: Excerpta medica.

Serratrice, G., Toga, M., Roux, H., Hassoun, J. and Aquaron, R. (1970). Étude anatomopathologique et biochemique des myopathies cortisoniques experimentales chez le lapin. *Proc. 6th Int. Congr. Neuropath.* pp. 1074–1075. Paris: Masson.

Shafiq, S. A. (1963). Electron microscopic studies on the indirect flight muscles of *drosophila melanogaster.* II. Differentiation of myofibrils. *J. Cell. Biol.* **17,** 363–373.

Shafiq, S. A., Dubowitz, V., Peterson, H. de C. and Milhorat, A. T. (1967). Nemaline myopathy: report of a fatal case with histochemical and electron microscopic studies. *Brain,* **90,** 817–828.

Shafiq, S. A. and Gorycki, M. A. (1965). Regeneration in skeletal muscle of mouse: some electron microscopic observations. *J. Path. Bact.* **90,** 123–127.

Shafiq, S. A., Gorycki, M. A., Asiedu, S. A. and Milhorat, A. T. (1969). Tenotomy. Effects on the fine structure of the soleus of the rat. *Archs Neurol., Chicago*, **20,** 625–633.

Shafiq, S. A., Gorycki, M., Goldstone, L. and Milhorat, A. T. (1966). Fine structure of fiber types in normal human muscle. *Anat. Rec.* **156,** 283–301.

Shafiq, S. A., Gorycki, M. A. and Mauro, A. (1968). Mitosis during postnatal growth in skeletal and cardiac muscle of rat. *J. Anat.* **103,** 135–141.

Shafiq, S. A., Gorycki, M. A. and Milhorat, A. T. (1967). An electron microscopic study of regeneration and satellite cells in human muscle. *Neurology, Minneap.* **17,** 567–574.

Shafiq, S. A., Gorycki, M. A. and Milhorat, A. T. (1969). An electron microscope study of fibre types in normal and dystrophic muscles of the mouse. *J. Anat.* **104,** 281–293.

Shafiq, S. A. and Milhorat, A. T. (1967). Some comments on the specificity of alterations in the fine structure in muscle disease. In *Exploratory Concepts in Muscular Dystrophy and Related Disorders*. Ed. Milhorat, A. T. Int. Congr. Ser. No. 147, pp. 268–273. Amsterdam: Excerpta medica.

Shafiq, S. A., Milhorat, A. T. and Gorycki, M. A. (1967a). An electron microscope study of muscle degeneration and vascular changes in polymyositis. *J. Path. Bact.* **94,** 139–147.

Shafiq, S. A., Milhorat, A. T. and Gorycki, M. A. (1967b). Fine structure of human muscle in neurogenic atrophy. *Neurology, Minneap.* **17,** 934–948.

Shafiq, S. A., Milhorat, A. T. and Gorycki, M. A. (1967c). Giant mitochondria in human muscle with inclusions. *Archs Neurol., Chicago*, **17,** 666–671.

Shafiq, S. A., Milhorat, A. T. and Gorycki, M. A. (1968). Crystals in muscle fibers in patients with diabetic amyotrophy and neuropathy. *Neurology, Minneap.* **18,** 785–790.

Sher, J. H., Rimalovski, A. B., Athanassiades, T. J. and Aronson, S. M. (1967). Familial centronuclear myopathy: a clinical and pathological study. *Neurology, Minneap.* **17,** 727–742.

Shimada, Y. (1970). Electron microscopic observations on the fusion of chick myoblasts in vitro. In *Proc. 7th Conf. Electron Microsc.* Ed. Favard, P. pp. 787–788. Paris: Société Francaise de Microscopie Electronique.

Shy, G. M., Engel, W. K., Somers, J. E. and Wanko, T. (1963). Nemaline myopathy. A new congenital myopathy. *Brain*, **86,** 793–810.

Shy, G. M., Gonatas, N. K. and Perez, M. (1966). Two childhood myopathies with abnormal mitochondria. I. Megaconial myopathy. II. Pleoconial myopathy. *Brain*, **89,** 133–158.

Shy, G. M. and Magee, K. R. (1956). A new congenital non-progressive myopathy. *Brain*, **79,** 610–621.

Shy, G. M., Wanko, T., Rowley, P. T. and Engel, A. G. (1961). Studies in familial periodic paralysis. *Exp. Neurol.* **3,** 53–121.

Simpson, F. O. and Oertelis, S. J. (1961). Relationship of the sarcoplasmic reticulum to sarcolemma in sheep cardiac muscle. *Nature, Lond.* **189,** 758–759.

Simpson, F. O. and Oertelis, S. J. (1962). The fine structure of sheep myocardial cells; sarcolemmal invaginations and the transverse tubular system. *J. Cell. Biol.* **12,** 91–100.

Siperstein, M. D., Unger, R. H. and Madison, L. L. (1968). Studies of muscle capillary basement membranes in normal subjects, diabetic and prediabetic patients. *J. clin. Invest.* **47,** 1973–1999.

Slotwiner, P., Song, S. K. and Maker, H. S. (1969). Myopathy resembling McArdle's syndrome. *Archs Neurol., Chicago*, **20,** 586–598.

Sluga, E. and Monneron, E. (1970). Über Feinstruktur und Topochemie von Riesenmitochondrien und deren Einlagerungen bei Myopathien. *Virchows Arch. path. Anat. Physiol.* **350,** 250–260.

Sluga, E. and Moser, K. (1970). Myopathy with glycogen storage and giant mitochondria (ultrastructural and biochemical findings). In *Proceedings International Congress on Muscle Diseases.* Ed. Walton, J. N., Canal, N. and Scarlato, G. Int. Congr. Ser. No. 199, pp. 116–119. Amsterdam: Excerpta medica.

Sluga, E., Seitelberger, F. and Moser, K. (1967). Über eine progressive Myopathie mit Muskelphosphorylasemangel und Riesenmitochondrien. *Wien. klin. Wschr.* **79,** 917–921.

Sluga-Gasser, E. (1965). Zur Ultrastruktur der neurogenen Muskelatrophie. *Proc. 8th Int. Congr. Neurol.* Vol. II. *Neuromuscular Diseases,* pp. 193–196. Vienna: Wiener Medizinische Akademie.

Smith, J. R., Burford, T. H. and Chiquoine, A. D. (1960). Electron microscopic observations of the ventricular heart muscle of man obtained by surgical biopsy during thoracotomy. *Expl Cell Res.* **20,** 228–232.

Smith, J., Zellweger, H. and Afifi, A. K. (1967). Muscular form of glycogenosis type II (Pompe). Report of a case with unusual features. *Neurology, Minneap.* **17,** 537–549.

Song, S. K. (1968). Electron microscopic study of terminal nerves, motor end-plates and sarcoplasmic reticulum in denervated skeletal muscle. *J. Neuropath. exp. Neurol.* **27,** 108.

Song, S. K. and Anderson, P. J. (1970). Submicroscopic abnormalities of neuromuscular junction induced by venom of black spiders. *Proc. 6th Int. Congr. Neuropath.* pp. 753–754. Paris: Masson.

Spiro, A. J. and Beilin, R. L. (1969). Human muscle spindle histochemistry. *Archs Neurol., Chicago,* **20,** 271–275.

Spiro, A. J., Prineas, J. W. and Moore, C. L. (1970). A new mitochondrial myopathy with salt craving. *Archs Neurol., Chicago,* **22,** 259–269.

Spiro, A. J., Shy, G. M. and Gonatas, N. K. (1966). Myotubular myopathy. Persistence of fetal muscle in an adolescent boy. *Archs Neurol., Chicago,* **14,** 1–14.

Stein, J. M. and Padykula, H. A. (1962). Histochemical classification of individual skeletal muscle fibers of the rat. *Am. J. Anat.* **110,** 103–124.

Stoebner, P., Sengel, A., Jesel, M. and Isch, F. (1970). Ultrastructure de certaines polymyosites myastheniformes. *Proc. 6th Int. Congr. Neuropath.* pp. 1078–1079. Paris: Masson.

Tello, J. F. (1917). Génesis de las terminaciones nerviosas motrices y sensitivas. I. En el sistema locomotor de los vertebrados superiores. Histogenesis muscular. *Trab. Lab. Invest. biol. Univ. Madr.* **15,** 101–199.

Teräväinen, H. (1968). Electron microscopic and histochemical observations on different types of nerve endings in the extraocular muscles of the rat. *Z. Zellforsch. mikrosk. Anat.* **90,** 372–388.

Teräväinen, H. (1969a). Electron microscopic localization of acetylcholinesterase in small multiple endings in the extraocular muscle of the rat. *Experientia,* **25,** 389.

Teräväinen, H. (1969b). Axonal protrusions in the small multiple endings in the extraocular muscles of the rat. *Z. Zellforsch. mikrosk. Anat.* **96,** 206–211.

Teräväinen, H. (1969c). Localization of acetylcholinesterase in the rat myoneural junction. *Histochemie,* **17,** 162–169.

Teräväinen, H. (1970). Satellite cells of striated muscle after compression injury so slight as not to cause degeneration of the muscle fibres. *Z. Zellforsch. mikrosk. Anat.* **103,** 320–327.

Theones, W. and Ruska, H. (1960). Über 'leptomere Myofibrillen' in der Herzmuskelzelle. *Z. Zellforsch. mikrosk. Anat.* **51**, 560–570.

Thiébaut, F., Gruner, J. E., Isch, F. and Isch-Treussard, C. (1963). Corrélations cliniques, électriques et histologiques en pathologie musculaire. *Revue neurol.* **108**, 575–596.

Thomas, P. K. (1963). The connective tissue of peripheral nerve: an electron microscope study. *J. Anat.* **97**, 35–44.

Thomas, P. K. (1964). Changes in the endoneurial sheaths of peripheral myelinated nerve fibres during Wallerian degeneration. *J. Anat.* **98**, 175–182.

Thomas, P. K. and Slatford, J. (1964). Lamellar bodies in the cytoplasm of Schwann cells. *J. Anat.* **98**, 691.

Tice, L. W. and Engel, A. G. (1967). The effects of glucocorticoids on red and white muscles in the rat. *Am. J. Path.* **50**, 311–333.

Toga, M., Berard-Badier, M., Gambarelli, D. and Pinsard, N. (1970). Ultrastructure des lésions neuromusculaires dans un cas de dystrophie neuroaxonale infantile ou maladie de Seitelberger. Communication to *II Journ. int. Path. Neuro-musculaire, Marseille.*

Tomé, F. and Mair, W. G. P. (1970). Electron microscopical and histochemical studies of muscle in a case of neuropathy with target fibres and laminar cytoplasmic structures. *Proc. 6th Int. Congr. Neuropath.* pp. 1070–1071. Paris: Masson.

Tomonaga, M. and Sluga, E. (1969). Zur Ultrastruktur der 'Target-Fasern'. *Virchows Arch. path. Anat. Physiol.* **348**, 89–104.

Tomonaga, M. and Sluga, E. (1970). The ultrastructure and pathogenesis of 'target fibres'. In *Proceedings. International Congress on Muscle Diseases.* Ed. Walton, J. N., Canal, N. and Scarlato, G. Int. Congr. Ser. No. 199, pp. 120–122. Amsterdam: Excerpta medica.

Toner, P. G. and Carr, K. E. (1968). *Cell Structure. An Introduction to Biological Electron Microscopy.* Edinburgh: Livingstone.

Urich, H. and Wilkinson, M. (1970). Necrosis of muscle with carcinoma: myositis or myopathy? *J. Neurol. Neurosurg. Psychiat.* **33**, 398–407.

van Bogaert, L., Kissel, P., Schmitt, J., Martin, J. J., Claes, C., Duc, M., Royer, R., Barrucand, D., Grignon, J. and Floquet, J. (1967). Syndrome myopathique au cours d'une maladie de Gamstrop. Étude anatomique. *Acta neurol. psychiat. belg.* **67**, 133–142.

van Breemen, V. L. (1952). Myofibril development observed with the electron microscope. *Anat. Rec.* **113**, 179–195.

van Breemen, V. L. (1960a). Ultrastructure of human muscle. I. Observations on normal striated muscle fibers. *Amer. J. Path.* **37**, 215–229.

van Breemen, V. L. (1960b). Ultrastructure of human muscle. II. Observations on dystrophic striated muscle fibers. *Am. J. Path.* **37**, 333–341.

van Vleet, J. F., Hall, B. V. and Simon, J. (1967). Vitamin E deficiency. A sequential study by means of light and electron microscopy of the alterations occurring in regeneration of skeletal muscle of affected weanling rabbits. *Amer. J. Path.* **51**, 815–830.

van Vleet, J. F., Hall, B. V. and Simon, J. (1968). Vitamin E deficiency. A sequential light and electron microscopic study of skeletal muscle degeneration in weanling rabbits. *Am. J. Path.* **52**, 1067–1079.

van Wijngaarden, G. K., Bethlem, J., Meijer, A. E. F. H., Hülsmann, W. Ch. and Feltkamp, C. A. (1967). Skeletal muscle disease with abnormal mitochondria. *Brain,* **90**, 577–592.

Virágh, S. (1968). Remarks on the leptofibrils of the cardiac muscle cells. In *Abstracts of*

4th European Regional Conference Electron Microscopy, pp. 295–296. Rome: Tipographia Poliglotta Vaticana.
Vital, C., Vallat, J. M., Martin, F., Le Blanc, M. and Bergouignan, M. (1970). Étude clinique et ultrastructurale d'un cas de myopathie centronucleaire (myotubular myopathy) de l'adulte. *Revue neurol.* **123,** 117–130.
Vracko, R. (1970a). Skeletal muscle capillaries in diabetics: a quantitative analysis. *Circulation,* **41,** 271–283.
Vracko, R. (1970b). Skeletal muscle capillaries in nondiabetics: a quantitative analysis. *Circulation,* **41,** 285–297.
Vye, M. V., Fischman, D. A. and Hansen, J. L. (1969). Ultrastructural localization of adenosinotriphosphatase activity in skeletal muscle by calcium precipitation at high pH. *Virchows Arch., Abt. B. Zellpath.* **3,** 307–323.
Wainrach, S. and Sotelo, J. R. (1961). Electron microscope study of the developing chick embryo heart. *Z. Zellforsch. mikrosk. Anat.* **55,** 622–634.
Walker, S. M. and Schrodt, G. R. (1965). Continuity of the T-system with the sarcolemma in rat skeletal muscle fibres. *J. Cell. Biol.* **27,** 671–677.
Walters, M. N. I., Papadimitriou, J. M. and Shilkin, K. B. (1967). Inflammation induced by dimethylsulfoxide (DMSO). I. Ultrastructural investigation of preinflammatory phase. *Expl molec. Path.* **6,** 106–117.
Walton, J. N. (ed.) (1964). *Disorders of Voluntary Muscle.* 1st ed. London: Churchill.
Walton, J. N. (ed.) (1969). *Disorders of Voluntary Muscle.* 2nd ed. London: Churchill.
Watanabe, I., Donahue, S. and Hoggatt, N. (1967). Methods for electron microscopic studies of circulating human leucocytes and observations on their fine structure. *J. Ultrastruct. Res.* **20,** 366–382.
Wechsler, W. (1966). Comparative electron microscopic studies on various forms of muscle atrophies and dystrophies in animals and man. *In* Experimental primary myopathies and their relationship to human muscle diseases. Ed. Bajusz, E. *Ann. N.Y. Acad. Sci.* **138,** 113–137.
Wechsler, W. and Hager, H. (1960). Elektronenmikroskopische Befunde am atrophischen quergestreiften Skelettmuskel der Ratte nach Nervdurchtrennung. *Naturwissenschaften,* **47,** 185–186.
Wechsler, W. and Hager, H. (1961a). Elektronenmikroskopische Befunde bei Muskelatrophie nach Nervendurchtrennung bei der weissen Ratte. *Beitr. path. Anat.* **125,** 31–53.
Wechsler, W. and Hager, H. (1961b). Elektronenmikroskopische Untersuchungen bei myotonischer Muskeldystrophie. *Arch. Psychiat. NervKrankh.* **201,** 668–690.
Wechsler, W. and Hager, H. (1962). Elektronenmikroskopische Befunde an der Skelettmuskulatur bei progressiver spinaler Muskelatrophie. *Arch. Psychiat. NervKrankh.* **203,** 111–122.
Wechsler, W. and Pabelick, W. (1966). Erbliche Muskeldystrophien beim Tier. In *Progressive Muskeldystrophie, Myotonie, Myasthenie.* Ed. Kuhn, E. pp. 165–177. Berlin: Springer.
Weinstein, R. B. and Hay, E. D. (1970). Desoxyribonucleic acid synthesis and mitosis in differentiated cardiac muscle cells of chick embryos. *J. Cell. Biol.* **47,** 310–316.
West, W. T. (1963). Muscular dystrophy of vitamin E deficiency. In *Muscular Dystrophy in Man and Animals.* Ed. Bourne, G. H. and Golarz, M. N. pp. 367–405. Basel: Karger.
Whisnant, J. P., Espinosa, R. E., Kierland, R. R. and Lambert, E. H. (1963). Chloroquine neuromyopathy. *Proc. Staff Meet. Mayo Clin.* **38,** 501–513.

Wigglesworth, V. B. (1957). The use of osmium in the fixation and staining of tissues. *Proc. R. Soc.* **B 147,** 185–199.

Wilkie, R. D. (1968). *Muscle.* London: Arnold.

Woolf, A. L. (1966). Morphology of the myasthenic neuromuscular junction. *Ann. N.Y. Acad. Sci.* **135,** 35–56.

Young, M. (1969). The molecular basis of muscle contraction. *Rev. Biochem.* **38,** 913–950.

Zacks, S. I. (1964). *The Motor End Plate.* Philadelphia: Saunders.

Zacks, S. I., Pegues, J. J. and Elliott, F. A. (1962). Interstitial muscle capillaries in patients with diabetes mellitus: a light and electron microscope study. *Metabolism,* **11,** 381–393.

Zacks, S. I. and Saito, A. (1970). Regeneration and *de novo* formation of mouse neuromuscular junctions. In *Proc. 6th Int. Congr. Neuropath.* pp. 647–649. Paris: Masson.

Zellweger, H., Afifi, A., McCormick, W. F. and Mergner, W. (1967a). Benign congenital muscular dystrophy: a special form of congenital hypotonia. *Clin. Pediat.* **6,** 655–663.

Zellweger, H., Afifi, A, McCormick, W. F. and Mergner, W. (1967b). Severe congenital muscular dystrophy. *Am. J. Dis. Childh.* **114,** 591–602.

Zellweger, H., Brown, B.I., McCormick, W. F. and Tu, J. B. (1965). A mild form of muscular glycogenosis in two brothers with alpha-1, 4-glucosidase deficiency. *Annls paediat.* **205,** 413–437.

Zenker, W. and Krammer, E. (1967). Unterschungen über die Feinstruktur und Innervation der inneren Augenmuskulatur des Huhnes. *Z. Zellforsch. mikrosk. Anat.* **83,** 147–168.

Zintz, R. (1966). Dystrophische Veränderungen in äusseren Augenmuskels und Schultermuskeln bei der sog. progressiven Graefeschen Ophthalmoplegie. In *Progressive Muskeldystrophie, Myotonie, Myasthenie.* Ed. Kuhn, E. pp. 109–114. Berlin: Springer.

Index

Roman numbers refer to text page and italic numbers to plates. L = lower, U = upper, UL = upper left, UR = upper right, LL = lower left, LR = lower right